Saphenous Vein-Sparing Strategies in Chronic Venous Disease

Paolo Zamboni
Erika Mendoza
Sergio Gianesini
Editors

Saphenous Vein-Sparing Strategies in Chronic Venous Disease

Springer

Editors
Paolo Zamboni
School of Vascular Surgery and
Vascular Diseases Center
University of Ferrara
Ferrara, Italy

Unit of Translational Surgery
AOU Ferrara
Ferrara, Italy

Sergio Gianesini
Translational Surgery Unit-Vascular
Disease Center
University of Ferrara Vascular
Disease Center
Ferrara
Italy

Erika Mendoza
Venenpraxis Wunstorf
Wunstorf
Niedersachsen
Germany

ISBN 978-3-030-09976-3 ISBN 978-3-319-70638-2 (eBook)
DOI 10.1007/978-3-319-70638-2

Softcover re-print of the Hardcover 1st edition 2018

Printed on acid-free paper

This Springer imprint is published by the registered company Springer International Publishing AG part of Springer Nature
The registered company address is: Gewerbestrasse 11, 6330 Cham, Switzerland

Foreword

During the 1970s and in the 1980s, we had more and more patients who needed a saphena bypass wherein the saphenous vein was unfortunately destroyed by a previous surgical or endovenous treatment. I was struck by our schizophrenic behaviour which consisted of, on the one hand, the saphenous vein destruction for the benign varicose disease and, on the other hand, lamenting for its absence when we needed it to perform a venous bypass for a critical or life-threatening arterial or coronary obstruction. So, as a former psychiatrist, I decided to confront and treat my insanity.

In addition to conservative treatments as foot elevation, bandaging and use of compression stockings, I tried to find a surgical treatment which could also preserve the saphenous capital. My observations of the varicose veins' disappearance when I lifted the feet of my patients combined with the Trendelenburg and Perthes manoeuvres' effects convinced me that the cause of the venous insufficiency and its symptoms was just a haemodynamic impairment of the venous flows and pressure control.

Then, from this basis and thanks to the studies of the venous pressure principally published by Bjordal and the revolutionary capability of recent echo-Doppler ultrasound devices, I could better figure out the better haemodynamic venous system and its anomalies. It resulted in proposals of venous pathophysiological haemodynamic principles as dynamic fractioning of hydrostatic pressure, various venous shunt patterns, re-entry concept, transmural pressure control as the target of any rational treatment, location of not yet individualized pelvic leak points, haemodynamic venous cartography, and finally the necessary conservation of the venous network for a correct drainage of the tissues and prevention of recurrence. These concepts were the basis of the CHIVA cure (French acronym for "cure Hémodynamique et Conservatrice de l'Insuffisance Veineuse en Ambulatoire") published in 1988.

As conservation is a pillar, CHIVA was received as provocative nonsense because, so far, the destructive paradigm was dominant. Indeed, for around a century, research, studies and devices where focused on killing the veins because the treatment failures and recurrences where attributed to the veins left behind. Indeed, CHIVA is based on dramatically different pathophysiological rational. Its concepts were verified by further experimental evidence. Thanks to hundreds of studies, some RCTs and a Cochrane review, achieved by various authors over Europe, CHIVA is today validated more successful than destructive methods and reaches, at the same time, both targets of treating efficiently the venous insufficiency and preserving the venous capital for future bypass.

CHIVA is also a scientific and intellectual challenge which demands a reconsideration of the mainstream knowledge and personal habits, a steep learning curve of the appropriate venous haemodynamics and its related duplex scan assessment. We cannot play a game of chess with the rules for checkers even if the board is identical. The same is for CHIVA. The rules of destructive methods cannot fit to the conservative CHIVA.

Conservative or ablative methods, as well as invasive and non-invasive or laser and other advanced devices, are powerful marketing arguments but not always medically fair. The conservative procedures are relevant only when they are better than the ablative in terms of risks/benefits ratio. Non-invasive procedures are not necessarily safe. CHIVA is feasible in outpatients with mini-invasive surgery.

Patient information should point out the risks/benefits based on medical evidence. That is like kicking down an open door if we refer to the Hippocratic oath "I am following that system of regimen which, according to my ability and judgement, I consider for the benefit of my patients, and abstain from whatever is deleterious and mischievous". Furthermore, the patient informed consent obliges to inform the patient about the nature and purpose and risks and benefits of the proposed treatment as well as the alternatives.

Unfortunately, reality is not so. Ignorance, cynicism, competition, greed and conflicts of interest are still to be taken into account.

I would like this book to revive the fair Hippocratic oath by permitting the phlebologist to better inform and treat the patient. Remind him that varicose veins are usually benign and may be treated or not according to his cosmetic or comfort expectation. In case of skin changes and ulcers, easy efficient procedures on transmural pressure decrease are available. In addition, the CHIVA concepts and strategy are applicable to deep venous diseases, particularly post-thrombotic, and also to venous malformations.

Many thanks and congratulations to the authors who are renowned world experts as researchers and practitioners in phlebology. They report and explain extensively and clearly the venous haemodynamic pathophysiology with the relevant contribution of other eminent colleagues, who improved the CHIVA strategy and tactics.

Claude Franceschi

Preface

Many phlebologists, surgeons and scientists were involved on the way that led to the writing of this book. The idea of venous-sparing surgery rests on the shoulders of these colleagues. Countless numbers of courses, meetings and discussion groups allowed us to sharpen our minds about the open questions. We deeply thank all the colleagues around the world who have contributed scientifically and practically to the development of the saphenous-sparing surgery and the underlying haemodynamics concepts.

We thank Dr. Kraemer, Heidelberg, for his support in starting this project, and Mr. Dhanapal Palanisamy, for his help along the writing and finishing of the book. Mr. William Barne translated some of the German texts which were supported financially by Dr. Hans-Jürgen Thomae and Bauerfeind (Zeulenroda). This was an invaluable help to the project.

We wish to acknowledge all the patients who trusted us giving us the possibility to learn and become experienced, thereby providing the foundations of this book.

As an introduction to one of his lectures, Claude Franceschi once said that it is important to empty a truck before storing new cargo. In a similar way, we would like to invite our readers to open up a free space in their minds to make room for new ideas. We anticipate that they will profit from the contents and that the information of the book will enrichen their professional life, as venous-saving strategies did with ours.

Ferrara, Italy — Paolo Zamboni
Wunstorf, Germany — Erika Mendoza
Ferrara, Italy — Sergio Gianesini
October 2017

Contents

Contributors

Massimo Cappelli, M.D. Office Surgery, Florence, Italy

Sylvain Chastanet, M.D. Riviera Veine Institut, Monaco, France

Roberto Delfrate, M.D. Responsible Surgery at Casa di Cura Figlie di San Camillo, Cremona, Italy

Sergio Gianesini, M.D., Ph.D. Vascular Diseases Center, University of Ferrara, Ferrara, Italy

USUHS University, Bethesda, MD, USA

Erika Mendoza, M.D., Ph.D. Venenpraxis, Wunstorf, Germany

Erica Menegatti, Ph.D. Vascular Diseases Center, University of Ferrara, Ferrara, Italy

Paul Pittaluga, M.D. Riviera Veine Institut, Monaco, France

Paolo Zamboni, M.D. School of Vascular Surgery and Vascular Diseases Center, University of Ferrara, Ferrara, Italy

Unit of Translational Surgery, AOU Ferrara, Ferrara, Italy

Part I

Background

1 Historical Background and Rationale

Paolo Zamboni

1.1 Historical Background

To ablate or not to ablate the saphenous vein: this has been the question along the last five decades. However, during the 1980s the debate appeared solved in favour of the ablation for the following evidence:

- The studies of the Lofgren group performed at the Mayo Clinic, who compared high ligation vs. stripping, seemed undebatable [1, 2].

Moreover, stripping was considered the cornerstone of chronic venous disease treatment, while whatever conservative treatment alone or in combination was taken into consideration only when saphenous ablation was withheld because of associated significant clinical problems.

- Although Quill [3] demonstrated the possibility of reversing sapheno-femoral refluxes with a correct combination of sclerotherapy and compression, the first randomized clinical trial in the history of varicose veins, by comparing ablation to sclerotherapy, Hobbs strongly recommended stripping especially in the long run [4].

The only discussed arguments opposed to the ablation procedure were essentially the nerve injury complication as well as the loss of the best available graft material.

Munn performed an interesting double-blind controlled investigation reporting a significantly higher incidence of paraesthesia and pain following stripping rather than sapheno-femoral junction ligation with incompetent tributary avulsion [5].

On a histological point of view, vein walls observed after extraction of varicose veins showed damages nobody could imagine recovering a normal structure, if the pressure and flow rate inside the vein were restored.

The paradigm shift began with the ultrasound technological improvement at the end of the 1980s. Particularly the possibility to couple in real time the information from Doppler haemodynamics with that of vein anatomy widened our ability to get deeper knowledge of venous pathophysiology. The introduction of colour-coded duplex ultrasound also opened out new questions related to the proper therapeutic strategies. Along the last two decades, the venous literature has been providing growing evidence supporting a saphenous sparing approach.

In 1988 Franceschi introduced CHIVA: the first structured saphenous sparing pathophysiological interpretation, with a related diagnostic

P. Zamboni, M.D.
School of Vascular Surgery and Vascular Diseases Center, University of Ferrara, Ferrara, Italy

Unit of Translational Surgery, AOU Ferrara, Ferrara, Italy
e-mail: zmp@unife.it

P. Zamboni et al. (eds.), *Saphenous Vein-Sparing Strategies in Chronic Venous Disease*,
https://doi.org/10.1007/978-3-319-70638-2_1

protocol and classification of hemodynamic impairment, leading to an innovative concept of restoration rather than ablation of the same saphenous system [6].

1.1.1 Anatomy and Physiology

In the following years, further scientific evidence pointed out the multifocal origin of venous reflux, in opposition to the more traditional vision of a simple descending saphenous incompetence starting at the sapheno-femoral junction [7–10].

Van Bemmelen, Somjen and Cappelli demonstrated that, despite a truncal saphenous reflux, almost 50% of the sapheno-femoral junctions are competent, thus requiring a more tailored procedure compared to stripping [11–13].

Different anatomic investigations demonstrated that there is an ascending evolution in the saphenous vein pathology, which is in contradiction to the classical convictions. Caggiati and Chastanet investigated cohorts of patients at different ages and compared the affection of tributaries and saphenous veins; Bernardini published a follow-up of non-treated patients with refluxive tributaries and partial refluxes in saphenous vein without affection of the sapheno-femoral junction. All three agreed to find that the younger patients had a lesser proportion in proximal affection of saphenous vein than the older ones; Bernardini could demonstrate an ascension in the parts of saphenous vein affected by reflux throughout the time [14–16].

1.1.2 Vein Wall Recovery

A mistaken belief was to consider the chronic pathology of the great saphenous vein as biologically irreversible in the course of primary chronic venous disease. This was a strong argument in favour of ablation, albeit was never proven.

On the contrary, already in 1990 the recovery of the vein wall elastic properties of the saphenous vein only with compression stockings was demonstrated [17].

In 1996 Recek publishes results after crossectomy and sclerotherapy of tributaries with reduction of calibre in saphenous veins and in 2000 with diameter reduction in re-entry perforating veins [18, 19].

In 1999 Creton reported the possibility of significantly reducing the great saphenous vein (GSV) calibre simply by ligating the incompetent tributaries [20].

Two years later, the possibility of restoring a great saphenous vein reflux by simple ligation of the incompetent tributaries was demonstrated by objective plethysmographic data [21]. Calibre reduction of great saphenous and also deep veins (common femoral vein) as well as plethysmographic improvement was also confirmed by Mendoza in 2011 (short-term) and 2013 (mid-term) after CHIVA [22, 23].

One of the major arguments in favor of ablation was represented by the biological impossibility of the saphenous vein to recover the tissue damage. In contrast, quite recently, it has been seen that the elimination of the oscillatory component of reflux allows both a reduction in the caliber and an improvement in the inflammatory profile of the venous endothelium. A demonstration that dismantles one of the major arguments against saphenous sparing surgery [24, 25].

1.1.3 Comparative Studies Between Ablative and Saphenous Vein Sparing Surgery

In 2003, in the first randomized trial between CHIVA and compression treatment, Zamboni proved the efficacy of sparing the saphenous trunk also in the most severe ulcer patients [26].

A first long-term randomized control trial was published by Carandina in 2008 demonstrating an odds ratio for recurrence at 10 years that almost doubled in stripping procedures compared to the saphenous sparing ones, analysing the recurrence sources in both groups [27].

In 2009, a new saphenous sparing theory was developed by Pittaluga and called ASVAL (ambulatory selective varicose vein ablation under local anaesthesia). According to the literature, ASVAL selective ablation of the incompetent tributaries is able to suppress saphenous reflux in more than 66% of cases at 4-year follow-up and 64% at 10-year follow-up [28, 29].

In 2010 Pares confirmed the smaller recurrence rate of a saphenous sparing approach compared to a traditional stripping with a 5-year follow-up [30].

A more practical case–control study gave the surgical indication to the treatment of the saphenofemoral junction or just of saphenous tributaries, as suggested by the first step of CHIVA 2 technique or ASVAL. Patients were assessed for the competence of the terminal valve of the GSV as proposed by Cappelli [11] and subsequently operated on simply detaching the incompetent tributary/tributaries from the GSV. The stratification of the results at 3 years revealed that the procedure is effective when it is performed in the presence of a competent terminal valve [31].

The results of the cited studies have confirmed and implemented the efficacy of a saphenous sparing strategy, so leading to a Cochrane validation in 2013 and to its confirmation in 2015 [32, 33].

Despite the renewed sparing surgery proposal, saphenous ablation became in the meantime more and more practiced thanks to the introduction of endovascular technology which permitted to minimize the ablative procedure. Classic stripping procedure was rarely performed on ambulatory bases. The introduction of endovenous techniques, such as laser or radiofrequency ablation of the saphenous veins, permitted to transform ablative surgery into an office surgical procedure. Thermal and nonthermal and tumescent and non-tumescent procedures for treating the insufficient saphenous veins became the current gold standard treatment. In performing this procedure, often the surgical indication and a careful selection of cases through a meaningful ultrasound selection of cases are lacking. Only in the last years, data have been gathered and published considering saphenous vein sparing surgery applying new endovenous technologies [34].

1.2 Rationale

Saphenous sparing rationale takes into consideration the pressure gradient overload occurring in case of venous reflux.

The rationale of the strategy is the application of the laws of physics with the aim of restoring physiological pressure gradients. This target can be reached by means of selective ligations (CHIVA, cure conservatrice et hémodynamique de l'Insuffisance veineuse en ambulatoire) after an accurate preoperative mapping guiding the treatment of the specific leaking points or ablation of incompetent tributaries (ASVAL, ambulatory selective varicose vein ablation under local anaesthesia).

Evolution in medicine throughout the twentieth century has undergone changes: First, large surgery was possible with implementation of good anaesthesia. Then proper imaging and screening methods allowed to discriminate and analyse which destruction could be avoided—and even in the oncologic surgery, the tendency to spare organs is obvious, even though it was supposed to induce recidives—in oncological cases mortal ones! Surprisingly this tendency to save organs found no acceptance in the phlebological world, even though the recidives would not put the patients' life at risk and even though studies demonstrated a reduction of recidives when organ saving.

A traditional reason to spare the saphenous trunk is to be found in its possible role as arterial bypass [35–41]. Moreover, vascular surgery is aimed to repair the vessels and/or restore the flow, something philosophically different from ablation.

At the same time, sparing the saphenous trunk leaves a potential flow route in case of thrombotic occlusion of the deep system.

Last but not least, saphenous sparing preserves a main conduit for tissue drainage: a hemodynamic scenario that is considered as the basis for reducing the recurrence onset [32, 33].

Literature

1. Lofgren EP, Lofgren KA. Alternatives in the management of varices. Geriatrics. 1975;30:111–3.
2. Lofgren KA, Ribisi AP, Myers TT. An evaluation of stripping versus ligation for varicose veins. AMA Arch Surg. 1958;76:310–6.
3. Quill RD, Fegan WG. Reversibility of femorosaphenous reflux. Br J Surg. 1971;58(5):389–93.
4. Hobbs JT. Surgery or sclerotherapy for varicose veins. Lancet. 1978;1(8074):1149.

5. Munn SR. To strip or not to strip the long saphenous vein? Br J Surg. 1981;68(6):426–8.
6. Franceschi C. Théorie et pratique de la cure Conservatrice et Hémodynamique de l'Insuffisance Veineuse en Ambulatoire. Precy-sous-Thil, France: Editions de l'Armançon; 1988.
7. Cooper DG, Hillman-Cooper CS, Barker SG, Hollingsworth SJ. Primary varicose veins: the sapheno-femoral junction, distribution of varicosities and patterns of incompetence. Eur J Vasc Endovasc Surg. 2003;25:53–9.
8. Engelhorn CA, Engelhorn AL, Cassou MF, Salles-Cunha SX. Patterns of saphenous reflux in women with primary varicose veins. J Vasc Surg. 2005;41:645–51.
9. Labropoulos N, Giannoukas AD, Delis K, et al. Where does venous reflux start? J Vasc Surg. 1997;26:736–42.
10. Labropoulos N, Leon L, Kwon S, et al. Study of the venous reflux progression. J Vasc Surg. 2005;41:291–5.
11. Cappelli M, Molino Lova R, Ermini S, Zamboni P. Hemodynamics of the sapheno-femoral junction. Patterns of reflux and their clinical implications. Int Angiol. 2004;23(1):25–8.
12. Somjen GM, Donlan J, Hurse J, Bartholomew J, Johnston AH, Royle JP. Venous reflux at the sapheno-femoral junction. Phlebology. 1995;4:132–5.
13. Van Bemmelen PS, Summer DS. Laboratory evaluation of varicose veins. In: Bergan JJ, Goldman MP, editors. Varicose veins duplex examination of the sapheno-femoral junction and telangiectasias, diagnosis and treatment. St. Louis, MO: Quality Medical Publishing; 1993. p. 73–84.
14. Bernardini E, DeRango P, Piccioli R, Bisacci C, Pagliuca V, Genovese G, Bisacci R. Development of primary superficial venous insufficiency: the ascending theory. Observational and hemodynamic data from a 9 year experience. Ann Vasc Surg. 2010;24:709–20.
15. Caggiati A, Rosi C, Heyn R, Franceschini M, Acconcia MC. Age-related variations of varicose veins anatomy. J Vasc Surg. 2006;44(6):1291–5.
16. Chastanet S, Pittaluga P. Patterns of reflux in the great saphenous vein system. Phlebology. 2013;28(Suppl 1):S39–46.
17. Hammersen F, Hesse G. Strukturelle Veränderungen der Varikösen Venenwand nach Kompressionsbehandlung. Phlebol Proktol. 1990;19:193–9.
18. Recek C, Karisch E, Gruber J. Veränderungen der Perforansvenen und tiefen Unterschenkelvenen nach Beseitigung des Saphena-Refluxes. Phlebologie (Stuttgart). 2000;29(1):37–40.
19. Recek C. Auswirkung der Krossektomie auf die venöse Zirkulationsstörung bei primärer Varikose. Phlebologie (Stuttgart). 1996;25(1):11–8.
20. Creton D. Diameter reduction of the proximal long saphenous vein after ablation of a distal incompetent tributary. Dermatol Surg. 1999;25(5):394–7.
21. Zamboni P, Cisno C, Marchetti F, Quaglio D, Mazza P, Liboni A. Reflux elimination without any ablation or disconnection of the saphenous vein. A haemodynamic model for venous surgery. Eur J Vasc Endovasc Surg. 2001;21(4):361–9.
22. Mendoza E, Berger V, Zollmann C, Bomhoff M, Amsler F. Kaliberreduktion der V. saphena magna und der V. femoralis communis nach CHIVA. Phlebologie. 2011;40(2):73–8.
23. Mendoza E. Diameter reduction of the great saphenous vein and the common femoral vein after CHIVA: long term results. Phlebologie. 2013;42:65–9. https://doi.org/10.12687/phleb2127_2_2013.
24. Tisato V, Zauli G, Gianesini S, Menegatti E, Brunelli L, Manfredini R, Zamboni P, Secchiero P. Modulation of circulating cytokine-chemokine profile in patients affected by chronic venous insufficiency undergoing surgical hemodynamic correction. J Immunol Res. 2014;2014:473765.
25. Zamboni P, Spath P, Tisato V, Tessari M, Dalla Caneva P, Menegatti E, Occhionorelli S, Gianesini S, Secchiero P. Oscillatory flow suppression improves inflammation in chronic venous disease. J Surg Res. 2016;205(1):238–45. https://doi.org/10.1016/j.jss.2016.06.046.
26. Zamboni P, Cisno C, Marchetti F, Mazza P, Fogato L, Carandina S, De Palma M, Liboni A. Minimally invasive surgical management of primary venous ulcers vs. compression treatment: a randomized clinical trial. Eur J Vasc Endovasc Surg. 2003;25(4):313–8. Erratum in: Eur J Vasc Endovasc Surg. 2003;26(3):337–8.
27. Carandina S, Mari C, De Palma M, Marcellino MG, Cisno C, Legnaro A, Liboni A, Zamboni P. Varicose vein stripping vs haemodynamic correction (CHIVA): a long term randomised trial. Eur J Vasc Endovasc Surg. 2008;35(2):230–7. Epub 2007 Oct 26.
28. Pittaluga P, Chastanet S, Réa B, Barbe R. Midterm results of the surgical treatment of varices by phlebectomy with conservation of a refluxing saphenous vein. J Vasc Surg. 2009;50:107–18.
29. Pittaluga P, Chastanet S. Treatment of varicose veins by ASVAL: results at 10 years. Ann Vasc Surg. 2017;38:e10. https://doi.org/10.1016/j.avsg.2016.07.021. Epub 2016 Oct 11.
30. Pares O, Juan J, Tellez R, Mata A, Moreno C, Quer FX. Varicose vein surgery: stripping vs. the CHIVA method. A randomized controlled trial. Ann Vasc Surg. 2010;251:624–31.
31. Zamboni P, Gianesini S, Menegatti E, Tacconi G, Palazzo A, Liboni A. Great saphenous varicose vein surgery without saphenofemoral junction disconnection. Br J Surg. 2010;97(6):820–5.
32. Bellmunt-Montoya S, Escribano JM, Dilme J, Martinez-Zapata MJ. CHIVA method for the treatment of chronic venous insufficiency. Cochrane Database Syst Rev. 2015;(6):CD009648.
33. Bellmunt-Montoya S, Escribano JM, Dilme J, Martinez-Zapata MJ. CHIVA method for the treatment of chronic venous insufficiency. Cochrane Database Syst Rev. 2013;(7):CD009648. https://doi.org/10.1002/14651858.CD009648.pub2.

34. Mendoza E, Amsler F. CHIVA with endoluminal procedures: LASER versus VNUS—treatment of the saphenofemoral junction. Phlebologie. 2017;46:5–12.
35. Hammarsten J, Pedersen P, Cederlund CG, Campanello M. Long saphenous vein saving surgery for varicose veins. A long-term follow-up. Eur J Vasc Surg. 1990;4(4):361–4.
36. Kniemeyer H, Rish H, Hakki H, Reber PU. Exigences pour les greffes veineuses destinees a la chirurgie des arteres peripheriques (Requirements for venous grafts destined for peripheral arterial surgery). Phlebologie. 1998;3:289–93.
37. Melliere D, Cales B, Martin-Jonathan C, Schadeck M. Necessity of reconciling the objectives of the treatment of varices and arterial surgery. Practical consequences. J Mal Vasc. 1991;16(2):171–8.
38. Melliere D. Why and when to preserve the saphenous veins of varicose patients to serve as an arterial bypass? J Mal Vasc. 1994;19(3):216–21.
39. Pennywell DJ, Tan TW, Zhang WW. Optimal management of infrainguinal arterial occlusive disease. Vasc Health Risk Manag. 2014;10:599–608. http://www.dovepress.com/article_18926.t34346121.
40. Royle JP, Somsen GM. Preservation of the long saphenous vein. J Cardiovasc Surg (Torino). 1991;32:7.
41. Samson R, 2013, Calling SOS—save our saphenous! http://www.mdedge.com/vascularspecialistonline/article/84109/calling-sos-save-our-saphenous. Accessed 21 Nov 2013.

2 Functional Anatomy of Leg Veins

Sergio Gianesini, Paolo Zamboni, and Erika Mendoza

2.1 Introduction

Lower limb venous anatomy knowledge is not necessary just for getting oriented inside the drainage routes. Rather it is fundamental for a proper comprehension of the architecture which influences haemodynamics law application.

Communicating vessel principle, Venturi's effect and Poiseuille law are just some of the many fundamentals in venous return determinants, all influenced by anatomy parameters like valve density, vessel calibre and length.

Moreover, the anatomical relationship among veins and muscle masses strictly influences the systolic push effect on the same vessels, so determining a velocity and pressure gradient moving from the most superficial towards the deepest compartments.

In conclusion, lower limb venous anatomy knowledge is necessary since itself is a determinant of the venous return pathophysiology.

Anatomy of leg veins is complex and described in various textbooks, to which we refer the interested reader (see Literature at the end of the chapter) [1–3]. In this chapter, the focus lays on those information concerning deep and superficial veins which are relevant to the non-ablating treatment of the saphenous veins. A detailed anatomical information necessary for the superficial vein exploration is included in Chap. 4, Ultrasound.

The venous system has been classically divided into two distinct parts. On the one hand, we find the **superficial system** which courses superficially to the muscular fascia and is responsible for carrying the blood away from the subcutaneous tissue and, on the other hand, the **deep or subfascial system** which is responsible for draining the muscles and bones. These two systems are separated anatomically by the muscle fascia. Both systems are connected by perforating veins.

Since the upcoming of duplex ultrasound devices and the new investigation possibilities of leg veins, the anatomical division of superficial leg veins into saphenous veins running between the muscular fascia and the saphenous fascia and epifascial veins was rediscovered [4]. Franceschi first described three different networks: "N1" for the deep veins, "N2" for the interfascial veins (saphenous veins) and "N3" for the epifascial veins [5]. Zamboni described the saphenous compartment in 1997 [6, 7], and Caggiati and

S. Gianesini, M.D., Ph.D. (✉)
Vascular Diseases Center, University of Ferrara, Ferrara, Italy

USUHS University, Bethesda, MD, USA

P. Zamboni, M.D.
School of Vascular Surgery and Vascular Diseases Center, University of Ferrara, Ferrara, Italy

Unit of Translational Surgery, AOU Ferrara, Ferrara, Italy
e-mail: zmp@unife.it

E. Mendoza, M.D., Ph.D.
Venenpraxis, Wunstorf, Germany
e-mail: erika.mendoza@t-online.de

P. Zamboni et al. (eds.), *Saphenous Vein-Sparing Strategies in Chronic Venous Disease*,
https://doi.org/10.1007/978-3-319-70638-2_2

Ricci investigated in corpses and ultrasound the relationships of saphenous veins and fasciae [8–12], and finally the fascia saphena and the saphenous compartment found their way into the nomenclatura anatomica [13].

The leg veins are furnitured with valves. These are thin connective tissue structures adherent to the vein wall and allowing blood flow only in direction to the heart, which mostly means from the foot to the groin.

> The wrapping of the saphenous vein in the fascial compartment is of fundamental importance in the venous sparing surgery.

2.2 Anatomical Compartments

In the description of the lower limb venous anatomy, three different compartments can be identified, based on their relationship to the muscular fascia: below the fascia, in-between the fascia layers and above the fascia [2, 6, 7, 13–15].

The *deep anatomical compartment* (N1) is located below the muscular fascia and includes the deep venous systems vessels (femoral, popliteal, soleal, gastrocnemial and tibial veins).

The saphenous system represents a separate anatomical compartment (N2), between the muscular and the saphenous fascia layers. The interfascial compartment (N2) includes the great saphenous vein (GSV), the small saphenous vein (SSV) and the interfascial segments of the anterior accessory saphenous vein (AASV) and Giacomini vein.

The third anatomical compartment (N3) is represented by the tributary system, between the fascia and the skin, being constituted by the veins surrounded just by subcutaneous fat.

More than 60 perforating veins connect the three anatomical compartments at the thigh, 5 at the knee level, 55 at the calf level and 28 at the foot level, by perforating the muscular fascia, so presenting interconnections for pressure gradient development and consequent drainage propulsion towards the heart [16, 17].

The anatomical nomenclature used throughout the book follows international convention. The saphenous trunks are the "great saphenous vein" (GSV) (Latin: *V. saphena magna*) and the "small saphenous vein" (SSV) (Latin: *V. saphena parva*). In international use, the **accessory veins** are called anterior, superficial and posterior accessory saphenous veins [13].

2.2.1 Muscular Compartment

The function of our legs is deambulation. Most of the leg mass is composed of bones and muscles, covered by the muscular fascia, which is embryologically derived from the mesodermal structures. In this compartment, we find the deep veins, as well as the intramuscular parts of the perforating veins. Even though veins do not have an own pump (like the heart) to drive the blood forwards, deep veins are directly influenced by the adjacent muscles in a way that expel the blood in direction to the heart with help of the valves.

The deep venous system consists of veins which run **inside the muscle fascia** (See Fig. 2.1). These are the:

At the *calf*

- Muscle veins inside the calf muscles
- Three calf veins, namely, the anterior and posterior tibial veins and peroneal veins

All these veins join at the *knee level* into the

- Popliteal vein

At the *thigh*

- Femoral vein (prolongation of the popliteal vein and formerly called superficial femoral vein)
- Deep femoral vein
- Common femoral vein (prolongation of the femoral vein after its junction with the deep femoral vein)

Along the leg, we find

- Deep parts of the numerous perforating veins

The deep veins of the leg accompany the arteries of the same name and are generally paired in the calf.

For further information, we recommend textbooks on venous anatomy (Fig. 2.1).

2.2.2 Epifascial Compartment

The functions of the skin and subcutaneous tissue are mainly two:

- Protection from external (biological, like bacteria or virus) as well as chemical (substances that would harm the body) aggressions
- Protection from heat and cold

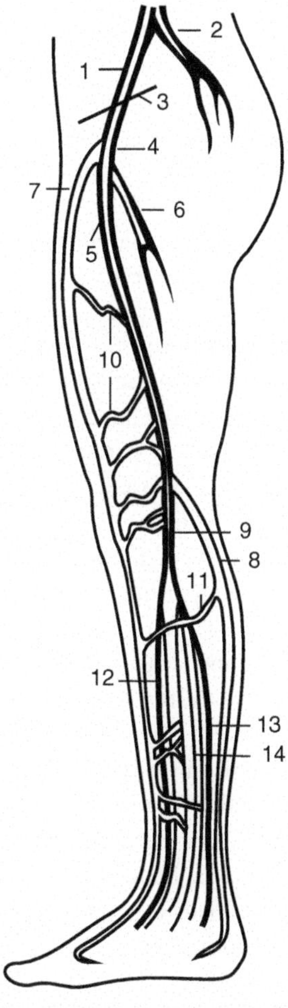

Fig. 2.1 Anatomy of the deep and superficial vein systems of the leg: (1) external iliac vein, (2) internal iliac vein, (3) inguinal ligament, (4) common femoral vein, (5) femoral vein (formerly superficial), (6) deep femoral vein, (7) great saphenous vein, (8) small saphenous vein, (9) popliteal vein, (10) perforating veins, (11) superficial communicating vein, (12) anterior tibial vein, (13) posterior tibial vein, (14) peroneal vein. With permission by [18]

The first function is provided by the skin, helped by the blood supply with antimicrobial cells (leucocytes). The second function is provided by the fatty tissue and a well-organized perfusion with blood in capillaries, able to regulate the temperature of the skin and thus the heat loss or the protection against cold environment. For this function, the subcutaneous tissue has a wide net of capillaries interconnected, drained by reticular veins. These run without any systematization in the fatty tissue, joining to other reticular veins and forming tributaries, which are defined as veins with diameters over 3 mm. Some of these are very constant and have their own names (arch veins, accessory veins).

The subcutaneous tissue is constructed around a skeleton of connective tissue, which is filled with fat (see Fig. 2.2). The external limit of the epifascial compartment is the skin. On ultrasound, this connective tissue is visible as white, echogenic layers which blend irregularly into the grey fat tissue in widely differing patterns (see Fig. 2.3a). In the deeper zone of the subcutaneous tissue, the connective tissue fibres thicken to form a membrane which usually lies directly on the muscle fascia and conforms the internal limit of the subcutaneous tissue.

In varicose disease, the varicose veins visible by the eye are the tributaries, which are the optically bothering aspect of the illness and often the reason for the patient to have a consultation. For many years, they never have been investigated or suspected to play any important role in the illness. Only in the last years, the role of the tributaries has come into focus: ASVAL is based on the role of tributaries as venous reservoir (see Chap. 12). Flow velocity investigations made it obvious that these veins play an important role (see Sect. 2.3). They also have valves and microvalves. In case of advanced chronic venous insufficiency, tributaries perform morphologic changes like demonstrated by Vincent—these changes being possibly responsible for the skin damage [19].

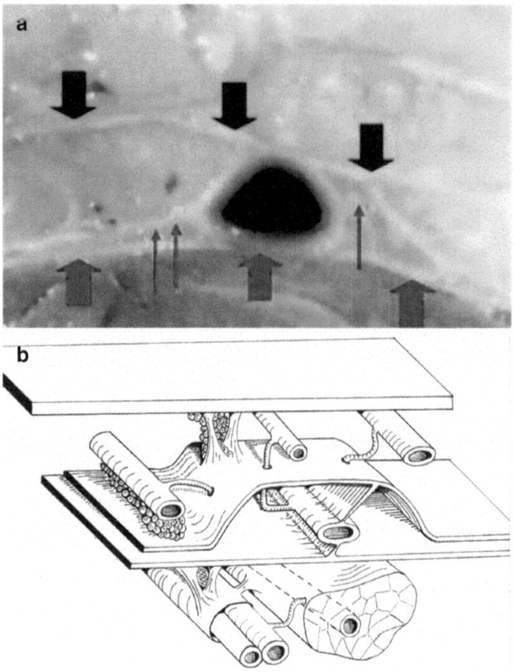

Fig. 2.2 (**a**) Section through the thigh in an anatomical preparation demonstrating layers of connective tissue separating cushions of fat around the great saphenous vein. (**b**) Sketch depicting the anatomical section with the muscle fascia and immediately above it the great saphenous vein in the fascial compartment. A connecting tributary is seen in the subcutaneous fatty tissue (Prof. A. Caggiati, Rome; by kind permission)

2.2.3 The Fascial Compartment of the Saphenous Veins

We have seen that the deep compartment is responsible for deambulation and standing position, the superficial compartment for temperature homeostasis, and defence from chemical and biological aggressors. The third compartment of the leg (saphenous compartment) has the very important function to wrap the saphenous veins, which serve as the main drainage pathway for the blood from the subcutaneous compartment.

The saphenous compartment is composed of the muscle fascia, as limit between the deep and superficial venous system and the saphenous fascia, which is a part of the membranous layer. Embryologically the muscle fascia originates from the mesodermal structures and the membranous layer from the ectodermal structures.

The muscle fascia and the membranous layer form a structural unit of connective tissue separating the muscle from the subcutaneous fatty tissue. In some parts of the leg, the two fasciae separate to form a tunnel for the veins and their accompanying arteries, nerves and lymphatic vessels. This tunnel is called the **compartment** of the great and small saphenous veins. In the upper part of the leg, it also contains the accessory saphenous veins, and it might be present at the posterior part of the leg along the way of the thigh extension of the small saphenous vein [13].

The membranous layer along the saphenous veins is seen as a white layer on ultrasound and can be distinguished easily from the surrounding echo-poor fat and muscle fascia. The characteristic ultrasound image of the saphenous veins between the two fasciae led to the description of the saphenous eye [20] (Fig. 2.3b).

In transverse view in ultrasound, two echogenic connective tissue streaks are visible which appear to anchor both sides of the saphenous trunks. They connect the adventitia of the saphenous vein, run relatively parallel to the membranous layer and the muscle fascia and finally merge into them (*white arrows* in Fig. 2.4).

The envelopment of the saphenous veins by the saphenous compartment between the membranous layer (saphenous fascia) and the muscle fascia, and their anchorage by the saphenous ligament, appears to be responsible for the lack of tortuosity observed when the saphenous veins become refluxive and dilated. This is in direct contrast to the behaviour of their refluxing tributaries. It might be also responsible for the retonisation observed in saphenous veins after reducing the volume overload, e.g. with saphenous vein sparing surgical principles.

2.2.4 Schematic Representation of Venous Networks

Throughout this book, we will use pictures to explain the different aspects of saphenous vein

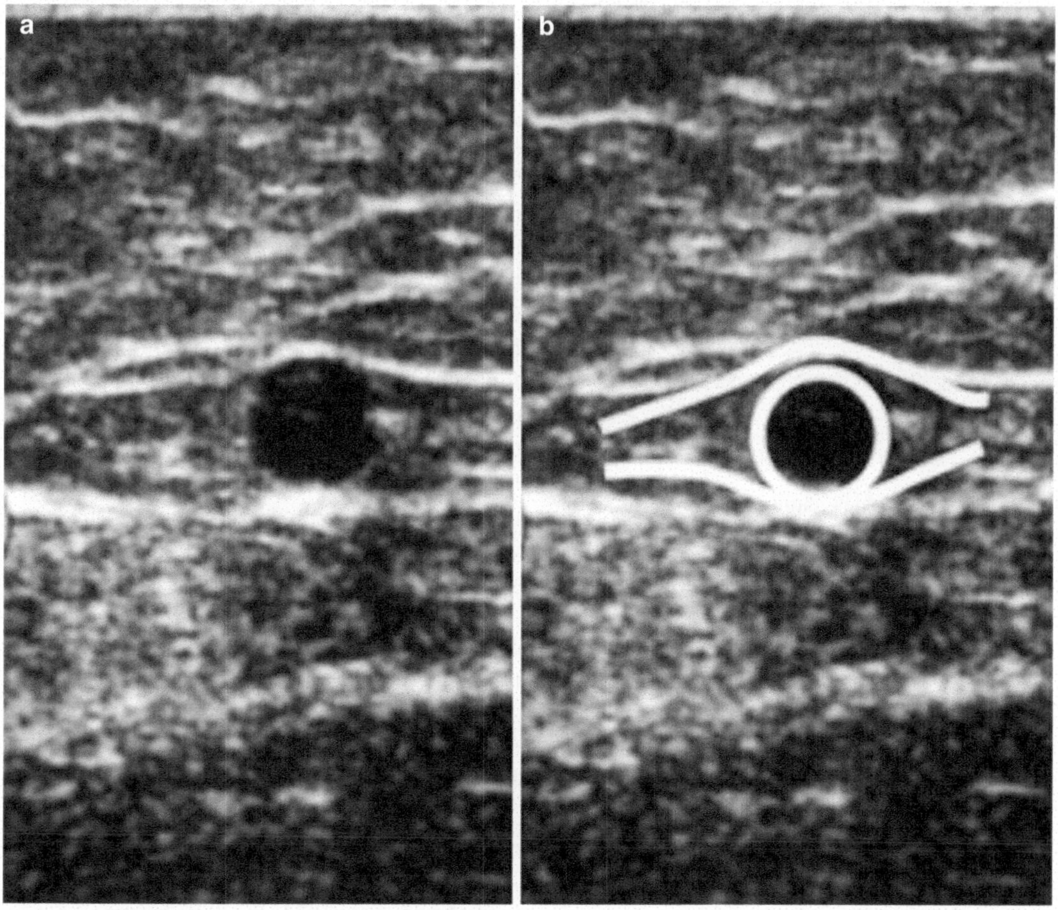

Fig. 2.3 (a) Transverse view through the thigh showing the great saphenous vein. (b) Overlay highlighting the "saphenous eye" where the upper lid is the saphenous fascia and the lower lid is the muscle fascia, and the iris is the great saphenous vein. In the upper half of both images, the structure of the lax subcutaneous connective tissue is visualized as white pattern in the grey fatty tissue. With kind permission by [21]

sparing strategies. They are based on the three networks and always kept as simple as possible to allow a better understanding. The deep veins (N1) are represented in dark blue as a line – one line representing all the deep veins as a system. In case the deep vein system has a special aspect, obviously, this can be implemented in the drawing, adding another line in dark blue to the deep veins. The saphenous veins (N2) are represented in light blue, also as only one line indwelling to the deep vein at the level of the junctions (see Fig. 2.5a). Giacomini vein and anterior accessory saphenous vein are only painted if directly involved in the pathology or haemodynamic situation (see Fig. 2.5b). Tributaries (N3) are only represented in case of pathology. In a tributary necessary for a drainage, it will be represented in orange. Refluxive vessels, independently of the level, are represented in red. Arrows next to the image indicate the main flow direction in the vessel (see Fig. 2.5c).

As the image is constant, the description of deep veins, great saphenous vein, small saphenous vein, Giacomini vein, etc. is not always represented to improve the comprehension of images. One "master" image with nomenclature will be displayed at the start of each chapter

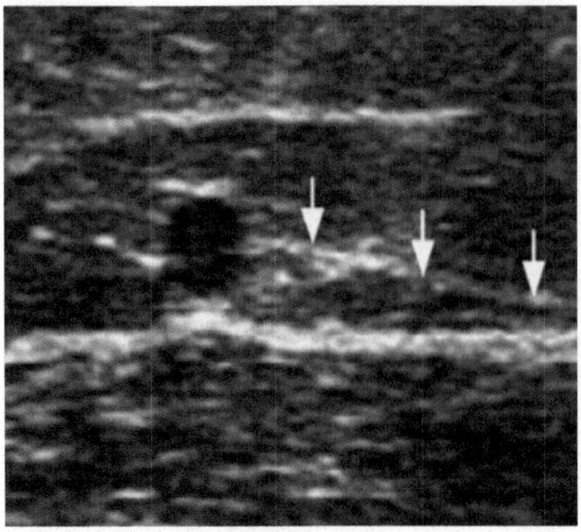

Fig. 2.4 Transverse view through the inner part of the thigh in an obese patient showing the great saphenous vein within its fascial compartment surrounded by fat. The arrows demonstrate the saphenous ligament. With kind permission by [21]

2.3 Hierarchical Order of Emptying

Normal blood flow is from the most distal lower extremity towards the heart and from the most superficial (N3) towards the deepest compartments (N2 and N1).

All the three networks are connected by perforating veins, physiologically draining from N3 and N2 to N1 (see Fig. 2.6). Schematically the order of draining can be represented as follows: N3–N2–N1. Whatever subversion of this hierarchical order of the venous networks, emptying can be considered as pathological. It would be represented as N1–N2–N3–N1 in the case of the reflux situation represented in Fig. 2.5c, d.

The above statement that even a reflux from a vein in N2 (saphenous vein) to a vein in N3 (tributary) represents a reflux with subversion of the physiological hierarchical order of the venous network emptying challenges the traditional view of superficial and deep venous reflux. N2 and N3 venous networks were traditionally considered the "superficial system". No anatomical and functional differences were contemplated if reflux flows backwards in one or both of N2 and N3 compartments [22].

2.3.1 Anatomical Aspects of the Venous Drainage

The anatomical features of the different compartments influence their haemodynamics:

The deep venous system, N1, is surrounded by the muscle, thus protected by excessive dilation and directly influenced by the pressure gradient that follows the muscle contraction and relaxation. In analogy to the heart contraction and relaxation, the leg muscle contraction exerts the function of a systole on the leg venous system, ejecting the blood back to the heart against gravitational forces. During leg muscle relaxation, the filling phase of the deep veins is allowed. For this reason, the leg muscular contraction is called systole and the leg muscular relaxation diastole of venous flow.

The saphenous or interfascial system, N2, is directly linked to the muscle mass by its laying on top of the muscle fascia, anchored to it with the saphenous ligament and covered by the saphenous fascia, which is firmly fixed to the muscular fascia on the edges of the compartment.

This feature indirectly transmits the muscular movements, the pressure during contraction and the fascial tone to the saphenous network, even if in a lower grade compared to the deep venous system.

At the same time, the two fascia layers wrap the saphenous system like a natural elastic stocking, limiting its excessive dilation under venous hypertension conditions and so impeding a tortuosity like the one observed in varicose tributaries.

Tributary veins of the N3 run outside the muscular fascia, surrounded just by subcutaneous fat, thus unprotected by neither muscular nor fascial structure. In this anatomical district, muscular systole and diastole have its minimum effect, while pressure gradients can exert their full action.

Tributaries do not seem to follow a precise anatomical structure. Apart from draining either into a saphenous vein or a perforator, they branch like a tree or they form networks. So, they can be structured according to the level of subdivision and named as first generation (the nearest to the saphenous vein), second generation after the first branching and third

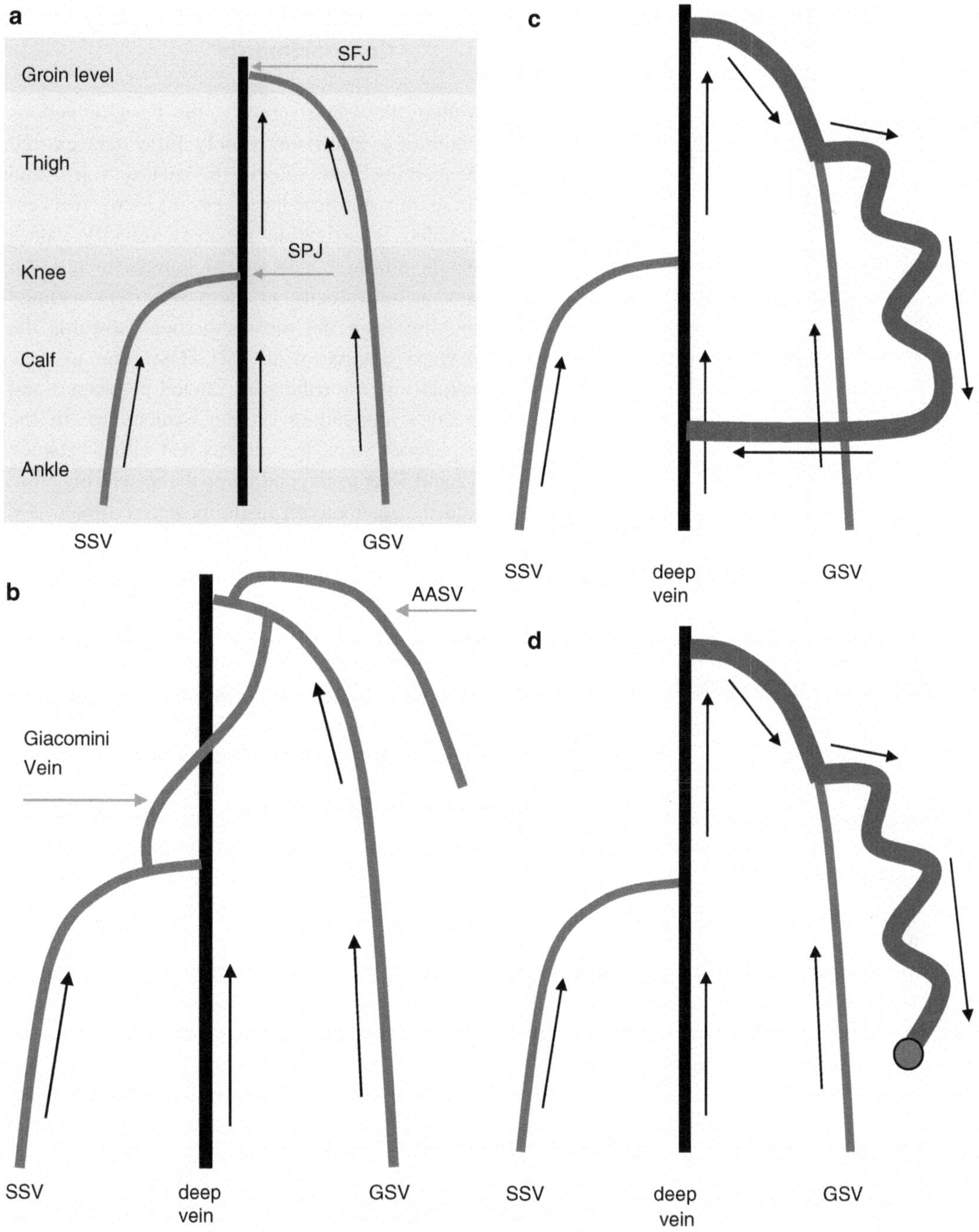

Fig. 2.5 Schematic representation of venous networks. (**a**) Deep veins (N1) and saphenous veins (N2), arrows indicating orthograde emptying of the veins. *GSV* great saphenous vein, *SSV* small saphenous vein, *SFJ* sapheno-femoral junction, *SPJ* sapheno-popliteal junction. (**b**) Same representation including (**a**) Giacomini vein and accessory anterior saphenous vein (AASV). (**c**) Representation of a refluxive sapheno-femoral junction with reflux in the great saphenous vein until mid-thigh, emptying into a tributary. This tributary drains through a perforator into the deep veins at the calf level. Note that in this representation the perforator line is crossing over the distal, sufficient saphenous vein. (**d**) To avoid lines crossing, perforators are represented as dots at the level of their drainage. Same image as **c**, the perforator line was replaced by a dot. As the perforator is draining the blood to the deep vein—that means the flow direction is orthograde—the dot is represented in blue. In case the perforator was refluxive, the dot would be represented in red. With kind permission by [21]

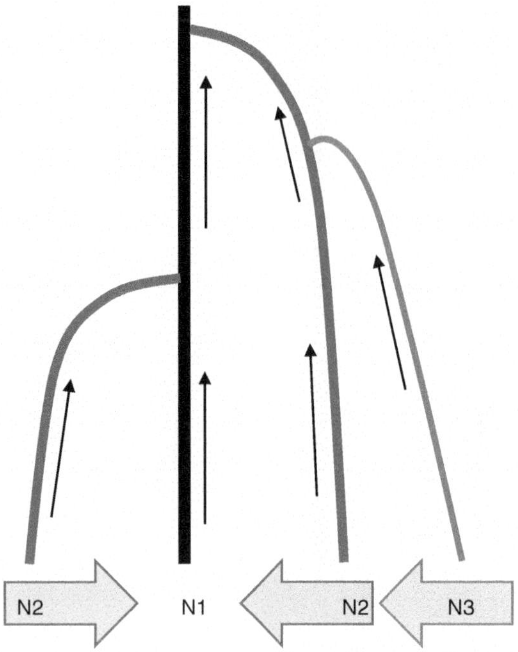

Fig. 2.6 Schematic representation of the hierarchical order of emptying. N3 (tributaries) drain into N2 (saphenous veins), and these drain into the deep veins (N1). With kind permission by [21]

generation after the next level of branching. Although this point of view is incorrect from the anatomical hierarchy, where the origin of the vein starts at the capillary level and follows the natural flow from the blood from distal to proximal, in phlebology often the veins are seen as refluxing pathways, so the first generation is the one "at the anatomic end" of the tributary, the one next to the saphenous vein or the perforator. Microvalves could be detected until the sixth generation of veins [19].

The anatomy-based consensus document has divided the superficial veins into *tributaries* (over 3 mm diameter) and *reticular veins* (less than 3 mm diameter) [13]. Reticular veins have a profile and are palpable, whereas thread veins or telangiectasia is only visible through the skin. Usually epifascial veins of the medial part or the thigh and leg and the dorsal part of the calf drain into the great and small saphenous veins, respectively, and are therefore called tributaries of these veins. The epifascial veins of the lateral aspect of the leg have no major vein to drain in and are called lateral plexus of the leg [13].

2.3.2 Blood Flow in the Different Compartments

Venous flow and reflux is the base of venous pathology. Surprisingly only little data existed concerning flow velocity in healthy veins, and these only consider large veins [23–26]. A recent detailed investigation reported velocity values inside all three anatomical compartments. An increasing velocity gradient was demonstrated moving from the most superficial towards the deepest compartment [27]. The time average velocity in the tributaries ranged between 5 and 9 cm/s, depending on the manoeuvre. In the saphenous veins, the velocity had values between 12 and 18 cm/s depending on the measuring point and the manoeuvre; in the posterior tibial vein, values between 15 and 18 cm/s were found. The deep venous system segments between the popliteal vein and the external iliac vein displayed values between 32 and 42 cm/s.

Comparing the flow velocities in each compartment, the femoral vein, popliteal vein, posterior tibial vein and short saphenous vein present significantly different velocity values compared to the other vessels of the same anatomical network. This feature requires further investigation. Possible explanations could be the fact that the posterior tibial vein is the only segment that was evaluated in the above reported analysis to be located above the plantar pump and below the calf pump. Moreover, posterior tibial vein is a usually duplicated vessel, in contrast to the other deep veins investigated [2, 28, 29].

The short saphenous vein presents a wide variability of anatomical junctions with the deep system: a fact that could influence its haemodynamics and blood flow velocity [30].

Femoral vein and popliteal vein belong to an intriguing anatomical site, whose valve presence and location variability could represent a clue for this result explanation [31, 32].

In fact, together with their anatomical variable distribution, valvular regions present potential confounding factors in the haemodynamics analysis, also due to the flow acceleration through the leaflet tract narrowing and to the valvular pocket turbulence [33, 34].

Independently by these considerations and different values between a compartment, the different anatomical venous networks result to be associated with different velocity values, which follow the drainage hierarchical order and are less in the tributaries and highest in the deep veins. The phenomenon introduces the possible aspiration effect from the slowest towards the fastest vessel, according to Venturi's effect.

a

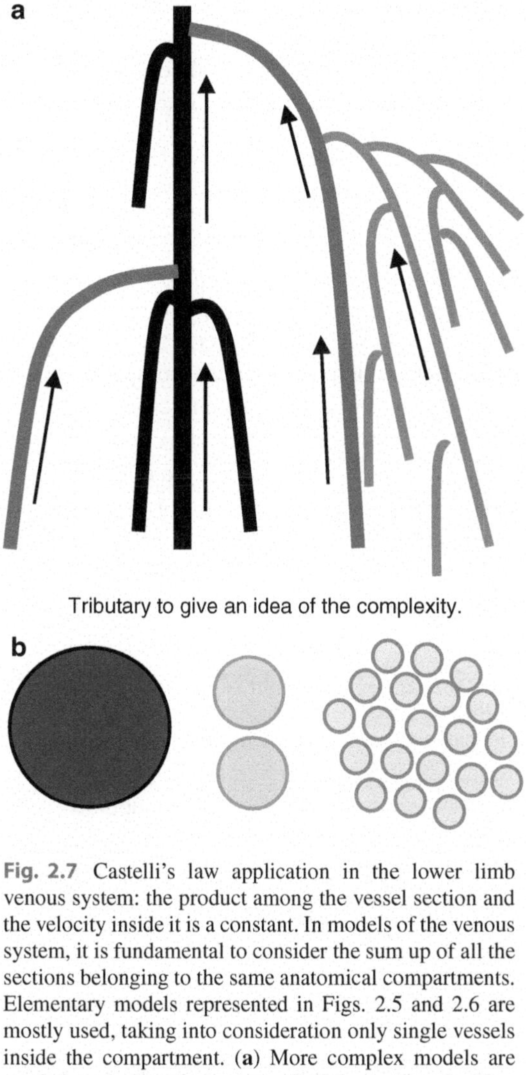

Tributary to give an idea of the complexity.

b

Fig. 2.7 Castelli's law application in the lower limb venous system: the product among the vessel section and the velocity inside it is a constant. In models of the venous system, it is fundamental to consider the sum up of all the sections belonging to the same anatomical compartments. Elementary models represented in Figs. 2.5 and 2.6 are mostly used, taking into consideration only single vessels inside the compartment. (**a**) More complex models are needed, evaluating the sum up of all the sections inside a specific anatomical compartment, like here, where all the deep veins are depicted, as well as the branching of one tributary to give an idea of the complexity. (**b**) Model of the section of the veins of each compartment, to be multiplied with the velocity in each vessel. With kind permission by [21]

Castelli's law (see also Sect. 3.1.3) states that the sum of the different vessel sections multiplied for the sum of the corresponding velocities is constant in a branching and closed tube system (see Fig. 2.5). For this reason, it will be mandatory to find out a way to assess not just a single vein segment of each network, rather the sum of all the different vessels that are localized inside the same compartment. The model will be more difficult, since at one level of the leg, different compartments are coexisting and interconnected. So, the number of vessels of every compartment must be adapted to the level of the leg considered (see Fig. 2.5c).

Interestingly, in case of superficial venous reflux, the velocity gradient is subverted, thus presenting a higher velocity in the incompetent tributary rather than in the saphenous trunk feeding the incompetent tributary. Further investigation on this topic is ongoing (Fig. 2.7).

Such kinetics component subversion leads to a lateral pressure drop and a potential Venturi's effect of aspiration from the saphenous system towards the incompetent varicose vein. This could be the fundament of the centripetal reflux propagation found by different authors [35–37].

Whenever considering velocity as guiding parameter for the venous network interpretation, it must be stated that a fundamental bias can rise by the same data acquisition tool. Even modern linear probes use large Doppler apertures to perform a proper beam steering and depth penetration. Consequently, these large apertures create a spectral spread that is unrelated to the blood cell velocity. The phenomenon is called intrinsic spectral broadening, and it occurs more or less in all the transducers, causing value overestimation [38, 39].

Recently, interesting technical instrumental innovations are offering the solution for a more precise assessment, paving the way for a more significant collection of data, also in settings that are like the ones herein presented [40–42].

2.4 Perforator Anatomy and Pathophysiological Significance

About 150 perforating veins could be found in anatomical studies of the legs [17]. Perforating veins are a group of a variable number of vessels (from 60 to more than 140) connecting the superficial (N2 and N3) and the deep lower limb venous system [17]. These vessels pierce the fascia and run in-between the muscular masses, almost always accompanied by a satellite artery. Functionally they play an important role, and surely the last word is not yet spoken about their implications in pressure balancing of the superficial and deep system, as well as evolution of varicose vein disease.

A comprehension of anatomic and functional aspects is important for the preoperative diagnostics in venous sparing surgery, which will be presented here and in the chapter for physiology (Chap. 3). Diagnostic aspects and their distribution along the leg are presented in Chap. 4.

2.4.1 Classification and Anatomy of Perforating Veins

Different classifications are described, without having been included in any anatomical consensus [2, 13].

Perforators depending on the compartment linked:

- N2–N1: Direct perforators link the saphenous system (N2) with the deep network (N1) (not to frequent).
- N3–N1: Indirect perforators are more frequent and link the subcutaneous veins (N3) with the corresponding vessel below the fascia (N1) by means of numerous scattered channels of communication.

Perforators depending on their path through the muscles:

- Direct perforators perforate the muscle fascia and course along intermuscular septa to reach deep axial veins.
- Indirect perforators are those which penetrate the muscle mass, to drain into intramuscular veins.

Perforating veins have been also discriminated according to their course with respect to the deep fascia in:

- Perpendicular when piercing the fascia in a right angle and running straight to the deep vein, also called direct or vertical perforators. Examples are Bassi, soleus perforating vein and Cockett (24 cm).
- Oblique or flexible if the course is not rectilineous. This form is the most often found in the leg.

A consensus about which classification should be applied uniformly is not yet found (personal information Prof. Caggiati, Rome).

From the haemodynamic point of view concerning venous sparing surgery, the differentiation after which anatomical compartment is linked seems to be the most interesting one. The pathology is different, if the reflux starts or ends in the saphenous vein (N2–N1) via a "direct" perforator or if the "indirect" perforator links the deep venous system (N1) with a tributary (N3). To keep it clear, throughout the book the veins connected by the perforators will always be mentioned.

We find direct perforators draining the great saphenous vein into the posterior tibial veins at the calf (paratibial perforators), seldom at the thigh, sometimes Hunter or Dodd, perforators of the medial thigh. The small saphenous vein shows two typical direct perforators, Bassi at the ankle level and May or soleus perforating vein in the middle third of the small saphenous vein. Further anatomical information about how to explore perforating veins is to be found in Sect. 4.7.

Anatomical studies show that perforating veins, particularly if of small calibres, are usually valveless or endowed with rudimental valves [43–45]. It is the combination of the valves and the muscles acting on the perforating vein, which results in the competence of the vein during muscular systole. At the calf level, pressure values up to 250 mmHg are achieved by muscle contraction (systole). No single valve would resist the pressure. Perforating veins often have an "S"-form way through the muscles until reaching the deep vein (see Sect. 4.7). This induces a compression of the perforating vein between the muscles during muscular systole, closing the lumen completely and avoiding a pathologic compartment change (reflux from deep vein N1 to superficial vein N2 or N3).

The large number of perforating veins suggests the importance of not considering just the single perforator in the haemodynamic role, rather the entireness of the perforating veins, of both small and large calibres, as multiple vessels connecting the deep and superficial compartments.

2.4.2 Flow Direction Through Perforating Veins

Direction of flow in perforating veins has started to be investigated after the upcoming of ultrasound. Prior to this era, every dilated perforator was defined as incompetent. This is a tendency still observed today among many phlebologists.

Already in 1992 investigations pointed out the presence of bidirectional flow in perforators, with an inward and outward orientation, so introducing the perforating veins' role as pressure equalizers among the deep and superficial veins. Sarin found that under distal compression (corresponding to systole), 21% of the medial calf perforators in limbs without superficial venous reflux reacted with outward flow, whereas during the relaxation phase (corresponding to the diastole), only legs with superficial venous reflux presented flow of any direction in 33–44% and none of the legs with no epifascial reflux [46]. During systole, an outward flow is pressure regulating, during diastole an outward flow is a sign of deep venous insufficiency, and an inward flow is a sign of superficial venous reflux draining through these perforators [47].

Since reflux duration in superficial veins was defined as pathologic above 500 ms, also in perforating veins, this value was adopted [48]. In the first measurement, inflow and outflow through the valves were evaluated independently of the systole or diastole phase of the provocation manoeuvre.

The correlation among the increased number of dilated and incompetent perforating veins and chronic venous disease severity testifies the haemodynamic role of these vessels, for which a dedicated, yet controversial, treatment has been proposed along the last decades [49, 50].

Even though the duplex techniques were getting better and the comprehension about inward flow and outward flow through perforators was described, any perforator with a flow lasting longer than 0.5 s was determined as incompetent perforator [51].

This was the reason why Delis reported a higher prevalence of perforating vein incompetence in the leg rather than in the thigh [49]. For sure the prevalence of dilated perforating veins is higher at the calf.

Since many years representants of saphenous vein sparing surgery claim that dilated perforating veins at the calf are mostly the re-entry pathway for the refluxive blood, rather than primary incompetent pathways. Also, some investigations measuring diameters of perforating veins after simple crossectomy and sclerotherapy of proximal saphenous veins confirmed that the diameter of perforating veins at the calf was significantly reduced [52].

Incompetent perforating veins feeding the refluxive saphenous vein (N1–N2) or the tributaries (N1–N3) are most often located at the thigh. On the contrary, draining perforating pathways N2–N1 or N3–N1 are mostly located at the calf [3, 16, 53] (see Sect. 3.4.1).

Large discussions have been held on the topic. The UIP consensus document on haemodynamics [14] summarizes as follows: "Most phlebologists now consider that thigh and calf perforating veins have a different hemodynamic behaviour. Thigh perforating veins are connected with the higher pole of the ambulatory pressure gradient; they become the source of reflux if incompetent and represent a pathological condition. In contrast to that, calf perforating veins are connected with the lower pole of the ambulatory pressure gradient and in the presence of normal deep veins IPVs are unlikely to be the source of the pathological refluxing flow, even if enlarged (IPV = incompetent perforating veins)."

So, the international phlebology community has changed their point of view – also those performing ablative techniques. Upcoming new techniques (see background information) are giving the opportunity to exactly measure the net in- and outflow through a perforating vein, giving the possibility to gather evidence-based information for a future consensus.

> Recent ultrasound investigations allow to assess the net flow direction in a vessel. This can be applied to the saphenous veins as well as to the perforating veins. Figure 2.8 shows an evaluation of flow in these vessels.
>
> This investigation could demonstrate the years-long defended hypothesis of venous sparing philosophy:
>
> There is a lack of overlapping among the traditional incompetence definition (diastolic outward flow lasting more than 500 ms) and the net flow direction.

In conclusion, rather than being just draining routes from the superficial towards the deep system, perforating veins can serve as pressure overload dissipators, draining the blood from the compartment at higher pressure towards the one at lowest values in healthy and in varicose vein legs. A typical example is the muscular systole of the calf, significantly increasing the pressure in the deep venous system, forcing the blood to move upwards but also laterally towards the saphenous system through a perforating vein without pathological implication. Perforating veins represent the best example of interaction among anatomical localization, structure and function in the contest of the intriguing topic of venous haemodynamics.

2.4.3 Perforating Veins as Equalizers Between the Compartments

During an investigation about the reflux duration in incompetent great saphenous veins and their calf tributaries, the simultaneous ending of reflux at the thigh and calf was demonstrated, independently of the fact that the reflux changed the compartment from N2 to N3 (from saphenous vein to tributary) in some of the patients or had an interfascial course from the groin to the mid-calf region in the saphenous vein [54]. Interestingly during this refluxing phase after standing up from recumbent position, no flow was detected at the popliteal vein, which could have been expected, if the superficial and deep veins were considered as non-compliant, rigid, interconnected tubes.

Shortly after the reflux cessation in the superficial vein and with a delay of 1–4 s, the orthograde flow in the popliteal vein started (non-published data). This leads to an interesting interpretation: Reflux in the superficial veins (N2 and N3) is possible as long as the pressure in the calf muscle capacitance veins filled through the perforators with the refluxing blood is lesser than the one in the saphenous vein. After the pressure equalizes, the reflux stops. Then it takes a little time, in which the pressure of the deep calf veins is increased by the arterial inflow until finally the pressure in the calf is higher than the one in the deep veins of the thigh provoking an orthograde emptying of blood of the calf veins through the popliteal vein. This illustrates the interconnection and teamwork of all three compartments, valves and muscles even in pathological circumstances.

2.4.4 Clinical and Therapeutical Implications of Incompetent Perforating Veins

There is still a huge lack of consensus and evidence concerning the diagnostics and the treatment implications of perforating veins. Coming from the radical ablative surgery with

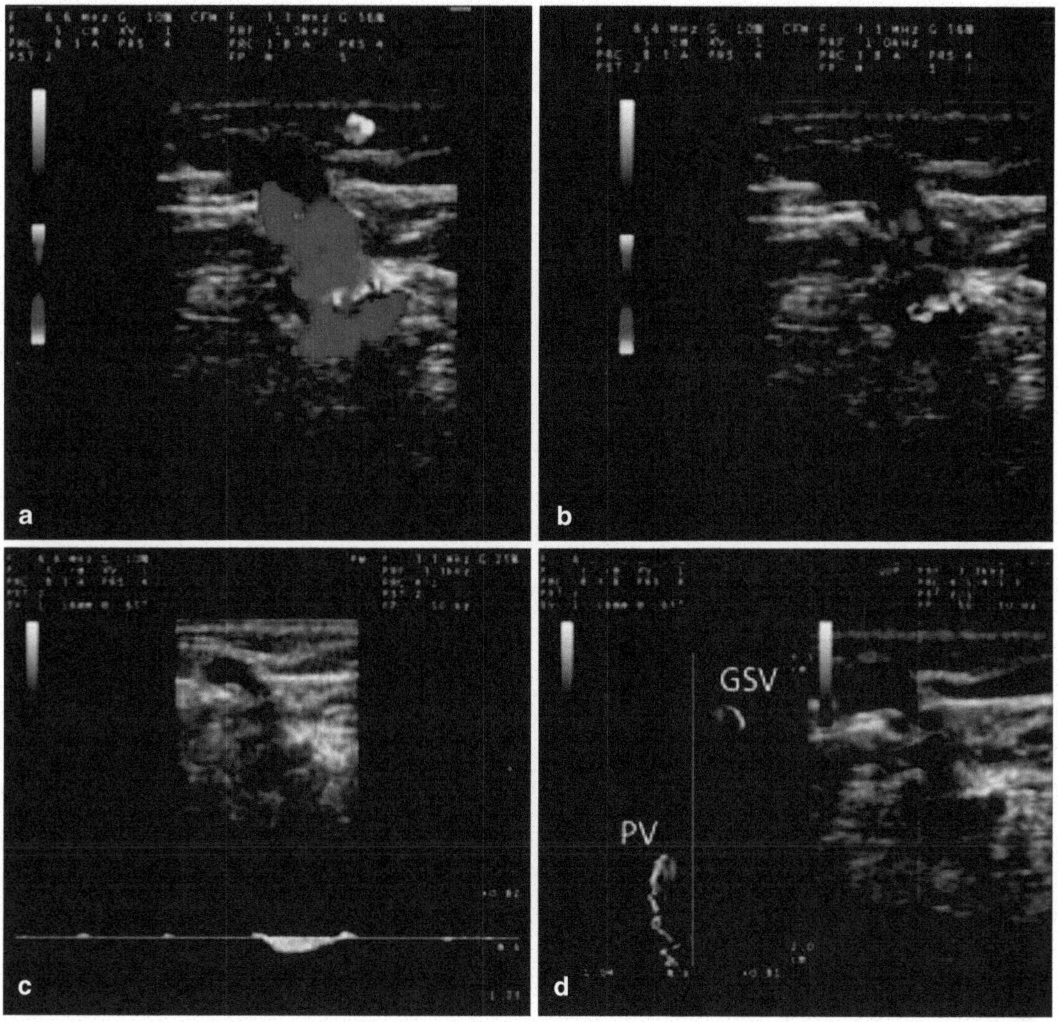

Fig. 2.8 Net flow analysis in a perforating vein: (**a**) Colour Doppler analysis showing the entire perforating vein flow moving away from the transducer (coded in blue) during diastole and (**b**) in red the flow towards the transducer during systole. (**c**) Pulsed wave spectral analysis reporting the flow inside the single spot of the perforating vein covered by the sample volume, displaying a little amount of outward flow (during systole) followed by a long-lasting inward flow (during diastole). (**d**) Great saphenous vein (GSV) and perforating vein (PV) net flow direction assessment by innovative softwares, showing the prevalent drainage direction of the entire perforating vein. Based on the localization of the curve on the baseline, it is possible to detect a net outward (right side of the baseline) or inward (left side of the baseline) flow. In this case it could be demonstrated that the great saphenous vein had a net reflux (right of the line) and the perforating vein a net inward flow (left of the line). Copyright: Sergio Gianesini

extraction of every refluxive superficial venous segment, as well as interruption of every dilated perforator detectable in the leg in the last century, even applying subfascial dissectors to perform this in a more radical way, things have changed until today, also in the ablative surgery:

According to the guidelines, elective treatment of incompetent perforating veins **is not** recommended in patients with simple varicose veins (CEAP C2) (Grade 1B). This means dilated perforating veins themselves were not to be interrupted, when treating varicose veins in CEAP Class C2. A perforating vein can be treated whenever presenting an outward flow lasting ≥500 ms, a diameter of at least 3.5 mm and a localization beneath a healed or open venous ulcer (Grade 2B) [55].

2.5 Venous Valves

The efficient functioning of the venous system depends upon the competence of valves. This thin endothelium-lined structures are so constructed as to support the venous return to the heart against action of gravity. Venous valves occur in many veins, both small and large, that conduct blood flow against the gravity. They prevent the backflow of blood from the heart. There are papers describing the anatomy of valve system of different anatomical district's veins [56, 57].

One important valve complex is the one located in the sapheno-femoral junction. Two main valves have been described at this position: the terminal valve at the junction outlet, which regulates the flow from the great saphenous vein to the femoral vein, and the preterminal valve, which is found in the saphenous arch, approximately 5–6 cm from the junction, located below the outlet of the main sapheno-femoral junction tributaries. While, in older anatomy studies, the terminal valve is almost constant being present in about 99% of individuals, the preterminal valve is present in 93–95% of the population [56–58]. In a more recent publication, the terminal valve was found only in about 70% of patients and the preterminal valve in about 90% of cases [59].

The valve leaflets are tiny, semilunar, pocket-like flaps formed by local folding of the intima. Each valve is usually composed of two leaflets positioned opposite each other, with their free edges directed towards the heart. When blood passes throughout the lumen between the leaflets, they flatten out against the wall of the vein. When blood begins to regurgitate, the pocket fills up, causing contact of the two leaflets and resulting in closing of the lumen of the vein.

2.6 Histology of the Venous Wall

2.6.1 Histology of the Saphenous Veins and Epifascial Branches

Like the arteries, the larger veins consist of three layers [60]. From inside to outside, they are the intima, media and adventitia. The intima is coated with an endothelium where the cells are orientated longitudinally and in direct contact with the blood. The valve cusps develop from horizontally orientated endothelial cells which arise from the intima in both the deep veins and the saphenous trunks.

Histologically, the saphenous trunks (N2) can be differentiated from the tributaries (epifascial branches, N3). The saphenous trunks consist of smooth muscle cells in all three layers of the vein wall. They are orientated longitudinally in the intima and adventitia with a circular orientation in the media. The thickness of the wall reduces from the foot upwards. There is a higher collagen content and a higher number of muscle cells in all three layers at the foot. These muscles are responsible for the fact that the saphenous vein is appropriate as arterial bypass material. And possibly they are also the reason why saphenous veins can reduce their diameter, which means to undergo "retonisation" after saphenous vein sparing surgery.

The adventitia of the saphenous vein contains very small supply vessels called vasa vasorum as well as terminal fibres of the sympathetic system. The intima and adventitia of the larger epifascial tributaries have scarcely any longitudinal smooth muscle cells. Under the endothelium there is only a thin layer of collagen and in the media a thin layer of muscle.

In case of aplasia of saphenous vein ("empty eye", see Sect. 4.5), a histological rudiment of a saphenous vein is always found. There are smooth muscle cells in all three layers of the wall but the lumen is absent.

In case of reflux, the venous wall changes are visible in light microscopy (see Fig. 2.9).

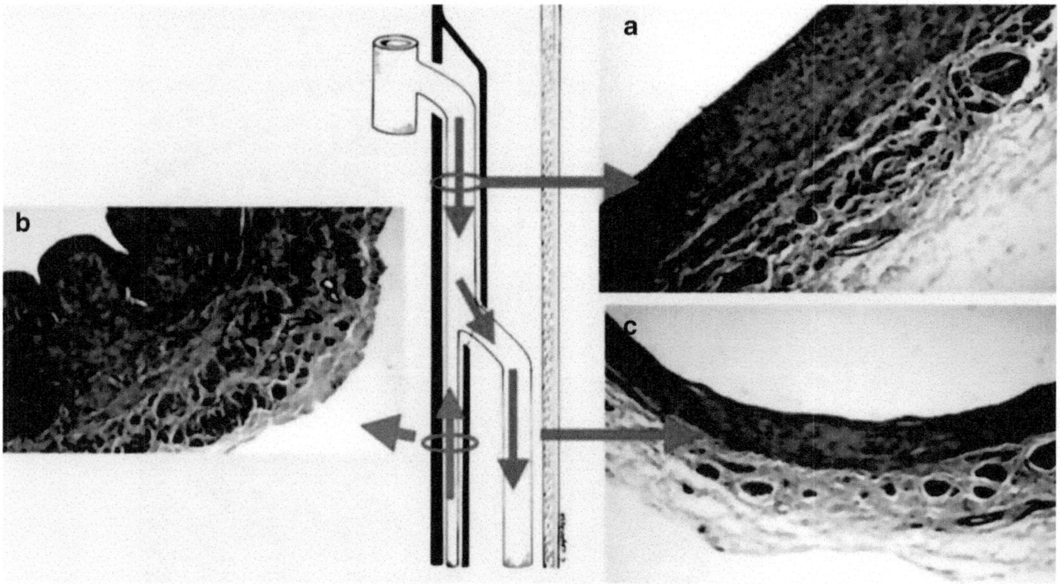

Fig. 2.9 Histology (Masson staining ×10) of (**a**) a refluxing great saphenous vein (N2) compared to (**b**) a healthy great saphenous vein (N2) in the same leg and (**c**) a refluxive tributary (N3). (Prof. A. Caggiati, Rome; by kind permission)

2.6.2 Histology of the Venous Wall and Physiological Implications

All blood vessels have an inner layer, the intima, lined by endothelium with subjacent connective tissue; a middle layer, the media, composed of smooth muscle, elastic tissue and collagen embedded in ground substance (see Fig. 2.10); and an outer layer, the adventitia, composed of elastic and fibrous tissue.

The endothelium of the great saphenous vein is a monolayer of elongated epithelium, with the individual cells oriented with the long axis in the line of blood flow. Adjacent cells are connected by tight and gap junctions, the number and proportion of each varying in different parts of the vascular system and in different segments of vessel (see Fig. 2.11 top). In course of chronic venous insufficiency, segments of great saphenous vein exhibiting reflux reflect the oscillatory and turbulent flow with a significant derangement of the endothelial cells and loss of the regular disposition in accordance with the laminar flow direction (Fig. 2.11 bottom).

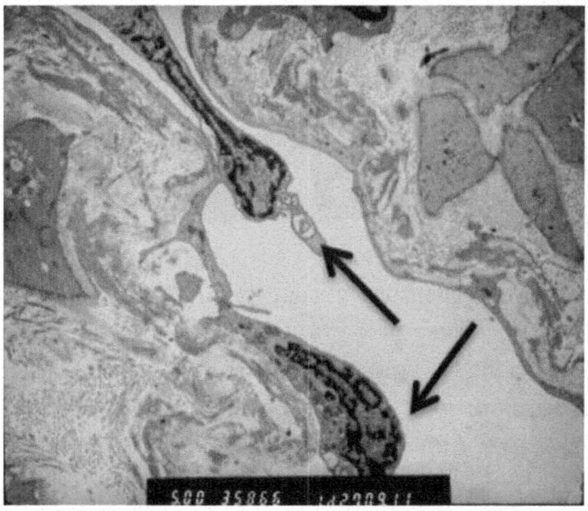

Fig. 2.10 Ultrastructure of the great saphenous vein lumen and wall at transmission electronic microscopy 5000×. The arrows in the lumen indicate the endothelial cell monolayer, with smooth muscle cells and fibres well visible in the media layer (Courtesy of Paolo Zamboni)

The ability of blood vessel to accommodate or influence changes in blood flow and intraluminal pressure by contraction or relaxation relies largely on the smooth muscle component of their wall, moderated by connective tissue elements and a complex of vasoactive substances and the

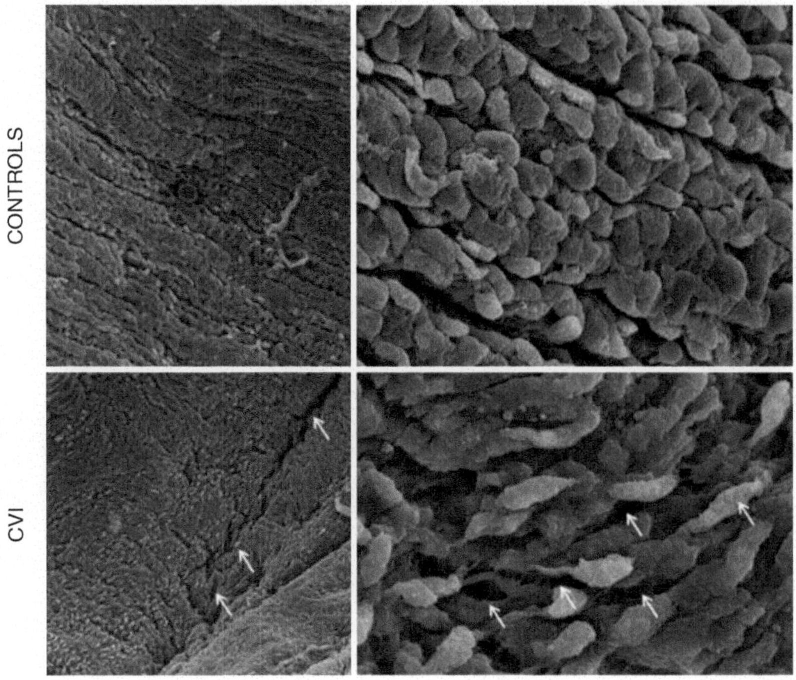

Fig. 2.11 Top panels: Scanning electron microscopy of the endothelial cells of a non-refluxive great saphenous vein (left 500× and right 3000×) harvested in course of an arterial bypass procedure. The endothelium appears very regularly arranged with the cells oriented along the flow direction axis. Bottom panels: Scanning electron microscopy of the endothelial cells of diseased great saphenous vein (left 660× and right 5000×) harvested in course of stripping procedure. Cell derangement with figures of the endothelial layer is indicated by the arrows. Abnormal white blood cells are visible on the surface of the vein lumen. The arrows show the endothelial lining. Copyright: courtesy of Sergio Gianesini and Paolo Zamboni

autonomic nervous system [61]. In this chapter the regulation of the different vasoactive substances on the smooth muscle tone will be further described.

At one time the smooth muscle was thought to be restricted to the media of vessels. With the advent of electron microscopy and other technological advances such as immunohistochemistry, it was established that so-called "transitional" or "myointimal" cells, a prominent component of the intima in normal adult blood vessels and also of arteriosclerotic lesions, are smooth muscle cells. The individual smooth muscle cell is spindle shaped and surrounded by a closely applied basement membrane; it contains thick myosin and thin actin filaments imparting contractile properties. The cytoplasm also contains noncontractile intermediate filaments of vimentin and desmin type as part of the cytoskeleton. In addition, fibronectin acts as regulator of smooth muscle cell contractility. Smooth muscle, in contrast to skeletal or cardiac muscle, will replicate and proliferate under appropriate stimuli as seen, for example, in the repair processes, in response to inflammation or in altered haemodynamic conditions such as venous hypertension and turbulent flow.

Collagen and elastic tissue, the main fibrous proteins, are embedded in a complex ground substance of proteoglycans. In the saphenous veins, the major fibrous proteins of the media are types I and III of so-called interstitial collagens; they are produced mainly by the fibroblasts of the adventitia, but it seems that they are also produced by smooth muscle cells of the media. These collagens provide the tensile strength of the saphenous veins and related tributaries, putting a constraint on its distensibility. Elastic tissue (the elastica) is composed of another fibrous protein (elastin). It is a prominent component of vessel walls, particularly well shown by appropriate staining methods where it is concentrated to form the fenestrated lamella (internal elastic membrane or lamina).

The elasticity inherent in all blood vessels is not determined by elastic tissue only, as the name of this tissue would seem to imply, but is a synergistic function of contractile smooth muscle with its associated elastic tissue and matrix. Collagen, which is much less elastic, is the tensile element that serves to prevent overdistension of vessels [58, 62, 63].

2.6.3 Compliance of the Venous Wall

The histology described above is closely linked with the mechanical wall properties of the veins and particularly with their compliance. Compliance (*c*) is a characteristic of every hollow system, but in veins perfectly fits with the venous function of drainage. Volumetric increase (d*V*) of the content is correlated with pressure increase (dP) inside the vein (the equation is compliance = volumetric increase/pressure increase, $c = dV/dP$) [64–67]. The components of the media layer of veins, described above, permit the venous system to achieve a higher compliance with respect to an artery.

This capability to receive fluid in the conduit and to maintain the gradient over time is expressed in physics as the "compliance" of the system. It depends on the elasticity or rigidity, the length and (to a lesser extent) the radius of the conduit and, also, on the degree of filling [1, 35, 68, 69]. The authors assessed in vitro and in vivo the mechanical wall properties especially by venous compliance in the great saphenous vein system and found out a very good correlation between venous compliance measured in vitro and that of the same vein measured in vivo by high-resolution B-mode ultrasound before great saphenous vein ablation [70, 71] (Fig. 2.12).

As the venous system has a high compliance, it can receive a significant volume of blood with a small increase in pressure; the correspondent curve will not be very steep [64–67] (see Class 4 in Fig. 2.12). Conversely, if the system has low compliance, even a small increase in blood volume within the system causes a significant increase in pressure, and the curve will be steeper (see Class 2 in Fig. 2.12).

Based on the correlation above, we introduced the ultrasound assessment of venous compliance in clinical practice. Ultrasound calculation on venous compliance is based on the assessment of the cross-sectional area (or diameter) of the great saphenous vein in a low-pressure situation (patient recumbent), and the diameter changes after standing up, by assuming the area reflects the blood volume and the pressure in the vein corresponds to the hydrostatic pressure. Cross-sectional area changes in

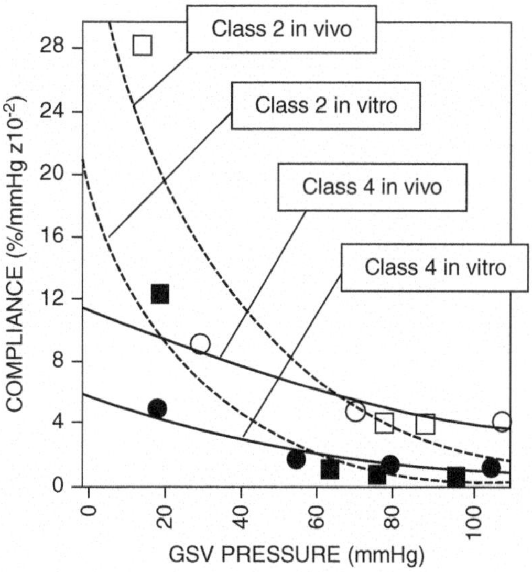

Fig. 2.12 Correlation curve expressing the percentage of variation of the cross-sectional area of the great saphenous vein (y-axis) in response to pressure variation (x-axis). The values were assessed in vitro and in vivo measuring the diameter of the vein with ultrasound and the pressure change. When the filling starts (0 pressure to 20 mmHg pressure), the change of the vein area is huge, showing it is capable to adapt lots of blood without inducing a higher intravenous pressure. The pressure gets higher, as more volume is introduced, because then the vein is no longer able to enlarge to fit the volume without pressure increase. The correlation of the curves is well apparent. Without surrounding tissue in the in vitro measurement, the compliance is worse [70, 71]

response to variation of the hydrostatic pressure represent a non-invasive measurement of venous compliance [67, 72, 73].

Moreover, by using the ultrasonographic assessment, the compliance of the great saphenous vein with respect to that of the varicose tributaries was also measured and compared and resulted in significantly different mechanical wall performance in the latter as compared to the great saphenous vein (see Fig. 2.13).

GSV tributaries showed a worsened compliance with respect to the GSV likely in consideration of the different wall thickness, which means less elastic components. In Fig. 2.13 tributaries with previous episodes of thrombophlebitis clearly show the worsened capability to accommodate and drain blood.

We know from classical physiology that the relationship between vein volume and pressure is characterized by a significant increase in volume with little change in pressure during the filling phase, in which the vein is distended by the increase in blood volume without experimenting

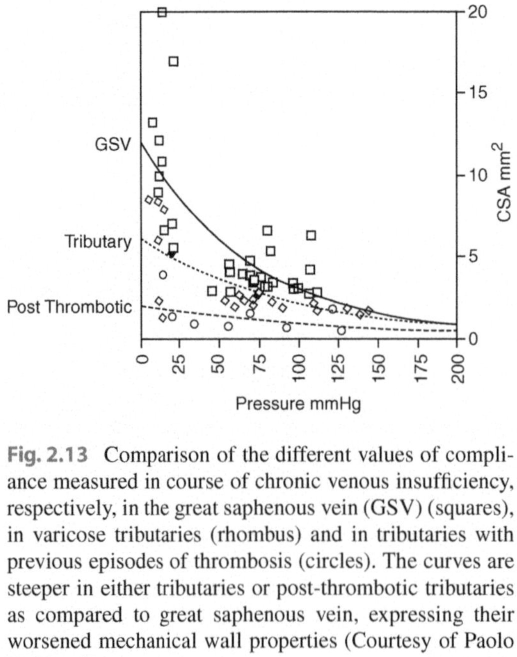

Fig. 2.13 Comparison of the different values of compliance measured in course of chronic venous insufficiency, respectively, in the great saphenous vein (GSV) (squares), in varicose tributaries (rhombus) and in tributaries with previous episodes of thrombosis (circles). The curves are steeper in either tributaries or post-thrombotic tributaries as compared to great saphenous vein, expressing their worsened mechanical wall properties (Courtesy of Paolo Zamboni)

an increase of pressure, just adapting to the volume [6, 7, 64–67, 72, 73]. In other words, during this first phase, the pressure and volume relationship is not linear. Instead, during the distension phase following the filling phase, further increases in volume are proportionally reflected by pressure increases, so that linearity of the volume/pressure relationship in veins can be demonstrated starting from pressure values around 20 mmHg (Fig. 2.14).

On the other hand, after completion of the filling phase, vein diameter is geometrically related to vein volume (provided that the vessel length is constant). This may explain the finding of a linear pressure/diameter relationship in the filled veins [6, 7, 65] (Fig. 2.14).

The mechanical behaviour of material subjected to tension is described by Hooke's law ($F = E \times dL$), which states that every material subjected to a force tends to develop a reactive force (F) proportional to the elongation produced (dL), in a linear ratio through a constant (E) (the Young modulus) which is characteristic of any material and represents the slope of the line ($E = dL/F$) [66].

Biological materials, however, do not obey this law and demonstrate a ratio between applied force (or developed force) and produced elongation that is curvilinear in form. The slope, called a tangential modulus, varies from point to point on the curve in proportion to the produced length and therefore is not a constant like the Young modulus.

By analogy with the tangential modulus of the force/elongation curve, compliance in biological systems (i.e. the slope of the pressure/volume curve) also varies from point to point in relation to the filling volume of the system.

The shape of the compliance curve is determined, therefore, by the physical characteristics of the material involved in the system. For such a reason, the great saphenous vein reservoir in standing is more efficient as compared to that of the tributaries (see Fig. 2.13). The curve depends also on the volumetric extension of the system

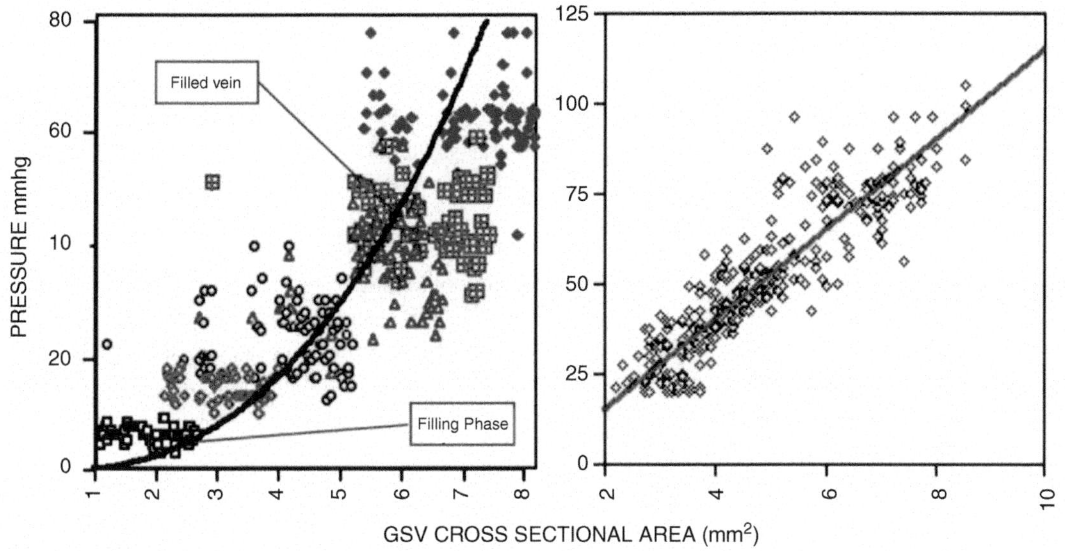

Fig. 2.14 Left: During the filling phase, increments of blood volume correspond to little or no pressure changes in the great saphenous vein (GSV). The filling phase was determined passing gradually by the means of a tilt bed from the supine to the standing posture. When the blood distends the great saphenous vein wall, the relationship becomes linear. Right: Starting from approximately 20–23 mmHg, the linear relationship between great saphenous vein cross-sectional area and pressure becomes very well apparent. Modified from [7]

and its geometric configuration. It is evident that the greater the volume of a container, the greater its capacity to receive the volume of the contents with a small increase in internal pressure until its capacity is reached. It is also evident that in a hollow spherical system, the extension of the system is correlated solely with the radius, while in a hollow tubular system, it is correlated principally with the length of the system and only to a small degree with the radius or diameter of the vein.

The actual value of compliance in the venous system is, instead, correlated, as we mentioned, with emptying capacity of the system. In the chapter devoted to the hierarchical order of emptying of the veins of the lower extremity, it has been shown that the great saphenous vein (N2) is connected to the deep veins (N1) and the tributaries (N3) via perforators. So, the transmission of the kinetic energy in the tributaries is reduced with respect to the deep veins and the great saphenous vein, thus further affecting the emptying capacity of the tributary system. Moreover, in hydrostatic condition, with the fluid in stasis like in standing or in sitting posture, the degree of filling in the system is influenced only by the volume; but in a hydrodynamic system, with the fluid in motion, the degree of filling in the system is influenced not only by the initial volume but also by the relation between the input rate and output rate.

The venous system needs high compliance because physiological postural changes determine big variations of hydrostatic pressure. The hydrostatic pressure of gravity is the major regulator of the volume content of the veins in the leg. In the sub-diaphragmatic veins, there are significant changes in volume according to the posture (see Fig. 2.14). In supine position the hydrostatic pressure is equalized within the venous system and the blood is equally redistributed in the upper and lower veins according to the principle of the communicating vessels. But when the subject is in standing posture, the veins of the lower extremity become enlarged to accommodate the redistribution of blood below the diaphragmatic line (see Fig. 2.15). From this point of view, it does not matter that the better mechanical performance of the great saphenous vein permits to accommodate more blood with a more rapid drainage during walking with respect to the superficial tributaries.

2.6.4 Wall Contraction of Control and Diseased Veins in Response to Physiologic Regulators of the Venous Tone

The dilatation of varicose veins appears to be a primary process that is initiated by unknown factors. There are several theories about the possible mechanisms that initiate the disease process [74]. One of the more often evoked theories concerns the weakness of the venous wall, which in turn leads to the separation of the valve cusps with consequent blood reflux. By acting on the vein wall, this haemodynamic change, and particularly high reverse flow velocity and turbulence, facilitates an extensive tissue remodelling. In support of this hypothesis, evidence is accumulating that implicates a deficient smooth muscle function in the pathogenesis of chronic venous insufficiency.

For instance, it was reported that the maximal responses of a varicose vein preparation to norepinephrine (NE) and/or to endothelin-1 (ET-1) are lower than those of control healthy tissues [68, 69, 75–80]. Whether these functional changes cause a multifocal impairment of vein smooth muscle and mediate the development of varicose veins or merely represent an epiphenomenon of the pathophysiologic process still remains a contentious issue. Contraction of the smooth muscle cells of the venous wall can be experimentally induced in vitro by a non-specific depolarization of the cell membrane. However, in physiology, the maintenance of the venous tone is expected to be largely controlled by the sympathetic nerves via norepinephrine (NE); by the autacoids, such as the endothelin (ET-1); and by the vasoactive hormones, such as angiotensin II (Ang II) [68, 69, 75–80].

All these stimulants are capable of inducing concentration-dependent contractions in healthy great saphenous vein tissues by acting through different mechanisms:

- KCl 100 mmol/L by inducing cell membrane depolarization
- NE, ET-1 and Ang II by activating specific receptors located in the smooth muscle cells of the great saphenous vein and their tributaries [37]

The authors assessed the maximal effects (maximum effect, grade of contraction), respectively, in control tissue, great saphenous vein in early stages of varicose vein illness (only visible veins, C2), great saphenous veins in later stages (skin changes, C4) and finally varicose tributaries, of dose-dependent concentrations, respectively, of norepinephrine (NE), endothelin (ET1) and angiotensin (Ang II). The maximum effect that could be evoked by the stimulants was reduced progressively with the increasing severity of the disease in the great saphenous vein as well as in tributaries, which raised the tributary assay to statistical significance for both NE and Ang II ($P < 0.05$). We also measured the affinity of, respectively, NE, ET1 and Ang II for their specific receptors (pEC50, the negative logarithm to base 10 of the molar concentration of the agonist, which produces the 50% of the maximal effect). Surprisingly, a marked reduction of Ang II apparent affinity was already evident in tissues that were taken from patients in an early stage of the disease ($P < 0.05$) and confirmed also in later stages and in the GSV tributaries (Fig. 2.15).

The decrease of affinity, specific for Ang II, may be interpreted by assuming, that in diseased tissues, changes occur at the Ang II receptor level. These receptors become more than tenfold less sensitive to the agonist, and their ability to induce contraction is not changed (the Emax in control tissues and in tissues of group 1 is not different). Such changes cannot be explained by a reduced accessibility of Ang II to its receptor because tissues of controls show little if any signs

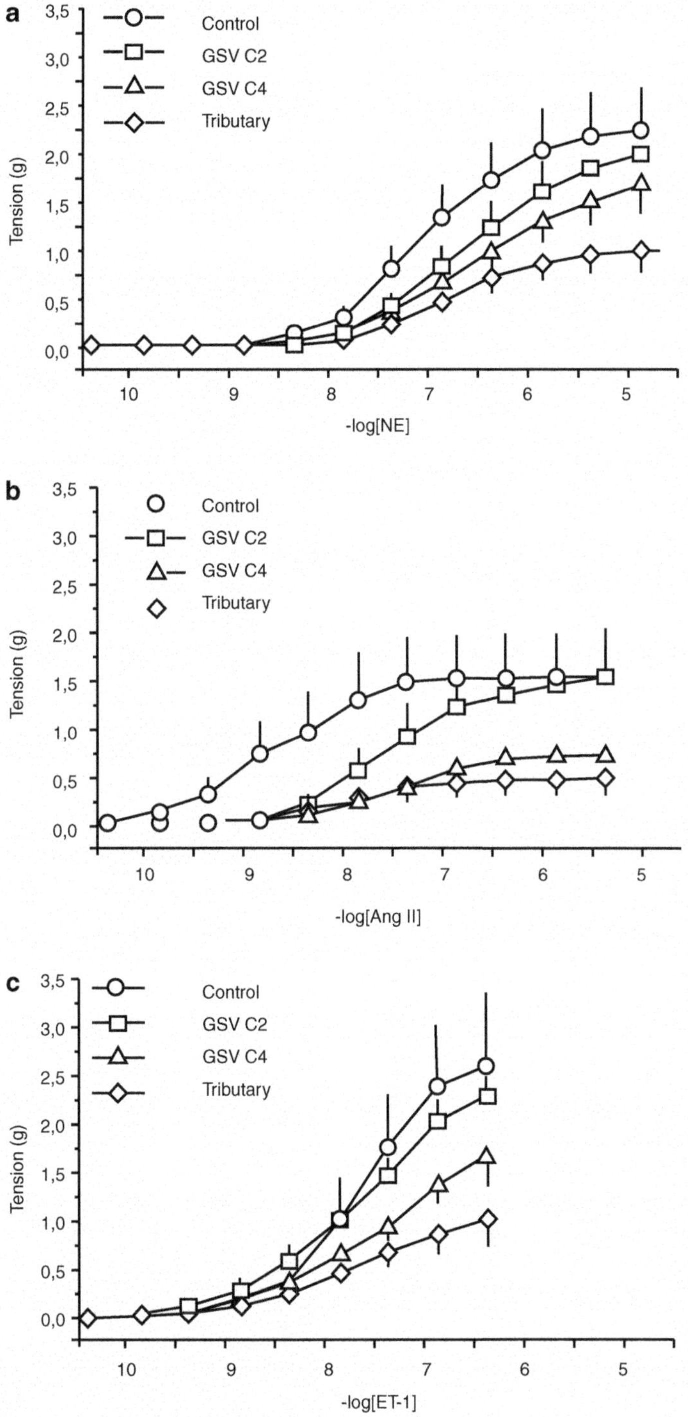

Fig. 2.15 Concentration response curves to (**a**) norepinephrine (NE), (**b**) angiotensin II (Ang II) and (**c**) endothelin-1 (ET-1) in human saphenous veins and tributaries from control subjects and from patients with primary varicose vein disease. Abscissa, logarithm of the molar concentration of agonist; ordinate, tension in g. The last value of each curve represents the maximal contraction, which appears to be significantly reduced in C4 GSV and in tributaries with respect to control tissue. We also evaluated the affinity of the smooth muscle cell receptors, respectively, for NE, Ang II and ET-1 (pEC50, the negative logarithm to base 10 of the molar concentration of the agonist, which produces the 50% of the maximal effect). The affinity for Ang II was lowered in all the diseased tissues. Modified from [79]

of remodelling. Accentuated local enzymatic degradation of Ang II seems unlikely, but no data are available to exclude this possibility. The intracellular smooth muscle machinery that subserves contraction appears to be efficient because NE and ET-1 and also high concentrations of Ang II evoke maximal contractions.

Although we did not measure control tributary veins, it is undebatable that varicose tributaries demonstrated reduced contractility in response to the physiologic vasoactive agents.

Taken together, the present findings support the intriguing hypothesis that a primary defective mechanism in the Ang II-mediated control of the venous tone could play a role in the pathogenesis of chronic venous insufficiency. In consideration of the primary role that is played by the renin-angiotensin system in cardiovascular pathophysiology, these findings could have important implications.

Conclusions

In this chapter reduced mechanical wall properties in vivo and in vitro were assessed in varicose tributaries with respect to diseased GSV. Venous compliance, a parameter reflecting the function of the venous system, is more efficient in the GSV. In addition, significant differences in the efficiency of venous tone control in response to NE, ET-1 and Ang II physiologic stimuli by comparing diseased great saphenous vein to varicose tributary have been demonstrated. Taken together such experimental data support the saphenous vein sparing strategies, pointing out the different structural and consequently also haemodynamics features of the great saphenous vein compared to the tributary network.

Literature

1. Bergan JJ. Common anatomic patterns of varicose veins. In: Goldmann MP, Weiss RA, Bergan JJ, editors. Varicose veins and telangiectasias. St Louis: Quality Medical Publishing Inc; 1999. p. 70–86.
2. Cavezzi A, Labropoulos N, Partsch H, Ricci S, Caggiati A, Myers K, Nicolaides A, Smith P. Duplex ultrasound investigation of the veins in chronic venous disease of the lower limbs—UIP consensus document. Part II. Anatomy. Eur J Vasc Endovasc Surg. 2006;31(3):288–99.
3. Mendoza E, Lattimer CR, Morrison N. Duplex ultrasound of superficial leg veins. Berlin: Springer; 2014.
4. Tillaux P. Traité d'Anatomie Topograpique avec applications a la Chirurgie. Neuvième ed. Paris: Asselin et Houzeau Editeurs; 1897. p. 1011–73.
5. Franceschi C. Théorie et Pratique de la Cure Conservatrice et Hémodynamique de l'Insuffisance Veineuse en Ambulatoire, Précy-sous-Thil 1988 (Armançon).
6. Zamboni P, Cappelli M, Marcellino MC, Murgia AP, Pisano L, Fabi P. Does a varicose saphenous vein exist? Phlebology. 1997a;12:74–7.
7. Zamboni P, Portaluppi F, Marcellino MG, Manfredini R, Pisano L, Liboni A. Ultrasonographic assessment of ambulatory venous pressure in superficial venous incompetence. J Vasc Surg. 1997b;26(5):796–802.
8. Caggiati A. Fascial relations and structure of the tributaries of the saphenous veins. Surg Radiol Anat. 2000;22:1–4.
9. Caggiati A. Fascial relationships of the short saphenous vein. J Vasc Surg. 2001;34:241–6.
10. Caggiati A, Ricci S. The long saphenous vein compartment. Phlebology. 1999;12:107–11.
11. Caggiati A, Ricci S. The caliber of the human long saphenous vein and its congenital variations. Ann Anat. 2000;182:1–7.
12. Ricci S, Caggiati A. Does a double long saphenous vein exist? Phlebology. 1999;14:59–64.
13. Caggiati A, Bergan JJ, Gloviczki P, Jantet G, Wendell-Smith CP, Partsch H. Nomenclature of the veins of the lower limbs: an international interdisciplinary consensus statement. J Vasc Surg. 2002;36:416–22.
14. Lee BB, Nicolaides AN, Myers K, Meissner M, Kalodiki E, Allegra C, Antignani PL, Bækgaard N, Beach K, Belcaro G, Black S, Blomgren L, Bouskela E, Cappelli M, Caprini J, Carpentier P, Cavezzi A, Chastanet S, Christenson JT, Christopoulos D, Clarke H, Davies A, Demaeseneer M, Eklöf B, Ermini S, Fernández F, Franceschi C, Gasparis A, Geroulakos G, Gianesini S, Giannoukas A, Gloviczki P, Huang Y, Ibegbuna V, Kakkos SK, Kistner R, Kölbel T, Kurstjens RL, Labropoulos N, Laredo J, Lattimer CR, Lugli M, Lurie F, Maleti O, Markovic J, Mendoza E, Monedero JL, Moneta G, Moore H, Morrison N, Mosti G, Nelzén O, Obermayer A, Ogawa T, Parsi K, Partsch H, Passariello F, Perrin ML, Pittaluga P, Raju S, Ricci S, Rosales A, Scuderi A, Slagsvold CE, Thurin A, Urbanek T, M VAN Rij A, Vasquez M, Wittens CH, Zamboni P, Zimmet S, Ezpeleta SZ. Venous hemodynamic changes in lower limb venous disease: the UIP consensus according to scientific evidence. Int Angiol. 2016;35(3):236–352. Epub 2016 Mar 24. PubMed PMID: 27013029

15. Meissner MH. Lower extremity venous anatomy. Semin Intervent Radiol. 2005;22(3):147–56.
16. Franceschi C, Zamboni P. Principles of venous haemodynamics. New York: Nova Science; 2010.
17. van Limborgh J. L'anatomie du systeme veineux de l'extremite inferieure en relation avec la pathologie variqueuse. Folia Angiol. 1961;8:240–57.
18. Strauss AL. Farbduplexsonographie der Arterien und Venen. Berlin: Springer; 1995.
19. Vincent JR, Jones GT, Hill GB, van Rij AM. Failure of microvenous valves in small superficial veins is a key to the skin changes of venous insufficiency. J Vasc Surg. 2011;54:62S–9S.
20. Bailly M. Cartographie CHIVA. In: Encyclopédie Medico-Chirurgicale. Paris: Editions Techniques; 1993. p. 43-161-B, 1–4.
21. Mendoza E. Handbuch CHIVA. Arrien GmbH; 2002.
22. Gianesini S, Occhionorelli S, Menegatti E, Zuolo M, Tessari M, Spath P, Ascanelli S, Zamboni P. CHIVA strategy in chronic venous disease treatment: instructions for users. Phlebology. 2015;30(3):157–71.
23. Coffman JD, Lempert JA. Venous flow velocity, venous volume and arterial blood flow. Circulation. 1975;52:141–5.
24. Fronek A, Criqui MH, Denenberg J, et al. Common femoral vein dimensions and hemodynamics including Valsalva response as a function of sex, age, and ethnicity in a population study. J Vasc Surg. 2001;33:1050–6.
25. Jamieson R, Calderwood CJ, Greer IA. The effect of graduated compression stockings on blood velocity in the deep venous system of the lower limb in postnatal period. BJOG. 2007;114:1292–4.
26. Nagahiro I, Watanuki Y, Sato S, et al. Venous velocity of the right femoral vein decreases in the right lateral decubitus position compared to the supine position: a cause of post-operative pulmonary embolism? Acta Med Okayama. 2007;61:57–61.
27. Gianesini S, Sisini F, Di Domenico G, Secciero J, Malagoni AM, Menegatti E, Gambaccini M, Zamboni P. Lower limbs venous kinetics and consequent impact on drainage direction. Phlebology. 2017:268355516688775. https://doi.org/10.1177/0268355516688775. [Epub ahead of print].
28. Broderick BJ. A haemodynamic study of the physiological mechanisms of the venous pump in the healthy human foot. Conf Proc IEEE Eng Med Biol Soc. 2008:1411–4. https://doi.org/10.1109/IEMBS.2008.4649430.
29. Broderick BJ. Venous emptying from the foot: influences of weight bearing, toe curls, electrical stimulation, passive compression, and posture. J Appl Physiol. 2010;109(4):1045–52.
30. Farrah J, Saharay M, Georgiannos SN, Scurr JH, Smith PD. Variable venous anatomy of the popliteal fossa demonstrated by duplex scanning. Dermatol Surg. 1998;24:901–3.
31. Moore HM, Gohel M, Davies AH. Number and location of venous valves within the popliteal and femoral veins – a review of the literature. J Anat. 2011;219:439–43.
32. Mühlberger D, Morandini L, Brenner E. An anatomical study of femoral vein valves near the saphenofemoral junction. J Vasc Surg. 2008;48:994–9.
33. Van Bemmelen PS, Beach K, Bedford G, Strandness DE Jr. The mechanism of venous valve closure. Arch Surg: Its relationship to the velocity of reverse flow; 1990.
34. Van Bemmelen PS. Regarding "The mechanism of venous valve closure in normal physiological conditions". J Vasc Surg. 2003;37(1):237. author reply 237–8
35. Bernardini E, DeRango P, Piccioli R, Bisacci C, Pagliuca V, Genovese G, Bisacci R. Development of primary superficial venous insufficiency: the ascending theory. Observational and hemodynamic data from a 9 year experience. Ann Vasc Surg. 2010: 709–20.
36. Caggiati A, Rosi C, Heyn R, Franceschini M, Acconcia MC. Age-related variations of varicose veins anatomy. J Vasc Surg. 2006;44(6):1291–5.
37. Chastanet S, Pittaluga P. Patterns of reflux in the great saphenous vein system. Phlebology. 2013;28(Suppl 1):S39–46.
38. Daigle RJ. Techniques in non-invasive vascular diagnosis: an encyclopedia of vascular testing. Littleton: Summer Publishing LLC; 2008.
39. Guidi G, Licciardello C, Falteri S. Intrinsic spectral broadening in US Doppler as a combination of transit time and local geometrical broadening. Ultrasound Med Biol. 2000;26:853–62.
40. Osmanski BF, Bercoff J, Montaldo G, Loupas T, Fink M, Tanter M. Cancellation of Doppler intrinsic spectral broadening using ultrafast Doppler imaging. IEEE Trans Ultrason Ferroelectr Freq Control. 2014;61:396–1408.
41. Boni E, Bassi L, Dallai A, Guidi F, Meacci V, Ramalli A, Ricci S, Tortoli P. ULA-OP 256: a 256-channel open scanner for development and real-time implementation of new ultrasound methods. IEEE Trans Ultrason Ferroelectr Freq Control. 2016. https://doi.org/10.1109/TUFFC.2016.2566920.
42. Tavoni V, et al. Conventional echo color Doppler versus ULA-OP in the assessment of venous flow model. Veins Lymphat. 2017. https://doi.org/10.4081/vl.2017.6841.
43. Barber RF, Shatara FI. The varicose disease. NY State J Med. 1925;25:16–24.
44. Hach W. Varicose veins of the deep perforating veins-DOUBLEHYPHENa typical phlebologic disease picture. Vasa. 1985;14(2):155–7.
45. Hadfield JIH. The anatomy of the perforating veins in the leg. In: The treatment of varicose veins by injection and compression. Stoke Mandeville Symposium, 1971, pp. 4–11.

46. Sarin S. Medial calf perforators in venous disease: the significance of outward flow. J Vasc Surg. 1992: Jul;16(1):40–6.
47. Zamboni P. Pathophysiology of perforators in primary chronic venous insufficiency. World J Surg. 2005;29(1):115–8.
48. Labropoulos N, Mansour MA, Kang SS, Gloviczki BH. New insights into perforator vein incompetence. Eur J Vasc Endovasc Surg. 1999;18:228–34.
49. Delis K. Leg perforator vein incompetence: functional anatomy. Radiology. 2005;235:327–34.
50. Ibegbuna V, Delis KT, Nicolaides AN. Haemodynamic and clinical impact of superficial, deep and perforator vein incompetence. Eur J Vasc Endovasc Surg. 2006;31(5):535–41. Epub 2006 Jan 4
51. Labropoulos N, Tassiopoulos AK, Bhatti AF, Leon L. Development of reflux in the perforator veins in limbs with primary venous disease. J Vasc Surg. 2006;43:558–62.
52. Recek C, Karisch E, Gruber J. (Changes of the perforating veins and deep calf veins after elimination of saphenous reflux) Veränderungen der Perforansvenen und tiefen Unterschenkelvenen nach Beseitigung des Saphena-Refluxes. Phlebologie (Stuttgart). 2000;29(1):37–40.
53. Mendoza E. CHIVA – ein Handbuch. Wunstorf: Arrien Verlag; 2002.
54. Lattimer CR, Mendoza E. Superficial venous reflux duration and cessation with two concurrent duplex probes. J Vasc Surg Venous Lymphat Disord. 2015;3(2):154–60.
55. Gloviczki P, et al. The care of patients with varicose veins and associated chronic venous diseases: clinical practice guidelines of the Society for Vascular Surgery and the American Venous Forum. J Vasc Surg. 2011;53(5 suppl):2S–48S.
56. Edwards JE, Edwards EA. The saphenous valves in varicose veins. Am Heart J. 1940;19:338–51.
57. Rose SS, Ahmed A. Some thoughts on the etiology of varicose veins. J Cardiovasc Surg (Torino). 1986;27:534–43.
58. Bassi GL. Le varici degli arti inferiori. Turin: Minerva Medica; 1962.
59. Mühlberger D, Morandini L, Brenner E. Venous valves and major superficial tributary veins near the saphenofemoral junction. J Vasc Surg. 2009;49:1562–9.
60. Caggiati A, Macchiarelli G, Familiari G. Topographical structural variations of the human long saphenous vein and its age-related remodelling as revealed by correlated light and scanning electron microscopy. Phlebology. 1998;13:156–62.
61. Dhital KK, Burnstock G. Adrenergic and non-adrenergic neural control of the arterial wall. In: Camilleri J-P, Berry CL, Fiessinger J-N, Bariety J, editors. Disease of the arterial wall. London: Springer; 1989. p. 97–126.
62. Mashiah A, Rose SS, Hod I. The scanning electronic microscope in the pathology of varicose veins. Isr J Med Sci. 1991;27:202–6. May;125(5):617-9. PubMed PMID: 2184798
63. Thulesius O, Ugaily-Thulesius L, Gjores JE, Neglen P. The varicose saphenous vein, functional and ultrastructural studies, with special reference to smooth muscle. Phlebology. 1988;3:89–95.
64. Baird RN, Abbott WM. Elasticity and compliance of canine femoral and jugular vein segments. Am J Physiol. 1977;233(1):H15–21.
65. Norgren L, Thulesius O, Gjöres JE, Söderlundh S. Foot-volumetry and simultaneous venous pressure measurements for evaluation of venous insufficiency. Vasa. 1974;3(2):140–7.
66. Norgren L, Thulesius O. Pressure-volume characteristics of foot veins in normal cases and patients with venous insufficiency. Blood Vessels. 1975;12(1):1–12.
67. Zamboni P, Marcellino MG, Portaluppi F, Manfredini R, Feo CV, Quaglio D, Liboni A. The relationship between in vitro and in vivo venous compliance measurement. Int Angiol. 1996;15(2):149–52.
68. Bax W, Bos E, Saxena PR. Heterogeneity of endothelin/sarafotoxin receptors mediating contraction of the human isolated saphenous vein. Eur J Pharmacol. 1993;239:267–8.
69. Biochl-Daum B, Schuller Petrovic S, Woltz M, Korn A, Bohler K, Eichler KG. Primary defect in alpha adrenergic responsiveness in patients with varicose veins. Clin Pharmacol Ther. 1991;49:49–52.
70. Zamboni P, Portaluppi F, Marcellino MG, Quaglio D, Manfredini R, Feo CV, Stoney RJ. In vitro versus in vivo assessment of vein wall properties. Ann Vasc Surg. 1998;12(4):324–9.
71. Zamboni P, Portaluppi F, Marcellino MG, et al. Ann Vasc Surg. 1998;12:324. https://doi.org/10.1007/s100169900162
72. Davies AH, Magee TR, Hayward J, Harris R, Baird RN, Horrocks M. Non-invasive methods of measuring venous compliance. Phlebology. 1992;7:78–81.
73. Nicolaides AN, Cardiovascular Disease Educational and Research Trust, European Society of Vascular Surgery, The International Angiology Scientific Activity Congress Organization, International Union of Angiology, Union Internationale de Phlebologie at the Abbaye des Vaux de Cernay. Investigation of chronic venous insufficiency: a consensus statement (France, March 5-9, 1997). Circulation. 2000;102(20):E126–63.
74. Clarke JH, Vadeskis SN, Hobbs JT, Nicolaides AN. Venous wall function in the pathogenesis of varicose veins. Surgery. 1992;111:402–8.
75. Barber DA, Wang X, Gloviczy P, Miller VM. Characterization of endothelin receptors in human varicose veins. J Vasc Surg. 1997;26:61–9.

76. Barker JE, Anderson J, Treasure T, Piper PJ. Influence of endothelium and surgical preparation on responses of human saphenous vein and internal thoracic artery to angiotensin II. Br J Clin Pharmacol. 1994;38:57–62.
77. Jenkinson DH, Barnard EA, Hoyer D, Humhrey PPA, Leff P, Shankley NP. International Union of Pharmacology Committee on receptors nomenclature and drug classification, IX: recommendations on terms and symbol in quantitative pharmacology. Pharmacol Rev. 1995;47:255–66.
78. Li Q, Feenstra M, Pfaffendorf M, Eijsman L, Van Zwieten PA. Comparative vasoconstrictor effects of Angiotensin II, II, and IV in human isolated saphenous vein. J Cardiovasc Pharmacol. 1997;29:451–6.
79. Rizzi A, Quaglio D, Vasquez G, Mascoli F, Amadesi S, Calò G, Regoli D, Zamboni P. Effects of vasoactive agents in healthy and diseased human saphenous veins. J Vasc Surg. 1998;28(5):855–61.
80. Sjoberg T, Norgren L, Andersson KE, Steen S. Comparative effects of the alfa adrenoceptors agonists noradrenaline, phenylephrine and clonidine in the human saphenous vein in vivo and in vitro. Acta Physiol Scand. 1989;136:463–71.

3 Venous Reflux Patterns

Sergio Gianesini, Paolo Zamboni, and Erika Mendoza

3.1 Venous Haemodynamics and Related Laws of Physics

Leg veins are interconnected tubes filled with flowing liquids, therefore reigned by laws of physics. But physics laws for fluids in tubes are usually described parting from noncollapsible tubes with regular walls without valves and with one single motor and known interconnections. This is truly not the case in leg veins. So, criticism of physics applied to phlebology is often heard. Nevertheless, without some physics, at least applied in analogy, a comprehension of venous haemodynamics and venous pathology is not possible, leaving the surgeon only with the possibility of applying an ablative method.

S. Gianesini, M.D., Ph.D. (✉)
Vascular Diseases Center, University of Ferrara, Ferrara, Italy

USUHS University, Bethesda, MD, USA

P. Zamboni, M.D.
School of Vascular Surgery and Vascular Diseases Center, University of Ferrara, Ferrara, Italy

Unit of Translational Surgery, AOU Ferrara, Ferrara, Italy
e-mail: zmp@unife.it

E. Mendoza, M.D., Ph.D.
Venenpraxis, Wunstorf, Germany
e-mail: erika.mendoza@t-online.de

3.1.1 Why Does Blood Flow in a Vein?

From a practical and simple observation point of view, venous behaviour varies depending on whether the subject is standing or lying. In the recumbent subject, the blood flows towards the heart slowly and continuously driven by arterial flow pushing from behind, called *vis a tergo*. After flowing through the capillaries, the blood has lost most or all of its pulsatility. In addition, respiration has the effect of augmenting the venous return. During inhalation, the negative intrathoracic pressure encourages venous flow upwards into the chest. The right heart atrium has a negative pressure after heart systole suctioning blood from the vena cava system during heart muscle diastole. In recumbent position gravidity plays no role; the venous valves and the muscle activity are not necessary to keep the system going.

When the subject stands up, gravidity takes part at the game. Even if the patient's leg muscles remain without movement like when the position of the patient is changed from recumbent to staying on a tilt table, the muscle veins in the calf fill with a reserve of around 350 mL of blood [1], meaning that at first no blood flows out of the leg. If the subject continues to stand still, the venous return resumes due to *vis a tergo,* the respiration

P. Zamboni et al. (eds.), *Saphenous Vein-Sparing Strategies in Chronic Venous Disease*,
https://doi.org/10.1007/978-3-319-70638-2_3

and the heart diastolic suction. This passive flow is enhanced substantially by the activity of the calf **muscle pump**. The combined action of the calf muscle pump and the valves propels the blood towards the heart during muscular contraction. The blood is forced in *one* direction through the openings of the venous valves which prevent retrograde flow towards the feet or outwards into the superficial veins in case of perforating veins. When the muscles relax, the blood normally cannot flow back because the venous valves close. This action results in a pressure drop in the deep veins which have just been emptied and so draws blood in from the superficial and muscle veins.

This pumping action can be compared to the heart using the terms **muscular systole** for muscle contraction and **muscular diastole** for muscle relaxation. Muscular systole pumps blood out of the deep veins, while muscular diastole fills them by draining the superficial veins.

In addition to the above described mechanisms, veins seem to develop an own pacemaker if chronically dilated, which has been called "saphenous pulse" [2]. This pulse starts after some time of dependency without any movements and is more frequent in advanced venous insufficiency.

3.1.2 Physics Laws Applying to Venous Haemodynamics

According to Poiseuille's law, in order to create a flow in a tube, a pressure gradient is needed.

The pressure gradient (ΔP) is directly related to the applied force (F) and the resistance (R).

$$\text{Poiseuille's law: } \Delta \text{P} = F \times R$$

The resistance to flow is directly related to the tube length (L) and viscosity of the fluid (η), while it's inversely related to its radius (r), according to the following formula:

$$R = 8\eta L / \Pi r4$$

Considering that pressure (P) can be defined as a force on a surface, many clinical implications follow this first formula already.

In fact, the pressure gradient is directly influenced by the force exerted by the heart systole, by the thoracic aspiration following the breathing act and by the peripheral muscle contraction.

At the same time, the pressure is inversely related to the vessel diameter and area, which leads to the implication of the venous tone and of the wall compliance: two variable factors able to influence the pressure gradient, thus the flow. The muscle contraction acts on the vein calibre, and the same vessel calibre influences the resistance formula, so adding another variable in the flow determination.

Together with an energy gradient, another important element in producing a flow in the venous system is the vessel capacity to receive a certain amount of fluid, adapting its diameter.

Considering the intrinsic collapsible vein nature, in a beginning filling phase, a great capacity variability is possible with little changes in venous pressure, turning the vein from an elliptical to a circular-shaped vessel: a property conferring the blood reservoir function to the venous system. So, in the first phase of filling, increased volume is not related to a pressure change but to a diameter change, depending on the compliance of the vessel, as has been explained in Sect. 2.6.3. Once the vessel has become circular, much more pressure is required to stretch the vessel.

The physical property of a vessel to increase its volume with increasing transmural pressure is known as compliance (C) and is expressed by the change in volume (ΔV) divided by the change in pressure (ΔP) [3].

$$\text{Compliance } C = \Delta V / \Delta P$$

Compliance is strictly linked not only to the filling degree but also to the geometric vessel properties (length and radius), together with its wall elasticity [4, 5].

Ultrasound introduction in clinical practice is permitted to measure in the clinical setting the venous compliance especially at the level of the saphenous vein to assess the mechanical wall properties before using it as an arterial conduit [6, 7].

Subsequently saphenous compliance was investigated as a pathophysiological parameter linked with chronic venous insufficiency.

A pressure-diameter curve highlights the nonlinear relationship in the initial filling phase, which is due to the great increase in vessel calibre following tiny pressure augmentations. On the contrary, in a distension phase, starting from pressure values around 20 mmHg, a volume/pressure linearity has been demonstrated (see Sect. 2.5.4) [8–10].

The pressure gradient is exerted both longitudinally along the vessel and transversally on the venous wall. This last energy development is associated to the so-called transmural pressure (TMP), and it represents a fundamental parameter both in haemodynamics and in fluid exchanges.

3.1.3 Relation of the Veins with the Surrounding Tissue

Not only is the vein a tube with variable dimensions adapting on the filling grade but the wall has a variable permeability to allow an exchange of nutrients with the surrounding tissue. The permeability is the highest at capillary level, descending towards higher levels of reticular veins, tributaries and saphenous or deep veins. The permeability is influenced by the vein diameter and the transmural pressure.

The transmural pressure is the difference between the internal venous pressure (IVP), acting on the internal vessel side to expand it, and the external venous pressure (EVP), pressing on the external parietal wall to collapse it (Fig. 3.1). Transmural pressure and vessels' permeability represent the intra-extravascular exchange determinants (Starling's law). The transmural pressure is the crucial parameter in tissue drainage and venous calibre regulation

$$\text{Transmural pressure TMP} = \text{IVP} - \text{EVP}$$

The intravenous pressure is determined by the lateral pressure, which is in relation to the blood flow velocity and the kind of flow present (laminar or turbulent, see below). It is also influenced by the hydrostatic pressure, which depends on the height of the fluid column above the measured point (see Sect. 3.1.4).

The external venous pressure is composed by the atmospheric pressure and the tissue pressure. This last factor is determined by lots of factors, as tissue characteristics, by oedema and by compression stockings and is modified by muscle contraction.

Another force playing an important role is the oncotic pressure. This is the pressure difference between the solved substances in the plasma of the vein and in the surrounding interstitial fluid. To make the equation easier, the oncotic pressure is taken as one value (which could be positive or negative) and added on the intravenous pressure side.

One fundamental component of the transmural pressure is composed by the lateral pressure. This follows the Bernoulli's principle, both in static and dynamic conditions. According to this law of physics, an increase in the speed of a fluid occurs simultaneously with a decrease in the fluid's potential energy, which is expressed as the lateral pressure and the gravitational pressure. This is a derivation from the principle of the conservation of energy, which states that, in a steady flow, the sum of all forms of energy in a fluid is constant. It requires that the sum of kinetic and potential energy remains constant.

The kinetic energy is determined by the fluid density and its velocity ($\rho v^2/2$; ρ represents the fluid density, v the fluid velocity). In ideal conditions, it states that the energy factors governing the venous haemodynamics are the kinetic energy together with the potential energy. This last one is constituted by the lateral pressure (lp), linked to the vessel wall elastic properties, and gravitational pressure (ρgh), produced by the blood column weight. The sum of them ($\rho v^2/2 + \text{lp} + \rho gh$) is constant at any point inside a tube or a vessel.

$$\begin{aligned}&\text{Bernoulli's principle: Kinetic energy}\\&+\text{lateral pressure}+\text{gravitational pressure}\\&=\rho v^2/2+\text{lp}+\rho gh=\text{constant}\end{aligned}$$

This means that thea higher the velocity of blood flow in a vein, the lesser the transmural

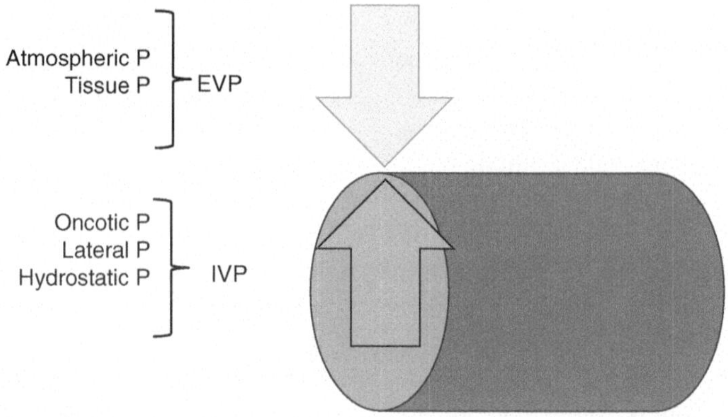

Fig. 3.1 Graphical representation of the transmural pressure. External venous pressure (EVP) is composed by the atmospheric pressure (AP) and tissue pressure (TP). The internal venous pressure (IVP) is composed of the lateral pressure (LP), the hydrostatic or gravitational pressure (HP) and the oncotic pressure (OP)

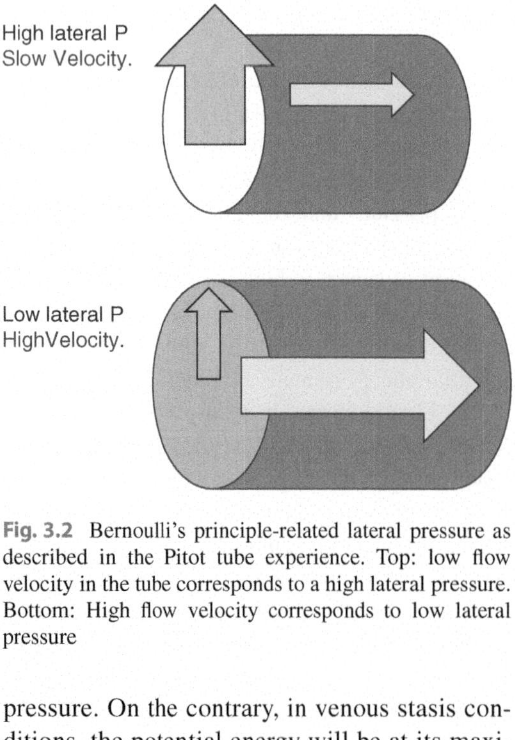

Fig. 3.2 Bernoulli's principle-related lateral pressure as described in the Pitot tube experience. Top: low flow velocity in the tube corresponds to a high lateral pressure. Bottom: High flow velocity corresponds to low lateral pressure

pressure. On the contrary, in venous stasis conditions, the potential energy will be at its maximum, while it will decrease proportionally to the flow velocity increase. The obvious and determinant consequence is that the lateral pressure, exerted on the venous wall, will decrease proportionally to the velocity reached by the fluid (Fig. 3.2).

According to Bernoulli's principle, in two communicating vessels, the one presenting a higher flow velocity will display a lower lateral pressure: a gradient will be created, and the blood will flow from the slower to the faster vessel. The aspiration effect performed by the higher velocity vessel is known as the Venturi's principle.

This last one is strictly linked to the Castelli's law (Fig. 3.3) which states that flow velocity (v) is inversely proportional to the vessel cross-sectional area (A). The same volume of blood through a vessel will be faster, if the diameter is less. Blood flow, which means blood volume changes in a given time frame, is defined by the area of the vessel and velocity of the blood flowing.

$$\text{Castelli's law}: A_1 v_1 = A_2 v_2 = \text{Flow}$$

This law applies to one tube changing its diameter, as well as in one tuber branching into tributaries. Whenever the vessel divides into several branches, if the sum of the area of the branches is smaller, an increased flow velocity will be expected; of course, the opposite will be the case if the sections' total area increases.

3.1.4 Flow and Hydrostatic Pressure

The third variable in the Bernoulli's principle is the potential energy, represented by the hydrostatic component, and it acts as a counterpart of the kinetic energy. In case of immobile persons on a tilt table, when reaching the standing

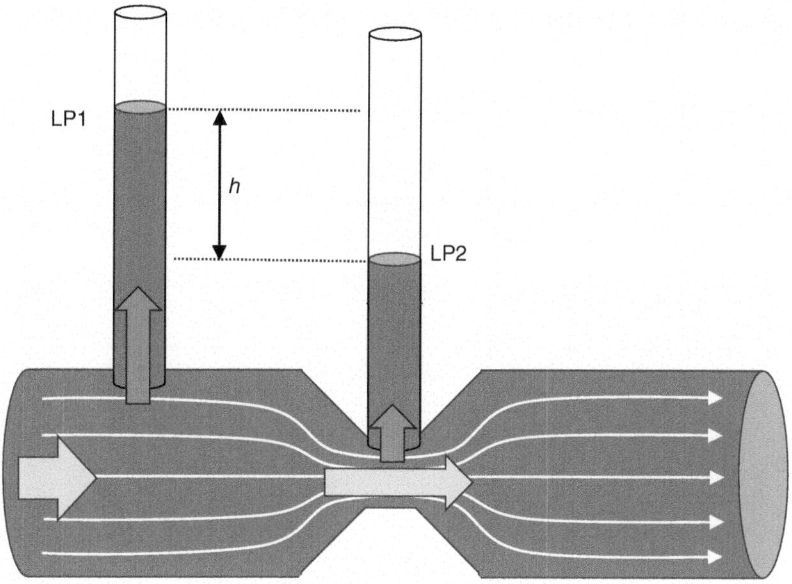

Fig. 3.3 Castelli's law and Venturi's effect. Flow velocity (violet arrows) is inversely proportional to the vessel cross-sectional area (Castelli's law), and consequently the lateral pressure is different. The lateral pressure is represented as red arrow and is larger in the wide segment and less in the narrow segment ($LP_1 > LP_2$) leading to the fluid aspiration determined by the Venturi's effect (corresponding to the difference in height between both lateral pressures represented with the black arrow "*h*")

position, the hydrostatic pressure along the leg will be determined by the distance between the measuring point and the right atrium. As soon as the muscle activity takes place, the competent valves in the venous system of the leg fractionate the hydrostatic column creating new pressure compartments in the vein.

The columns present different energy states, which vary just according to the same column height.

In fact, in a static situation without flow (no lateral pressure) and without vein wall permeability (no oncotic pressure), the only energetic level determinant of the transmural pressure is the potential gravitational energy value, which is expressed by the following formula:

$$\text{Potential gravitational energy} = r^{*} g^{*} h$$
$$= \text{fluid density}^{*}\text{gravity constant}$$
$$^{*}\text{height of the column}$$

(ρ represents the fluid density, g the gravity constant, h the height below the surface)

The principle of communicating tubes says that whenever the different tubes are in communication (Fig. 3.4), the pressure will be equalized. The height of the fluid column in all connected tubes will be the same. So, the fluid will flow from the part of the tube with the higher fluid column to the one with the lower column, and finally settling into a balanced common energetic state, in which all the column heights are equal.

In the leg vein system, this phenomenon is translated into a blood flow from the system presenting a higher distance between valves and in consequence a higher blood column to the one with a smaller column, due to a lesser distance between valves.

Different valve density in the deep versus the superficial system gives a rationale to such blood movement during the diastolic phase as represented in Fig. 3.5, where the height of the blood column is represented as if an air bubble would be found below the valve level to make the height more evident.

Certainly, up to this point, all the described physics law applications have been made considering the vessel and the blood as an ideal conduit and liquid, respectively. To the contrary, in the human body environment, the vessel wall produces friction through blood contact, while this last one possesses complex visco-elastic properties due to its composition with fluids, proteins, fats and blood cells.

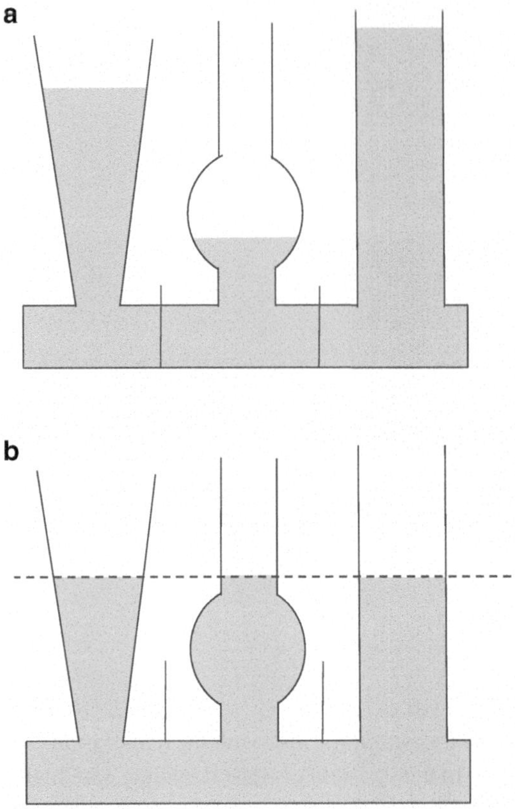

Fig. 3.4 The communicating vessel principle. (**a**) Noncommunicating hydrostatic columns presenting different heights, which leads to different energetic states (the column at the right presents the highest energetic value). (**b**) Communicating columns in which the flow moves from the higher to the lower energetic state systems, until a common energetic balance is reached. The dotted line represents the horizontal level that equalizes the hydrostatic pressure for the whole system

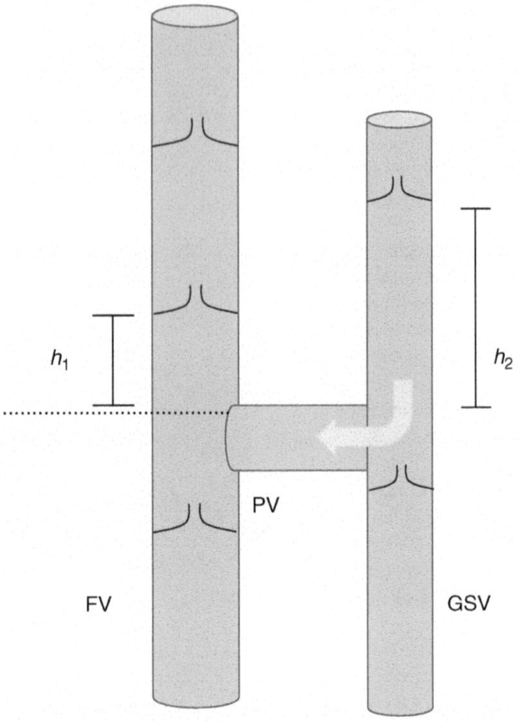

Fig. 3.5 Valve density and hydrostatic pressure: considering that the hydrostatic pressure is directly related to the only variable of the column height (h), during the diastolic phase, the venous blood flows from the higher to the lower column, moving from a system with higher energy values to one at a lower energy state. As the distance between the perforating vein (PV) and the valve is higher in the great saphenous vein (GSV) than in the femoral vein (FV), the hydrostatic pressure is higher in the great saphenous vein (h_2) provoking a flow from the saphenous vein to the deep vein (h_1), represented as a yellow arrow

An extension of the thermodynamics' second principle, the entropy law, states that in case of not ideal conduits or liquids, part of the energy is dissipated as heat generation, so increasing the amount of no more available energy (entropy). The human body solution to counteract this energetic dissipation has been the creation of the several pump mechanisms placed in series all along the cardiovascular system [11].

3.1.5 Laminar and Turbulent Flow

The principles of blood flow are derived experimentally from the behaviour of liquids in rigid tubes. However, blood vessels are not ideal tubes as they are collapsible, and the flow within them is not exposed to a constant pressure [12].

The flow through a straight rigid tube depends on two factors:

1. The pressure difference between the ends of the tube.
2. The resistance of the tube to flow. This is influenced by the viscosity of the liquid, the properties of the wall and the diameter of the tube.

If the tube walls are smooth, the liquid inside will flow in an orderly way, within a certain range of velocities. The layer in immediate contact with the wall flows very slowly due to friction. The next layer flows faster over the first and so progressively towards the centre of the pipe where the flow is the fastest. This is known as **laminar flow** which is a property of a Newtonian fluid. In laminar flow, no additional pressure is exerted on the venous wall. Under the following conditions, this flow will start to be turbulent:

- If bends are introduced into the tube.
- At the site of impediments (like venous valves).
- The pipe diameter is very small.
- The velocity is very high.

This causes the blood to divert from its parallel path and flow in all directions, even towards the wall. This results in an increase in friction and resistance. Consequently, the forward velocity is reduced and the pressure on the wall increases.

In analysing the flow in the veins by analogy, we find optimal laminar flow conditions in the following situations:

Sufficient deep and saphenous veins run straight forwards, as tubes without bends (excepting for the junctions of the saphenous veins), with little diameter variations and no impediments: Open valves adapt to the vein wall and do not hinder the antegrade flow.

As soon as an incompetent valve plays a role and a pathologic compartment change takes place, turbulences are programmed: At the point of the compartment jump (N1 → N2) through a perforator or the junction, blood flow changes direction. The incompetent valves are obstacles in the way of the reflux. This provokes turbulences (see Fig. 3.6b). The consequences of turbulent flow are discussed in Sect. 3.2.3.

3.2 Characteristics of Blood Flow in Leg Veins

3.2.1 Definitions of Flow and Reflux

Pressure gradients are usually considered physiological or pathological inside the venous network based on the flow direction they determine.

Blood flow in leg veins in standing position challenges gravity. Different mechanisms are involved (see Sect. 3.1.1), like the vis a tergo, the heart suctioning, the aspiration effect by respiration and above all the muscle pump. Combined with the valves, the connections between the veins (junctions, perforators) are a complex system of draining mechanisms and venous flow results. Classically this flow direction was called antegrade flow. Considering the vein compartments, physiological flow direction is defined by the following compartment jumps:

- N3–N1: Tributaries drain into the deep veins.
- N3–N2: Tributaries drain into saphenous veins.
- N2–N1: Saphenous veins drain into deep veins.

If this order is reverted, we find a pathological flow, a reflux, with pathological compartment jumps from deep to superficial veins (N1 → N2 or N1 → N3) or from saphenous veins to tributaries (N2 → N3).

The standard definition for venous reflux is focused on the inverted direction of a flow lasting more than a specific cut-off (0.5 s in the superficial venous system, 1 s in the deep venous system). This value was defined by Labropoulos et al. [14] after analysing the flow in healthy persons. They found, that in healthy legs the inverted flow always lasted less than 0.5 s. When analysing reflux duration in patients with venous insufficiency, a reflux duration of longer than 1 s either with manual compression or with toe elevation manoeuvre was found, as well as refluxes of less than 0.5 s in all healthy control subjects. So, the definition of competent veins in case of reflux duration of less than 0.5 s was consistent with Labropoulos et al., but possibly a reflux is not just the flow duration of above 0.5 s but above 1 s [15].

Classical concepts of physiologic flow in leg veins in standing position implied that it was represented by the flow directed upwards, from the foot to the knee, to the groin, against

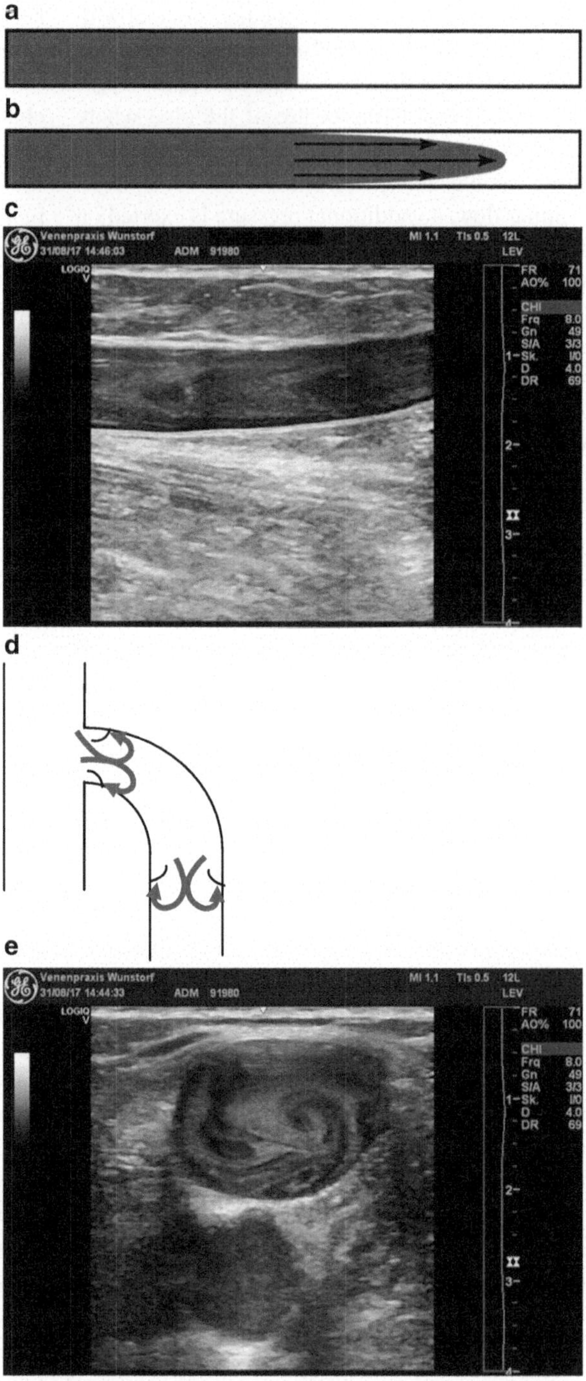

Fig. 3.6 A diagram of a tube containing two different coloured fluids to demonstrate laminar flow: (**a**) no flow, (**b**) a velocity profile is created as the red fluid begins to flow. The flow is faster at the centre of the tube compared to the periphery. (**c**) Dilated GSV with slow antegrade flow in B mode—the erythrocyte sludge moves forwards in laminar shape (compare with **b**). (**d**) Schematic vision of turbulent flow: reflux through the sapheno-femoral junction with turbulence of the blood at the incompetent valve site. (**e**) Longitudinal representation of the proximal aspect of the great saphenous vein. Turbulent flow in a proximal, dilated great saphenous vein can be observed in B mode by the formations of the erythrocyte sludge during muscular diastole forming circles in the vein lumen. With kind permission by [13]

gravity. After the introduction of duplex ultrasound, downward-directed flows were found and recognized as non-pathological. This is the case of the flow in the cranial branches of the sapheno-femoral junction (epigastric and circumflex veins, see Sect. 4.4) and of the flow in the Giacomini vein draining into the small saphenous vein. In addition, flow between valves in the muscular diastole is directed footwards, for example to drain a saphenous vein segment into the deep vein during muscular diastole. So, the flow direction itself did no longer determine the discrimination of antegrade flow and reflux. The terminus "centripetal" flow was introduced to define the flow from periphery (organs/skin) to draining vessels and then to the heart and "centrifugal" if this direction is inverted [16].

Then the concept of muscular systole and diastole in perforating veins made the question more complex: It has been shown that perforating veins might be a pressure-equalizing system during muscular systole with flows directed from the deep veins (N1) to the superficial veins (N2 or N3) during systole but with a "net flow" draining from N2 or N3 to N1 if considering the sum of systolic and diastolic flows. This is the reason why the diastolic flow is the one determining the pathology of perforating veins (see Table 3.1).

3.2.2 Velocity-Curve Shapes of Flow and Reflux

Since the upcoming of duplex ultrasound, the flow curves can be represented inside the veins. For an easier understanding, we will just consider the effect of systole and diastole only in one vein without interconnections.

Applying manual compression to the calf or dynamic provocation manoeuvres, e.g. toe elevation manoeuvre (see Sect. 4.3.2) to one segment of the vein, we provoke a so-called muscular systole,

Table 3.1 Analysis of flow in perforators involved in a recirculation in systole and diastole, different pathological significance

Description	Blood flow in PW, schematic representation	Pathological significance
During muscular systole inflow, during muscular diastole: inflow	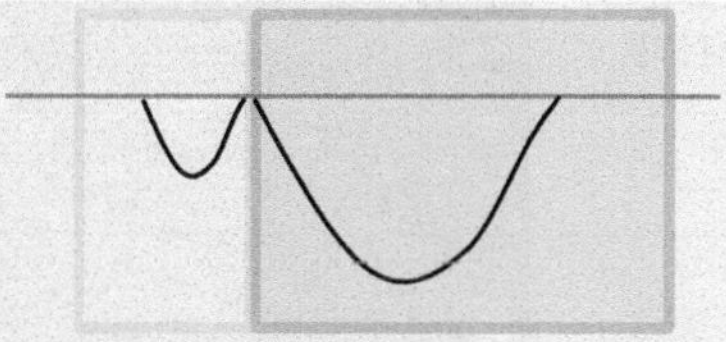	Re-entry perforator, because during diastole we find a draining flow
During muscular systole no flow, during muscular diastole: inflow	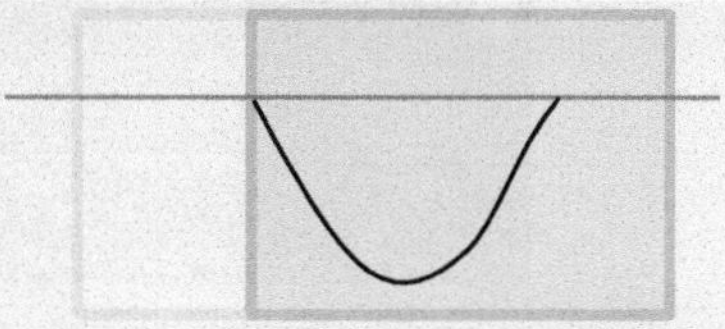	Re-entry perforator, because during diastole we find a draining flow
During muscular systole outflow (typical in case of dilated re-entry perforators), during muscular diastole: inflow	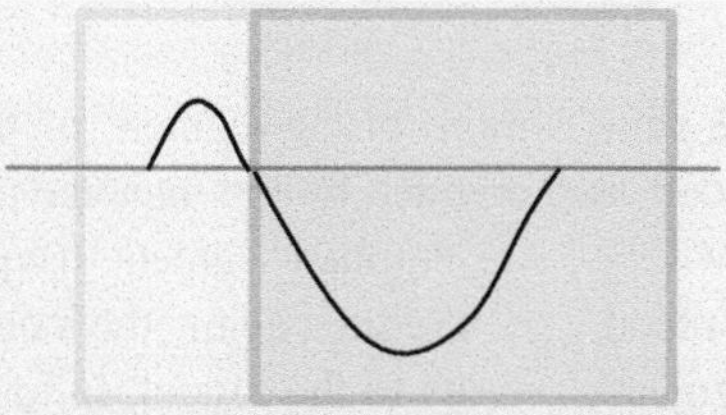	Re-entry perforator, because during diastole we find a draining flow. The outflow during systole does not implicate pathology. Dilated re-entry perforators on the calf can serve as pressure equalizers during systole
During muscular systole in- or outflow (in this case inflow), during diastole outflow	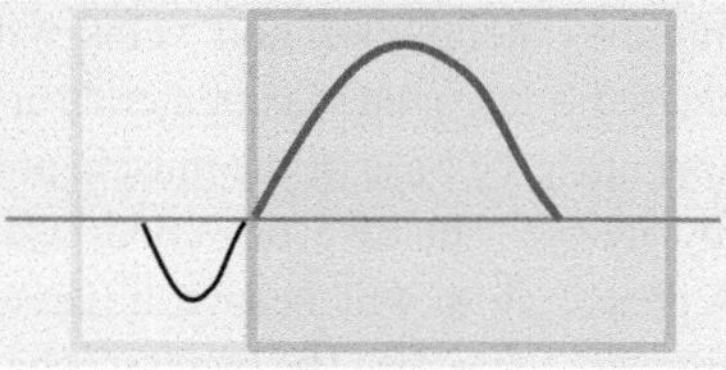	Incompetent perforator. This shape is most often indicating that the perforator is the start of the recirculation, the one point responsible for the superficial venous insufficiency and the place where blood changes the compartment pathologically
During muscular systole and diastole outflow	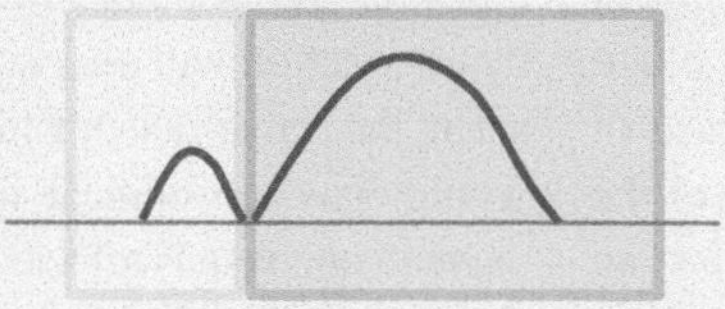	If an outflow is found in systole and diastole, an incompetent deep venous system has to be suspected

Inflow, flow from superficial to deep veins; outflow, flow from deep to superficial veins. Schematic representation of blood flow in PW: yellow field, systole; green field, diastole; red line, reflux. With kind permission from [34]

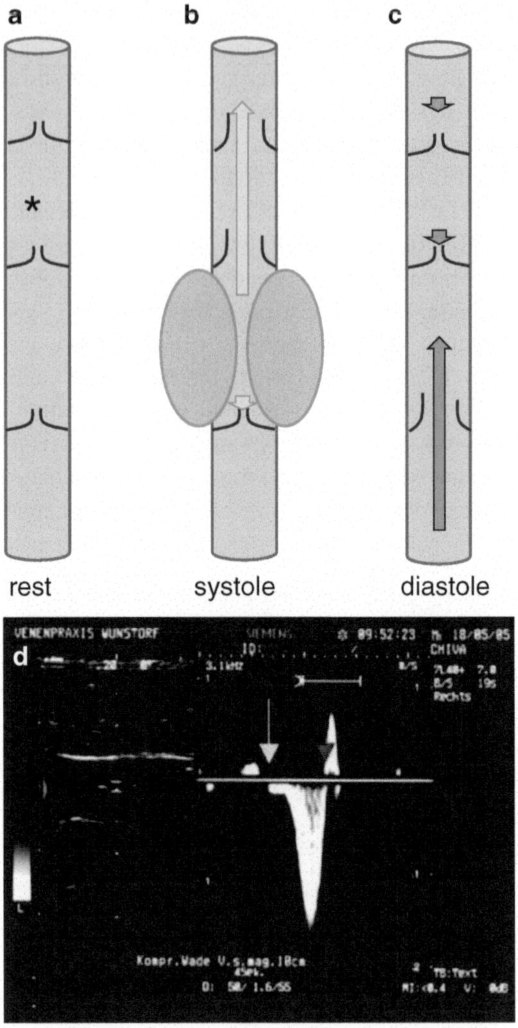

Fig. 3.7 Blood flow through a single vein with valves. (**a**) Vein with valves and no blood flow. The asterisk shows the place, where duplex measurement is taken in (**d**). (**b**) Compression of a segment of the vein (muscular systole). The pressure in this segment turns high and the blood tends to move to equalize with neighbourhood segments: Downwards a closed valve impedes the flow, upwards the valves open and a flow is possible (yellow arrows). (**c**) Release of the external pressure (diastole). The blood of the upward segments tends to flow back, finding a closed valve. The blood from the downward segment follows pressure gradients and fills the emptied segment (green arrows). (**d**) Blood flow in the vein (PW mode, saphenous vein at the thigh, cross section), measured in the segment above the compression (* in image **a**) at rest, during systole (starts at yellow arrow) and diastole (starts at red arrow). We observe a strong "upward" flow during systole, a short retrograde flow at the start of diastole, stopped by the closing of the valves. Note: Blood flow in PW mode is encoded as to the bottom of the image when the flow is advancing away from the transducer and to the top of the image if the flow is directed towards it. The transducer is held in inclined position, with the tip of the probe to the head of the patient, so that antegrade flow in veins will be encoded as curve to the bottom of the curve and flow to the foot as curve to the top (see Sect. 4.2). With kind permission by [13]

which will induce a centripetal flow in the vein: The proximal valves open allowing the blood to ascend towards the heart. The distal valves will be closed by the retrograde pressure of the blood, impeding a retrograde flow to more distal segments (see Fig. 3.7a). This will be followed by the muscular diastole in the very moment the hand is released from the calf or the toe is relaxed. In this moment, the pressure in the vein segment exerted by the hand or the muscle contraction is released. A pressure gradient towards the emptied vein segment exists. Following gravity, the just expelled blood column will tend to flow back again. In case of competent valves, this will induce a closure of the valve with the display of an inverted flow lasting less than 0.5 s (see Fig. 3.7b, c). The blood from the more distal segment of the vein, which was not emptied by the manoeuvre, will be flowing inside the emptied segment to equalize blood pressures.

Adding again the collaterals and perforating veins to the model, following pressure gradients, neighbourhood veins will fill the emptied vein segment via collaterals or perforating veins; this is the base of the muscle pump action (see Fig. 3.8).

In case of venous valve incompetence, blood flow will behave differently during the muscular diastole. The blood that has been moved proximally by contraction will afterwards flow back in the vessel if the valve doesn't hinder it by closing. This would have no clinical implications, if only one valve in one vein is affected. It will provoke a reflux, if the backflow involves two different veins

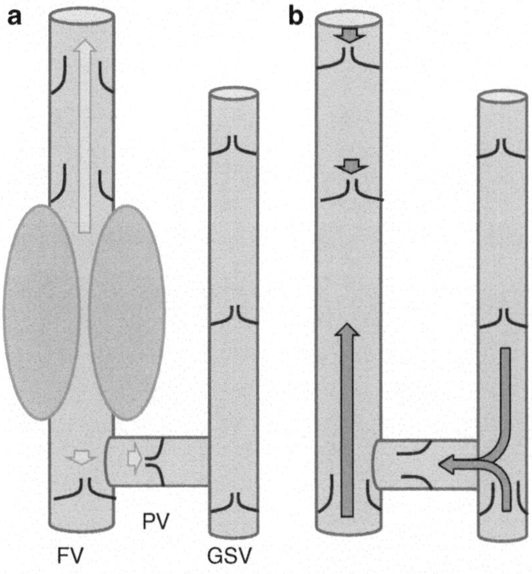

Fig. 3.8 Model of flow in two veins interconnected with a perforating vein (PV), supposing that only the left vein (femoral vein, FV) is exposed to muscular contraction and the right vein (superficial vein, SV) is not. Bottom of the image = distal, top = proximal. (**a**) Muscular systole compressing one segment of the femoral vein, the blood is expelled in direction of the heart following the pressure gradient: High at the contraction point and lower in comparison in the proximal segment, the valves distal to the contraction are closed, in the femoral vein as well as in the perforating vein. (**b**) Muscular diastole, the segment of the deep vein that had been compressed has now a lower pressure. Blood cannot flow back from the proximal segments, because the valves close, but can follow the pressure gradient filling the emptied segment from the distal segment of the deep vein and from the superficial vein through the perforating vein, now with opened valve

(e.g. two different veins of the deep calf venous system). And it will be part of a varicose vein reflux, if there is a jump of compartments, like a reflux from the deep vein to the saphenous vein (N1 → N2). A model of this situation is represented in Fig. 3.9.

3.2.3 Draining Versus Refluxing Flow

As described above, blood flow interacts with the vein wall. Laminar flow has little interaction, turbulent flow the most. By its shear stress on the vessel wall, venous reflux is considered responsible for the venous inflammation associated with cytokines release from the same endothelium [17]. So refluxive flow patterns associated with turbulent flow have shown to release inflammatory-mediating cytokines from the vein wall. Particularly the oscillatory character of reflux with quick changes of direction in the same vessel (see Fig. 3.9) seems to act as cytokine releaser.

Further studies have shown that the biosignaling among physical forces and biochemical release is not directly related to the reflux duration but rather to several haemodynamic aspects [18, 19].

Cytokines were analysed in refluxive veins and then in veins after haemodynamic flow correction: Saphenous veins after saphenous vein sparing techniques (CHIVA) often are perfused from the groin to the knee—which would classically be considered the wrong direction. But after an interruption of the reflux source, this flow in the saphenous vein (N2) is only composed by blood of tributaries (N3) physiologically draining through this vein. No reflux from deep veins, no volume overload is present.

Cytokine analysis after saphenous-sparing procedure demonstrated that in procedures restoring normal pressure gradients but keeping an inverted flow direction, the inflammation component is no longer detectable: a possible demonstration of the fact that a physiological flow can be also directed towards the more distal part of the limb, as long as it finds a draining route through a perforating vein towards the deep venous system [20]. This flow has been called “draining flow”. The restoration of the cytokine level demonstrates that this draining flow does not harm the vessel.

A draining flow presents small diastolic velocity and laminar features, independently of the length of its duration. To the contrary, reflux is characterized by higher peak diastolic velocities and turbulence.

It has been demonstrated that it is the oscillatory component of reflux which acts as a chronic inflammatory stimulus on the endothelial cells. CHIVA haemodynamic correction, while maintaining the saphenous conduit, restores a monodirectional flow. It can be directed upwards or downwards as the reader may better understand in the subsequent chapters. Approximately 6 months after the procedure, the cytokine profile is completely changed.

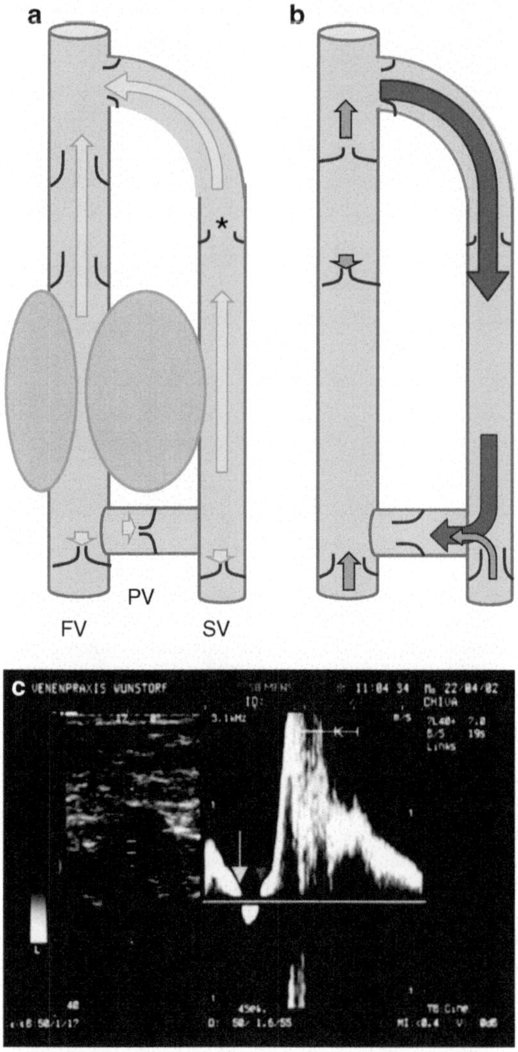

Fig. 3.9 Model of flow in the femoral vein (FV) is exposed to muscular contraction and the saphenous vein, also exposed to contraction, but to a lesser extent (SV). Bottom of the image = distal, top = proximal. (**a**) Muscular systole compressing one segment of the femoral vein and of the saphenous vein. The blood is expelled in direction of the heart following the pressure gradient in both veins (yellow arrow = flow in systole). The valves distal to the contraction are closed, in the femoral vein as well as in the perforating vein. (**b**) Muscular diastole, the segment of the deep vein that had been compressed has now a lower pressure. Blood follows the pressure gradient filling the emptied deep segment from the distal segment of the deep vein (green arrow) through the perforating vein from the distal part of the saphenous vein following the hydrostatic pressure, which is much higher in the saphenous vein, as the valves are not closing. Refluxing blood will follow this pressure gradient, and the saphenous vein is filled out of the proximal deep vein against the rules of the compartments. This is a reflux. Thus, the arrow is red. (**c**) Flow measurement in the great saphenous vein at the position of the *: systole starts at the yellow arrow. Little amount of antegrade flow. Red arrow: start of diastole with high velocity and long-lasting reflux. With kind permission by [13]

Tumour necrosis factor alpha (TNFα) and interferon gamma-induced protein 10 (IP-10) even returned inside a physiological range after CHIVA suppression of the oscillatory component of reflux. Both cytokines showed a significant correlation with flow parameters, indicating how reflux represents an inflammatory stimulus not when it is directed downwards but when it is oscillating upwards and downwards and with components of turbulent flow. The vision of the oscillatory component of venous reflux challenges the current view above reported, which considers venous reflux as an inverted direction of a flow lasting more than a specific cut-off.

In addition, the lesson learned is that the great saphenous vein can be recovered when surgery corrects the abnormal haemodynamics [21].

A cornerstone of ablative strategy is represented by the never proved statement that an incompetent great saphenous vein cannot be recovered to normal function because the biology of chronic venous insufficiency cannot be corrected. This dogma, repeated for years, should have been revised since the first results of venous sparing surgery were published. But now, with cytokine evidence as the base of vein wall recovery, the dogma should no longer be repeated, even though further investigations are needed.

3.3 Pathological Compartment Jumps

The actual anatomical and physiological interpretation of the lower limb venous network indicates a draining direction from the most superficial to the deepest lower limb compartments: from the tributary network (N3), towards the saphenous system (N2) and the deep venous system (N1). In this interpretation reflux can be defined as whatever subversion of the above reported hierarchical order of emptying [22, 23] (see Sect. 2.3).

According to Poiseuille's law, a pressure gradient is needed among two points in order to create a flow or a reflux. This means that whenever there is a reflux in a vein, a leaking point and a so-called re-entry point must be identified. While the leaking point can be whatever junctional point presenting a pathologically inverted flow (sapheno-femoral or sapheno-popliteal junction, incompetent perforating vein), a re-entry point can be defined for example as the perforator draining the refluxing blood back into the deep system.

The identification of the leaking and re-entry points is fundamental in venous insufficiency treatment: a mistake in the reflux source or re-entry point selection invariably leads to an incorrect diagnosis and treatment, potentially leading to the creation of a non-draining system and thus to venous stasis and thrombosis.

The reflux always induces higher volume of blood in the filled vein: As an example, in case of a reflux from the femoral vein (N1) into the saphenous vein (N2), a much larger vessel empties blood into a vessel with a lesser diameter. This extra volume overloads the N2 vessel, and we find a dilatation—classical in superficial vein insufficiency. The same occurs with jumps from N2 to N3. This volume is drained through re-entry points again to the compartment where it arose from, closing a recirculation circle and, by the way, overloading the deep venous pathways with this extra blood.

As already described by Trendelenburg [24] and later by Hach [25], superficial venous insufficiency is part of a blood flow circle, with an escape point (where the blood changes the compartment from deep to superficial); a refluxive segment, where a blood volume not usually present in a superficial vein flows retrograde and turbulent; a re-entry point where the blood finally is brought back to the original compartment; and a drainage through the deep veins back in its physiological course.

These recirculations have been stratified by Franceschi after analysing that they always follow certain patterns into so-called shunts [16, 22, 23, 26–28]. A shunt is a venous pathway that carries not only the physiological drainage but also the pathologically deviated blood. The flow overload inside the shunt leads to a transmural pressure excess and to the related clinical consequences. To understand the shunts, it is necessary to have a closer look at the reflux or insufficiency points and the re-entry points. General definitions around the shunts can be found at the start of Chap. 6.

The central point in superficial venous insufficiency is the volume overload of a saphenous vein or tributary by blood from the deep veins. Despite this overload, the vessel continues to drain the blood of the tributaries with blood flowing from the tributaries (N3) through the refluxive saphenous vein and into the deep veins. Even though filled pathologically, the vein still fulfils its function of a draining pathway for lots of tributaries. Finally, the net blood flow is out of the leg through the deep veins, but this is constantly hampered by the recirculation.

3.4 Reflux Sources

The reflux source is the point, where the blood flow changes the compartment in a pathological way, as described in Sect. 3.3. We distinguish the following:

- Reflux from deep veins to saphenous veins (N1 → N2)
- Reflux from deep veins into epifascial veins (N1 → N3)
- Reflux from saphenous veins to epifascial veins (N2 → N3)
- Reflux from pelvic networks into saphenous

or epifascial veins

- Reflux from bone perforators

3.4.1 Reflux Sources from Deep Veins into Saphenous Trunk (N1 → N2)

In case of refluxing saphenous veins, the blood source frequently is the deep vein. To be defined as "N1 → N2" jump, blood flow has to arise directly from a deep vein into a saphenous vein:

- From the femoral vein into the great saphenous vein through the sapheno-femoral junction (Fig. 3.10a). Note that a "conditio sine qua non" is an incompetent terminal valve. The reflux must be observed through the ostium level emerging from the deep vein (see Sect. 4.4.2).
- From the popliteal vein into the small saphenous vein through the sapheno-popliteal junction (Fig. 3.10b).
- From the deep veins into the great saphenous vein through perforating veins (Fig. 3.10c).
- From the deep veins into the small saphenous vein through muscle veins or perforating veins (Fig. 3.10d).

The further down the leg a perforating vein is located, the less likely it is to act as a reflux source and the more likely it is to act as a re-entry point. The

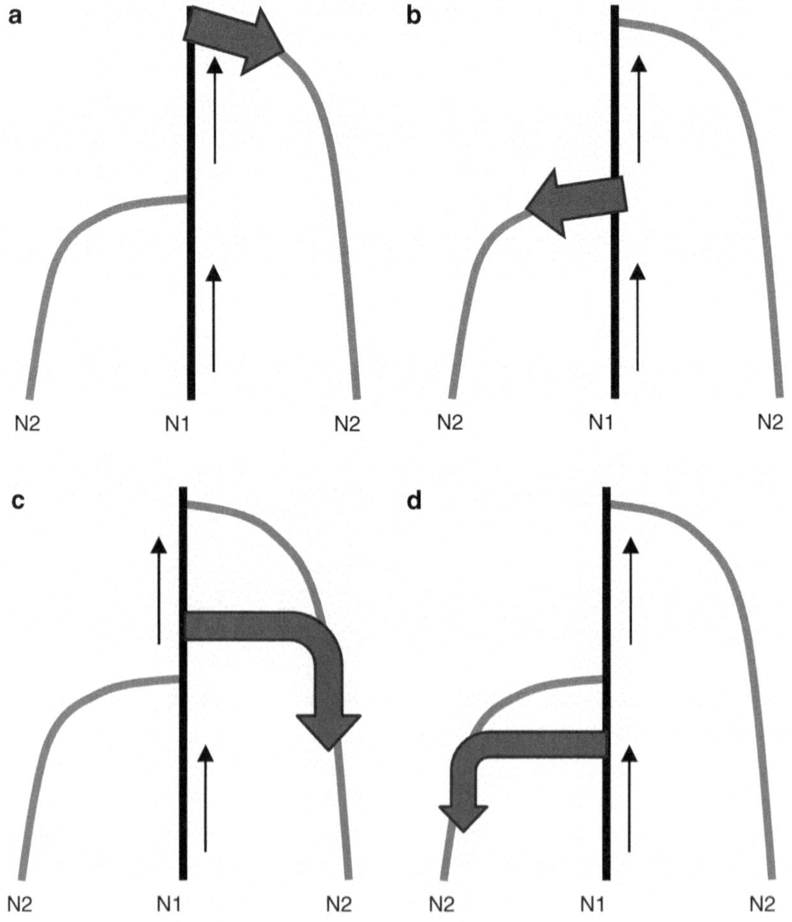

Fig. 3.10 Reflux source from the deep vein (N1) to the saphenous trunks (N2): (**a**) Reflux from the deep vein into the great saphenous vein through the sapheno-femoral junction. (**b**) Reflux from the deep vein into the small saphenous vein through the sapheno-popliteal junction. (**c**) Reflux from the deep vein into the great saphenous vein through a thigh perforator. (**d**) Reflux from the deep vein into the small saphenous vein through a calf perforator. With kind permission by [16]

fact, that a perforating vein is dilated, is not demonstrating, that it is refluxive (see Sects. 2.4 and 4.7).

These reflux sources (N1 → N2) are found in shunt types 1 and 3 according to Franceschi.

3.4.2 Reflux Sources from Deep Veins into Varicose Tributaries (N1 → N3)

In this case, the reflux from the deep veins (N1) escapes through a perforating vein and fills a tributary (N3). The tributary can be the only varicose refluxive vessel, or it can—in its further course—fill a saphenous vein with reflux.

Such a primary reflux source is frequently observed in the **back of the thigh** where the dorsal thigh perforating vein originates (Hach perforator) (Fig. 3.11a).

In athletes, especially footballers, it is not unusual to find several refluxive muscle veins which fill the lower leg tributaries through perforating veins (Fig. 3.11b). These patients may have various reflux sources. The origin of these incompetent perforators is not clear. It might be that the pressure on muscle veins or perforating veins is too high during repeated exercise or the perforators could be destroyed by a direct trauma damaging the valve leaflets and leaving these veins permanently incompetent.

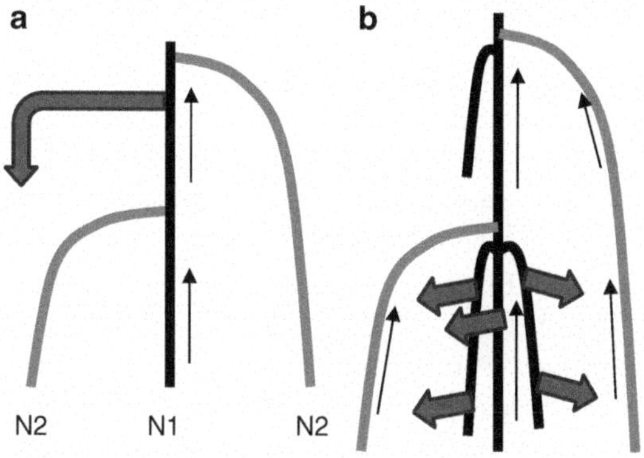

Fig. 3.11 Reflux source from the deep vein (N1) to tributaries (N3) via perforating veins: (**a**) Reflux through a dorsal thigh perforator (Hach). (**b**) Multiple refluxing perforators at the calf. With kind permission by [16]

3.4.3 Reflux Sources from Saphenous Trunks into Tributaries (N2 → N3)

An antegrade flowing saphenous vein can be the origin of a reflux into a tributary. This occurs when blood flows out of a competent saphenous trunk vein into a varicose tributary (N2 → N3). In these cases, reflux is confined to the epifascial veins. The saphenous vein carries blood upwards, draining its healthy tributaries. At a certain point, one tributary is not competent and is filled reversely from the saphenous trunks getting pathologically dilated. The saphenous trunks in this case are not filled from the deep veins or from pathologically refluxive pelvic or superficial inguinal veins.

Varicose veins without saphenous reflux are generally a cosmetic problem. They do not cause any chronic venous incompetence, since they do not increase the total volume flowing through the leg.

Following the reservoir theory, this situation is the precursor of chronic venous insufficiency (see Chap. 12). Many phlebologists advocate treatment for these because they could be precursors of saphenous reflux.

3.4.4 Retrograde Flow in Saphenous Veins with No Proximal Reflux Source

In many patients with saphenous retrograde flow, the examiner is unable to find a reflux source from the deep vein on duplex ultrasound [13, 29]. The junctions and tributaries are competent as are the perforating veins and the proximal saphenous vein. Further down a discreet retrograde flow may be found as successive healthy tributaries join in. The rather discreet volume of this flow towards the foot increases with each joining tributary, but it is still the blood that belongs into the saphenous vein—the one drained from tributaries (N3–N2). Further down, this retrograde blood flow feeds a refluxing tributary. This is the pathological **compartment jump**, where the blood from N2 fills N3. This reverse flow without a prior reflux source is very often found by chance in the contralateral leg which has minimal or no signs of clinical venous disease. It has been called shunt type 0 in the current shunt classification (see Sect. 3.7).

Ascending and Descending Theories of Varicose Vein Progression

Whether reflux originates near the foot and progresses upwards or arises from an incompetent junction and progresses downwards is important. If the direction of progression can be predicted, then treatments can be more focused. If an ascending pathology is interrupted, this may prevent subsequent incompetence of the upper end of the great saphenous vein and the sapheno-femoral junction [30]. In a standing patient, a refluxive vein is constantly retrogradely filled with blood by the force of gravity. Suction into the deep veins caused by calf diastole will suck blood out of the varicose vein. This in turn will result in a downward **Venturi** force in the tributary in addition to the effect of gravity. If these forces continue, then the valves in the upper saphenous vein may begin to fail leading to the slow development of a retrograde flow. When the suction reaches the sapheno-femoral junction, this may create a reflux source and the formation of a recirculation loop now involving the deep veins [16] (see Fig. 3.12). Interestingly, the saphenous veins of many patients can regain competency after the interruption of refluxive tributary. This can be observed after saphenous conservation approaches like CHIVA [11] (see Sect. 6.4.1) and ASVAL (see Chap. 12, [31, 32]).

3.4.5 Reflux Sources Above the Inguinal Ligament

Pelvic networks can be the reflux source of varicose veins in the legs. This is deeply explained in Chap. 8. This reflux can join the superficial leg veins via some variable pathways:

- A tributary of the great saphenous vein in the groin especially the pudendal vein from medial and the epigastric or circumflex vein from cranial
- Refluxive network over the labia in the inner thigh joining or not any saphenous vein
- Refluxive network on the abdominal wall with flow into the subcutaneous venous network on the front of the thigh
- Refluxive network on the medial aspect of the thigh, joining or not any saphenous vein
- Refluxive network at the posterior aspect of the thigh fed by gluteal perforators, joining or not the saphenous veins

A common element in all these variants is that the refluxive blood **does not come from the leg nor from a deep vein** but is draining blood from the abdominal skin, the scrotum/labia or from inner organs in the pelvis, like via the ovarian vein. Thus, considering the anatomic compartment concept, these veins are collectors from capillaries and would correspond to venous network 3. But as they are not part from the leg veins, but from a completely different anatomical compartment normally not draining into leg veins, a compartment jump is certainly occurring, being the substrate of a varicose vein insufficiency. To avoid misunderstandings with leg venous networks, this reflux source will be represented as "P" in our schemes.

In clinical practice recirculation from reflux sources above the inguinal ligament is a frequent source of **recurrence** after treatment of the leg veins. This is because the actual reflux point is not eliminated by normal interventions for varicose veins.

Pelvic venous reflux can be demonstrated using transvaginal ultrasound and a Valsalva manoeuvre.

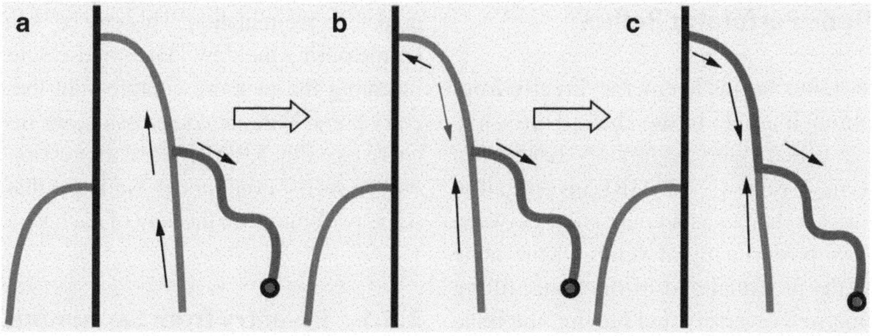

Fig. 3.12 Ascending progression theory. (**a**) Varicose tributary with a competent great saphenous vein; (**b**) varicose tributary with a suction (Venturi) effect on the proximal saphenous vein causing the start of a retrograde flow out of part of the saphenous vein and into the varicose tributary (**c**) further ascending progression to complete incompetence of the great saphenous vein and the sapheno-femoral junction. With kind permission by [13]

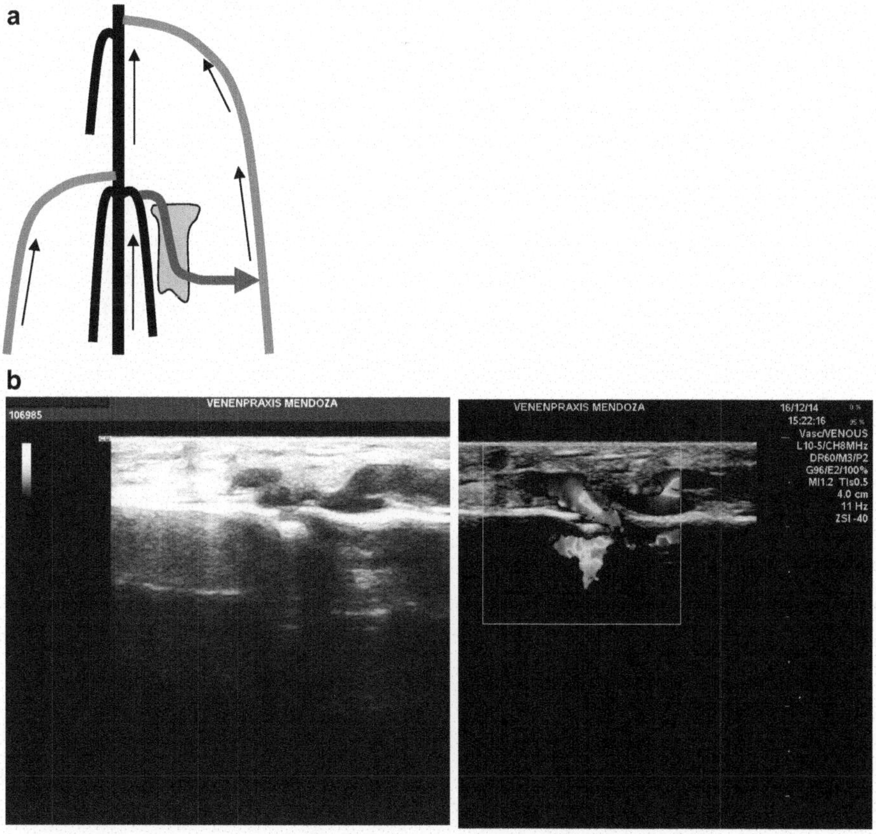

Fig. 3.13 Bone perforators. (**a**) According to MRI images, a reversed flow from the posterior tibial vein into the bone marrow at the proximal end of the tibia could be demonstrated. The blood flows backwards through the bone and fills the bone tributary through a distal hole. These perforators have contact either to the saphenous vein or to a refluxive tributary. (**b**) Longitudinally scan of the tibia with ultrasound image of the hole in the tibia left in B mode with a part of the cortex displaced inside the bone. Right in colour duplex with emerging flow from inside the bone

3.4.6 Bone Perforator Reflux

Sometimes reflux seems to emerge directly from the tibia through a hole in the shaft. Thirty-five cases of so-called bone perforators have been published in a review. An MRI investigation could show that there was a connection between the proximal posterior tibial vein and the bone marrow at the proximal end of the bone, filling the bone marrow reversely and feeding the bone perforator at the distal end ([33], see Fig. 3.13). So, it looks like the order of emptying of the bone marrow had been reversed. It was no more drained through the tibial collateral, but reversely filled by it, blood escaping from the bone through a distal hole feeding a tributary, which could or not connect to the saphenous vein (see Fig. 3.13). The flow followed the order: N1 → Bone → N3 (–N2). Further investigations are necessary to enlighten the pathophysiology of these cases. In the authors' experience, the five known cases in the own office all had a prior major tibial trauma accounting for the hole in the bone.

3.5 Re-entry Points

The point where an incompetent superficial vein is drained into the deep vein is called re-entry point. It can be drainage from N3 to N1 or N2 to N1. Also, a drainage from a refluxive tributary (N3) to a saphenous vein (N2) is a re-entry point. Always, when refluxing blood starts following the compartment rules, we find a re-entry point.

Re-entry points complete the recirculation circuit. While there is normally only one reflux source for every recirculation loop, the number of re-entry points is generally greater than one. Different types of re-entry points may occur in the same leg.

The furthest distal re-entry point in the circuit is the **terminal perforating vein** (Zamboni 1998). When varicose veins are clinically visible and dilated, there is always a terminal perforating vein marking the point where the reflux ends.

Only those **perforating veins** which have suffered secondary dilatation from re-entry flow will serve as re-entry points for a recirculation. Non-dilated perforating veins are present but do not participate in recirculation. This can be demonstrated by measuring the flow in a varicose vein and then repeating the measure compressing the distal re-entry point. Without compression, we find a reflux curve (see Fig. 3.9c). Under compression no reflux will be seen—even though we know that there are some perforators on the way of each vein.

3.5.1 Re-entry from Saphenous Trunks (N2–N1)

Perforating veins draining reflux from an incompetent great saphenous vein must be sufficiently wide for the blood volume involved. Therefore, perforating veins which are not dilated in B scan (<3 mm) are unable to accommodate this drainage and are not significant for the recirculation.

The re-entry point from the refluxive saphenous vein may be a perforating vein in the middle of its refluxive segment (Fig. 3.14, single red arrow) or a terminal perforating vein below which the flow in the great saphenous vein is anterograde (Fig. 3.14, double red arrow). The terminal perforating vein is not only draining the refluxing blood but is also the drainage point for the distal part of the great saphenous vein, through which the blood flow is anterograde. In addition to this draining perforating vein, there are usually refluxive tributaries which drain the recirculation volumes from the great saphenous vein to the deep veins through other perforating veins.

3.5.2 Re-entry from Refluxive Tributaries to the Deep Veins (N3–N1)

The blood from refluxive tributaries can find various drainage routes into the deep veins, always through a perforating vein. The tributary can

- Wind for a long stretch until it finally joins a terminal perforating vein (Fig. 3.15a)
- Wind without dividing and drain through several perforating veins, the last one the terminal one (Fig. 3.15b)

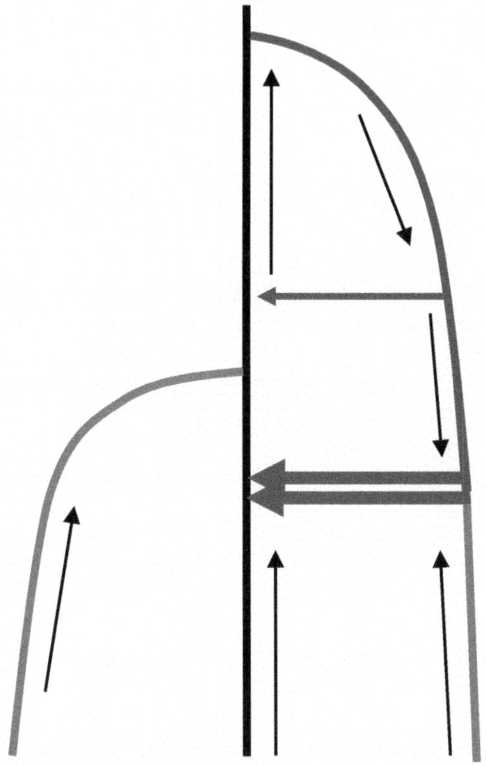

Fig. 3.14 Refluxive great saphenous vein (GSV) from the sapheno-femoral junction until a perforator below the knee (double red arrow) that drains the blood to the deep vein (DV). Another re-entry perforator from the saphenous vein into the deep vein is seen at the thigh (single red arrow). The lower one (two arrows) is a terminal perforating vein through which the below knee part of the competent great saphenous vein drains in anterograde flow. This condition, with two draining perforating veins and no visible tributaries, is not very often found. With kind permission from [16]

- Divide into further refluxive tributaries drained by the possibilities described above (Fig. 3.15c)

3.5.3 Flow Analysis in Perforating Veins

As seen in Sect. 2.4, not every dilated perforating vein is a refluxing one, as supposed in the beginnings of modern phlebology. It is known that lots of perforators are present in the path of a varicose vein, but only the enlarged perforators can efficiently drain a refluxive blood volume or act as escape point feeding a varicose vein with refluxing blood.

We have seen in this chapter that most of the perforators are draining the recirculation, thus taking part in the pathological flow, but not as "creators" of reflux but as equalizers of pressure and draining pathways, as consequence of pathology.

The possibilities of flow in systole and diastole are presented in Table 3.1 [34].

3.5.4 Re-entry from a Tributary into a Saphenous Vein (N3–N2)

There are several possible variants:

- The tributary drains into the same saphenous vein from which it has received the reflux. The saphenous segment between the proximal and distal end of the refluxive tributary can be competent or not, as well as the distal segment of the saphenous vein. A reflux can escape and re-enter a saphenous vein twice (117 from 770 legs, 15.2% of cases in great saphenous vein) or three times (5 from 770 legs, 0.7% of cases in great saphenous vein) [35] (Fig. 3.16).
- A refluxive tributary drains into the other saphenous vein (usually the small saphenous vein) which is not the original source of the reflux. In this case the draining saphenous vein may itself become incompetent (Fig. 3.16), but it may also carry the reflux volume antegrade into the deep veins through its junction. This may be the precursor of the situation described above with reflux through both saphenous junctions.

Refluxive connections between the saphenous trunks are confusing when trying to assess haemodynamics. Special attention must be paid to these connecting veins between small and great saphenous veins during examination.

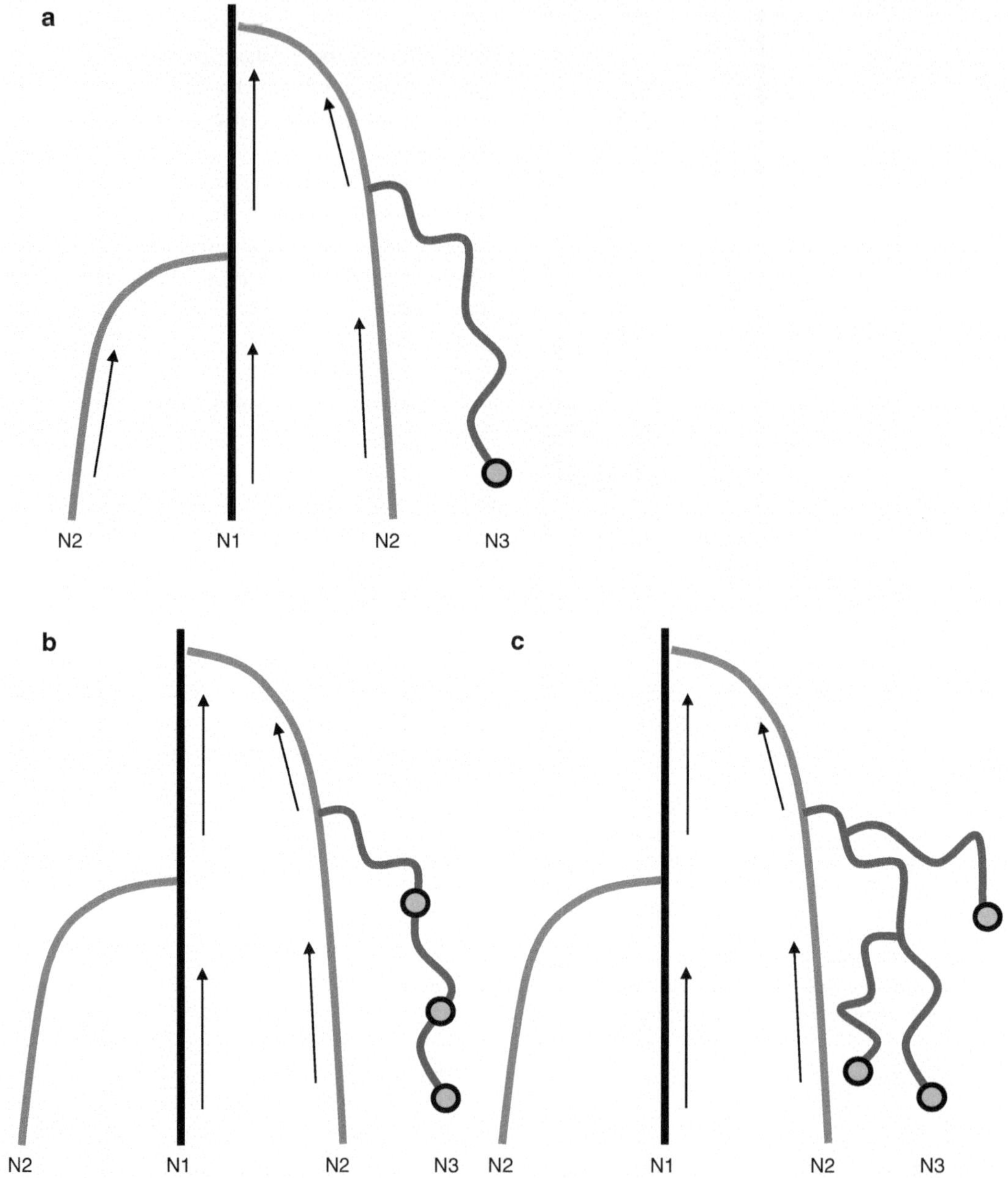

Fig. 3.15 Varicose tributary showing the different drainage possibilities via the perforating veins (shown as a blue dot): (**a**) Through a single terminal perforating vein. (**b**) Through several perforating veins; the last one is the terminal perforating vein. (**c**) Through several tributaries, with terminal perforating veins at the end. With kind permission from [16]

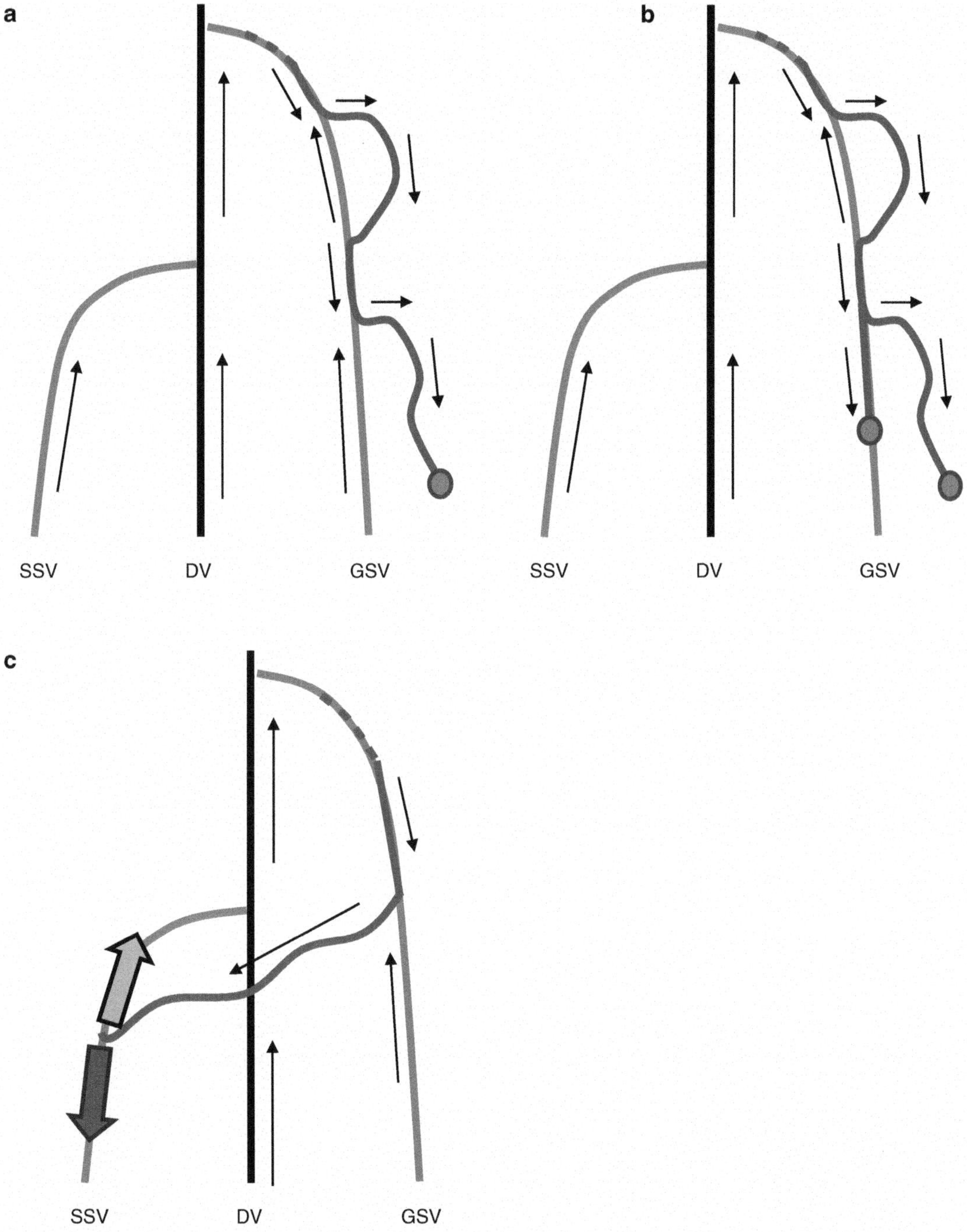

Fig. 3.16 Reflux from the great saphenous vein (GSV) into a tributary (N2–N3), draining back to the same GSV, which again is refluxive after the joining of the refluxive tributary. Then the reflux drains (**a**) Through a further tributary and a perforator (N2 → N3–N1). (**b**) Through a perforator on the GSV itself (N2–N1), as well as through a further refluxive tributary and a perforator (N2 → N3–N1). (**c**) Reflux from the great saphenous vein into a tributary (N2 → N3) draining into the small saphenous vein (SSV). This can drain the blood via the junction (antegrade flow, blue arrow) or can be filled pathologically by the reflux (reflux, red arrow). With kind permission from [16]

3.5.5 Re-entry from a Tributary Through a Poorly Drained Venous Network

Occasionally a dilated perforating vein cannot be identified at the end of a varicose tributary. This is common with **reticular varices** which are remote from the anatomical distribution of the saphenous trunks, for example, the lateral and posterior sides of the thigh and the lateral side of the calf. Reticular varices are partially intradermal, very little veins and form an unsightly venous network. They drain into perforating veins which are not visible either clinically or on ultrasound. Flow and reflux in reticular veins are very slow and barely measureable on ultrasound with usual devices.

A poorly drained re-entry can also be the consequence of venous treatment, if too much re-entry paths are disconnected, leaving a saphenous vein or tributary without sufficient drainage (see Sect. 6.10.2).

3.5.6 Drained and Poorly Drained Systems

The flow rate in a refluxive vein depends on three main variables:

- The reflux source
- The compliance of the refluxive vein
- The calibre of the re-entry perforating vein

Compliance is the capacity of the vein wall to adapt incoming volume (see Sect. 2.6.3). If the patient has been standing for some time, the veins become quite full regardless of their compliance. The **calibre of the re-entry perforating veins** then has a considerable influence on the flow curve. During muscular diastole, only so much blood will flow towards the foot as can pass back into the deep veins through the perforating vein. Thus, the perforating vein acts like a gatekeeper throttling the rate of recirculation.

3.5.6.1 Drained System

Because of their capacity to stretch, varicose veins receive more blood than their diameter at rest allows. This excess of blood then flows down to drain through the large calibre perforating veins, allowing the vein to collapse. The flow curve in PW mode will rise steeply and then fall again over a few seconds during a stimulation manoeuvre. These patients generally have large calibre, very winding varicose tributaries, but little distress.

3.5.6.2 Poorly Drained System

If, however, the vein wall is rigid and stiff, with no stretch capacity, only a small amount of blood will be received proximally at the start of muscular diastole. Small calibre perforating veins also hamper drainage. Only so much blood will be able to enter the vein as can be drained distally. A further cause of a poorly drained system is an impaired muscle pump. If the deep veins are not properly emptied during systole, no pressure drop can be generated during diastole to allow the superficial veins to empty.

The blood will flow very slowly in the varicose vein demonstrated by the curve in PW duplex which is long and flat. In many instances, the flow may be too slow to measure even after adjusting the machine settings. Slow flow results in higher transparietal pressure leading to the formation of an oedema or matting after surgery. This group often includes patients with scarcely visible varices but suffer the distress associated with chronic venous insufficiency [16].

3.6 Combination of Reflux Sources and Re-entry Points

As we have seen above, different possibilities of reflux sources and re-entry points can be combined to create a pathologic flow in leg veins, a recirculation or a veno-venous derivation (shunt according to Franceschi).

Before explaining the shunt concept according to Franceschi, the possible participation of each network is summarized:

The deep veins (N1) can feed the interfascial veins (N1 → N2) and the epifascial veins (N1 → N3) pathologically. They can drain the blood from saphenous veins (N2–N1) and from tributaries (N3–N1).

Table 3.2 Combination of reflux sources and re-entry points

Reflux Type	N1	P	B	N3	N2	N3	N2	N3	N1	Description	Shunt Type	Figure
N1 – N2										N1 – N2 – N1	1	3.19a, 3.22
										N1 – N2 – N1 N3 – N1	1+2	3.25
										N1 – N2 – N3 – N1	3	3.26a
Pelvic Reflux										P – N2 – N1	4 Pelvic	3.27a
										P – N3 – N2 – N1		3.27b
										P – N2 – N3 – N1	5 Pelvic	3.29a
										P – N3 – N2 – N3 – N1		
N1 – N3										N1 – N3 – N2 – N1	4 Perforator	3.27c
										N1 – N3 – N2 – N3 – N1	5 Perforator	3.29b
										N1 – N3 – N2	6	3.30
N2 – N3										N2 – N3 – N2	2	3.23, 3.24
Bone Perforator										(N1) – B – N3 – N1	6	3.13
										(N1) – B – N3 –N2 – N1	4 Perforator	
										(N1) – B – N3 – N2 – N3 – N1	5 Perforator	
Two Sources	1									N1 – N2 – N3 ↘	3	3.17a
	2									N1 – N3 – N2 – N3 – N1*	5 Perforator	

N1 deep veins, N2 interfascial veins (saphenous veins), N3 tributaries, P reflux from pelvic networks, B bone perforator reflux

* Path 1: Reflux from the deep vein through the great saphenous vein, draining in a tributary, that joins the small saphenous vein and mid-calf

Path 2: Reflux through a dorsal thigh perforator into a tributary, that fills the short saphenous vein below the knee fold

Draining path: Reflux leaves the small saphenous vein through a tributary, that drains into the deep veins through a perforator

The interfascial veins (N2) can be pathologically fed by the deep vein directly (N1 → N2) or via a refluxing tributary (N1 → N3–N2) or a bone perforator (N1 → B → N3–N2). Saphenous veins can be fed by the pelvic network in the groin (P → N2) or via a superficial thigh tributary (P → N3–N2). Competent interfascial veins can feed tributaries with reflux (N2 → N3). Interfascial veins can drain their pathologically refluxing blood to the deep veins through a perforator (N2–N1) or via a tributary (N2 → N3–N1).

The epifascial veins can be fed pathologically by a competent saphenous vein (N2 → N3), by a refluxing saphenous vein (N1 → N2 → N3 or P → N2 → N3), by a perforating vein (N1 → N3), by the pelvic network (P–N3) or by a bone perforator reflux (N1 → B → N3). It can drain via a perforator (N3–N1), via a competent saphenous vein through its junction or a perforator (N3–N2–N1). Depending on these possible combinations (see Table 3.2), the shunt type classification was created.

More than one reflux source may occasionally be found in a leg when there is retrograde flow from the deep veins at several independent points, or two independent tributaries are filled refluxively from a saphenous vein with antegrade flow. In these cases, the higher reflux source is generally more important, for example,

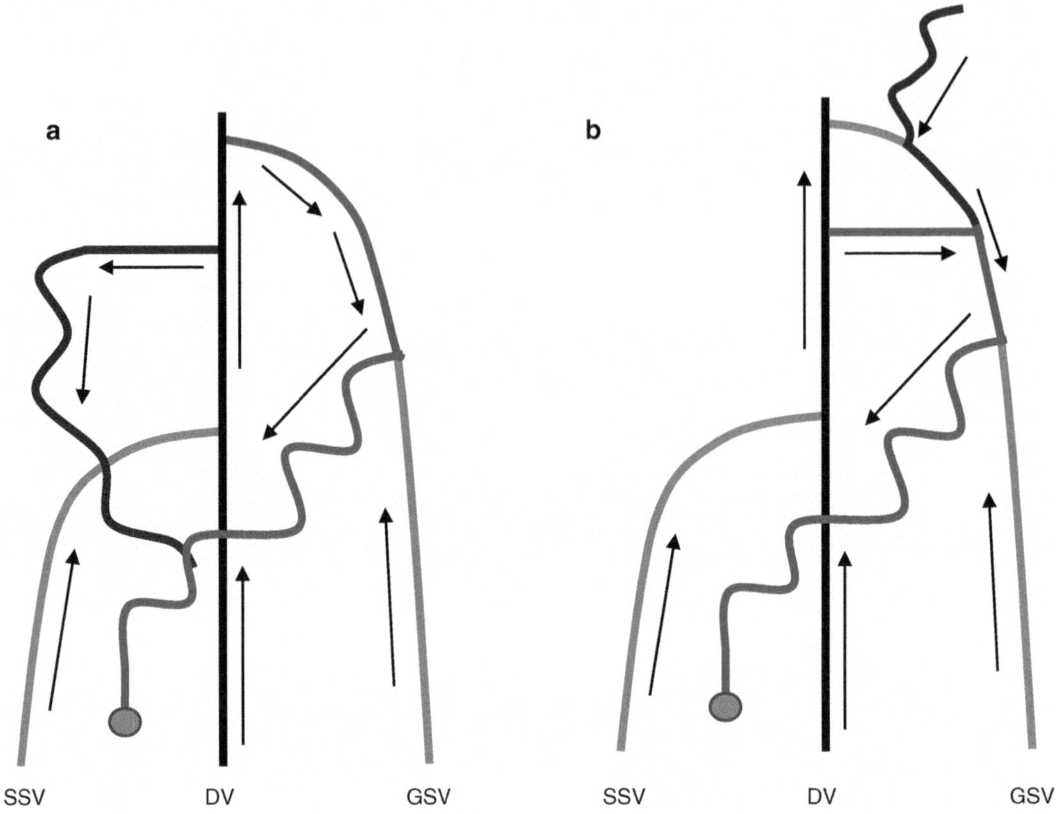

Fig. 3.17 Examples of coexisting reflux sources in recirculation (principal reflux source, light red), with an additional recirculation (lesser reflux source, dark red). (**a**) Recirculations flow through the sapheno-femoral junction perforating vein. (**b**) Slight reflux from the pelvis with the principal recirculation from a perforating vein in the adductor canal (formerly Dodd). With kind permission from [16]

a refluxive sapheno-femoral junction and a refluxive perforating vein in the back of the thigh (Fig. 3.17a). However, the reverse may occur, for example, if there is minor reflux from the pelvis through the pudendal vein which fills the great saphenous vein in retrograde flow, but the latter is only really dilated and refluxive from a perforating vein in the adductor canal (formerly Dodd) (Fig. 3.17b). Evaluation of the flow curves in PW mode is particularly important in prioritising the relative importance and contribution of a reflux source. Diagnostic problems arise when **both saphenous junctions are refluxive** and the saphenous trunk veins are connected by a tributary (ramus communicans). In this case it cannot always be clearly established whether the small saphenous vein suffered the primary incompetence or if it started as the drainage route of the great saphenous vein and at some point was so volume overloaded that it subsequently became incompetent (Fig. 3.18).

It is also possible for two independent disconnected recirculation circuits to occur.

3.7 Shunt Concept and Classification

Depending on the reflux source and the draining pathways, Franceschi developed the concept of shunt as a veno-venous derivation [27, 28, 36]. After gaining more information and experience in 2002, the shunt types were restructured [16, 22, 26].

As reported in the section Anatomy (Chap. 2), the hierarchical order of venous emptying is from

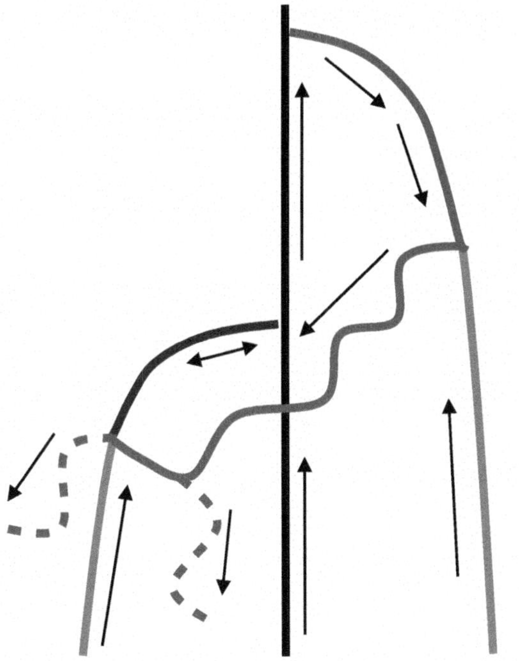

Fig. 3.18 Reflux in the great saphenous vein with drainage through a tributary into the small saphenous vein. The proximal section of the small saphenous vein is dilated but not significantly refluxive at first. Instead there is an oscillating flow pattern refluxing upwards on calf muscle diastole. Later, tributaries may also carry some of the reflux and offer a drainage route from the great and small saphenous veins (dotted lines). Thus, both veins are refluxive, even though the small saphenous vein was not refluxive at the start. Nevertheless, the principal reflux source is from the great saphenous vein. With kind permission from [16]

network 3 (N3 = epifascial veins) to network 2 (N2 = interfascial veins, saphenous veins) and to network 1 (N1 = deep veins). Other veins relevant for the shunts are the supra-inguinal veins filling the leg vein system with blood. In this chapter, these vessels are summarized as "P" for pelvic reflux. In this model, a shunt is defined as a flow pattern with whatever subversion of the hierarchical order of venous drainage. A shunt is a venous pathway that carries not only the physiological drainage but also the pathologically deviated blood. The flow overload inside the shunt leads to a transmural pressure excess and to the related clinical consequences of chronic venous insufficiency. (See also start of Chap. 6 for definitions.)

There are different groups of shunts, depending on the circumstance the flow changes the anatomical compartment:

- At rest (permanent)
- During muscular contraction (systole)
- During muscular relaxation (diastole)

These conditions can appear alone or in combination, so that three main types of shunts are haemodynamically described, according to their anatomical constitution, and their overloading flow feature (permanent, systolic or diastolic) [22, 26–28, 36]:

- Closed (CS)
- Open deviated shunts (ODS)
- Open bypassing shunts (OBS), originally called open vicarious shunts (OVS)

3.7.1 Closed Shunt

A closed shunt (CS) derives its name from the fact that it forms a "closed" circuit among the escape point and the re-entry point, as described by Trendelenburg's "private circulation" [24] and by Hach's "recirculation" [25].

During the muscle pump diastole, a closed shunt is overloaded through the escape point with flow from a deeper compartment to a more superficial compartment. The pressure gradient feeding the reflux is provided by the venous muscle pump during diastole and by the height of the incompetent hydrostatic column into the shunting vein (see Fig. 3.9). Most of the superficial venous insufficiencies, involving N2 and N3, are closed shunts, and their types are described in Sect. 3.8.

3.7.2 Open Deviated Shunt

An open deviated shunt (ODS) is not associated with a recirculation, and the blood changing the anatomic compartment is not returning to the start, as in the closed shunts. It is just a deviated drainage pattern leading to a venous pressure increase in the N3 vessel that is overloaded only

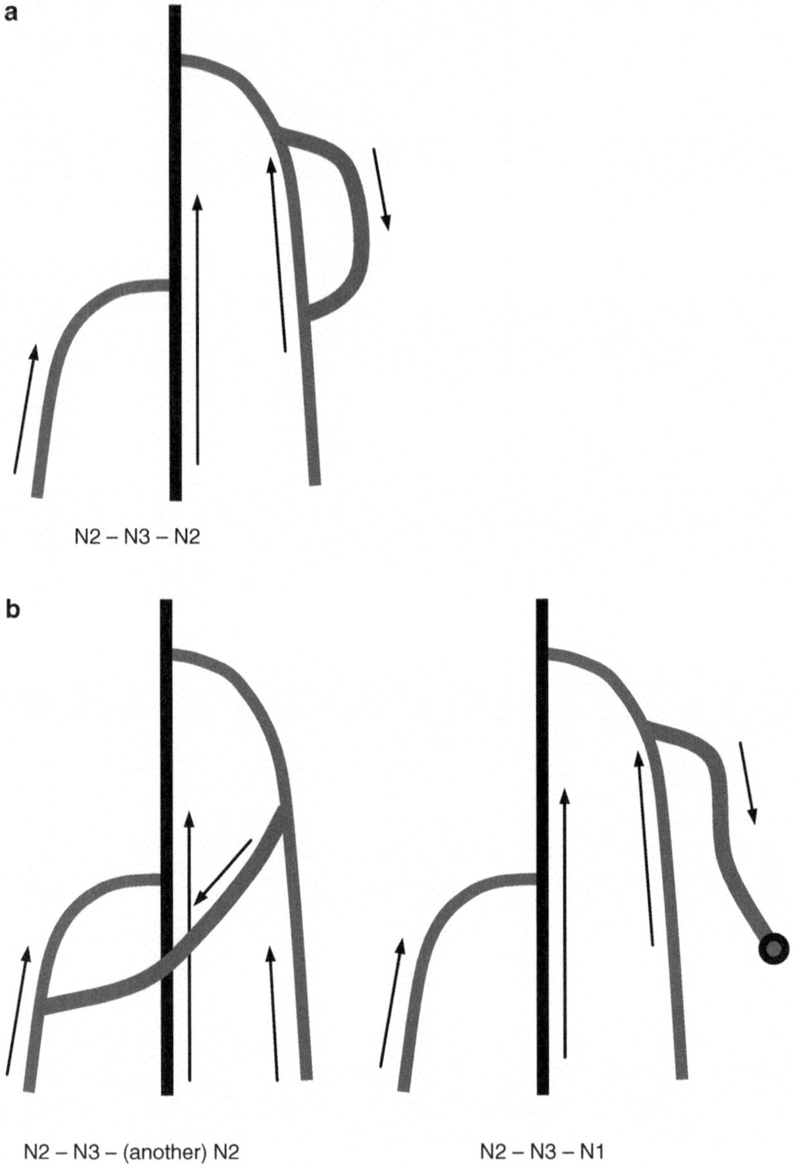

Fig. 3.19 Closed and open deviating shunt type 2. (**a**) Closed shunt type 2: The blood from the competent great saphenous (N2) vein feeds a refluxing tributary (N3), which drains again into the same saphenous vein, so the blood closes a recirculation circle. N2 → N3–N2. (**b**) Open deviating shunt, open shunt type 2: The blood emerges from the great saphenous vein. Reflux through N3 (Tributary) drains into the short saphenous vein (N2 → N3–different N2, left image) or a perforator (N2 → N3–N1, right image). The blood in the refluxive segment doesn't return to the start of the recirculation; that is why it is called open shunt. With kind permission by [16]

by the blood coming from a saphenous vein. There is no refluxing N1 → N2 connection nor any footward flow in the saphenous veins fed by physiologically draining veins (see shunt type 2, Sect. 3.8.2). Its clinical implications are very little, only the visible tributary can be bothering.

This is the case when a tributary is retrogradely fed by a competent saphenous vein and the drainage of the tributary is either through the other saphenous vein or through a perforator directed to the deep vein, so that no recirculation circle is closed (see Fig. 3.19). It is different to the closed shunt 2, described in Sect. 3.8.2. An open deviating shunt is only active in muscular diastole; during systole all involved veins drain towards the heart and following the compartment rules.

3.7.3 Open Bypassing Shunt (Franceschi: Open Vicarious Shunt)

An open bypassing shunt bypasses venous obstructions, like thrombotic or post-thrombotic changes or functional muscle compression of veins. Claude Franceschi used the term open vicarious shunt based on the fact that a vicar is a substitute and the shunt is a substitute for an obstructed pathway. As this wording has provoked criticism in those persons not understanding the meaning of vicarious, in this book we offer an alternative terminology to vicarious, introducing the term bypassing shunt.

Usually the escape point is distal to the obstruction, filling a more superficial compartment with the blood from the closed or (partially) obstructed segment. The return to the original, deeper compartment through a re-entry point occurs proximal to the obstacle.

This open bypassing shunt is fed by the residual pressure increased by the resistance due to the venous obstruction, so diverting the flow in a more superficial channel in order to bypass the obstacle (Fig. 3.20).

As a consequence of the obstruction, a transmural pressure increase occurs so dilating the distal veins, hampering the drainage and forcing the blood to shunt usually towards a more superficial compartment where the resistance is lower. The progressive dilatation of the open bypassing shunt reduces this resistance, and the upstream transmural pressure decreases in proportion.

Contrary to a closed shunt and an open deviated shunt, the open bypassing shunt is NOT activated during the diastole, but only during the venous muscle pump systole and sometimes permanently when the bypassed obstacle is hemodynamically very important, even at rest.

The open bypassing shunt (open vicarious shunt) is a "natural defence mechanism" to bypass a closure and make sure that the distal leg veins are drained. So, the open bypassing shunt has to be spared. For that reason, it is very important to distinct the shunt types during the examination, as open bypassing shunts have to be respected and not confused with closed shunts or open deviating shunts.

On the other hand, this phenomenon explains the part of the varicose recurrence after ablation of superficial veins. Indeed, due to the residual pressure in tributaries left in the leg without draining pathway, the ablated veins are progressively bypassed by varicose collaterals. This could provide a rationale for the better long-term outcome that is observed comparing CHIVA versus ablative strategies [37, 38].

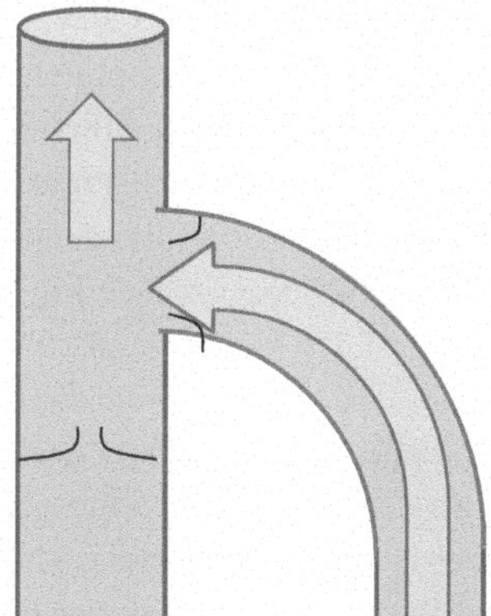

Fig. 3.20 Open bypassing shunt with an obstruction in the femoral vein. Distal to it, the pressure in the deep vein is high, thus finding an escape point through a perforator, filling the great saphenous vein and draining back into the proximal common femoral vein. The shunting blood flows in systole, thus the arrows are yellow

Anatomic example: In the presence of a proximal thigh femoral vein occlusion by an organised thrombus, a perforating vein distally connecting the same femoral vein to the great saphenous vein can reverse its drainage direction, allowing flow from the deep vein (N1) towards the more superficial N2 network. If the saphenous vein valves are competent, this shunted blood drains in a cardiopetal direction, so bypassing the femoral obstruction and then finding its re-entry point at the saphenofemoral junction, as depicted in Fig. 3.20.

Another example is a femoral vein obstacle diverting the blood from the popliteal vein (N1) through the sapheno-popliteal junction into the Giacomini vein and thus into the great saphenous vein, in order to get back into the deep system by the sapheno-femoral junction (see Fig. 3.31).

Also in case of left iliac venous obstacle, the hindered femoral flow (N1) can force a reflux through the sapheno-femoral junction as escape point, then proceeding through the great saphenous vein arch, its upper tributaries (N3) will get dilated. The flow will fill the pelvic net or more frequently the subcutaneous plexus at the level of the pubis and finally join the opposite femoral vein (N1) through the opposite great saphenous vein and its sapheno-femoral junction as re-entry point. A spontaneous femoro-femoral anastomosis, so-called Palma anastomosis, is formed. This is a typical open bypassing shunt.

It is evident how an open bypassing shunt is actually a natural defence against venous hypertension. In the above depicted scenario, no aggressive indications are requested: just an appropriate elastic stocking compression, an anticoagulant scheme depending on the history of thrombosis and risk factors and an accurate sonographic follow-up.

3.7.4 Reflux Without Escape Point: Shunt Type 0

A footward flow but without pathological compartment jumps can be observed sometimes, when a reflux in the great saphenous vein is not fed by an escape point nor a refluxive tributary is found. It could be defined by: (?)–N2–N1. That means after a thorough exam of the saphenous vein, no refluxive perforator or junction or groin tributary with reflux under Valsalva manoeuvre can be found feeding the refluxive saphenous vein. And no refluxive tributaries drain the vein, but a perforator connecting the saphenous vein to the deep vein. As there are no pathological compartment jumps, the definition of shunt is not fulfilled. But as the definition of reflux (diastolic flow in opposite direction as the physiologic flow) lasting longer than 0.5–1 s is fulfilled, this situation was defined as shunt type 0 (see Fig. 3.21) [16]. The retrograde is originated by physiologically draining vein that feeds the saphenous vein. Thus, the question mark can be substituted by N3: N3–N2–N1. No compartment jumps to be found, so this downward flow does not overload the system. The amount of blood is exactly the one the great saphenous vein is designed to drain, coming from tributaries and directed towards the deep vein—via a distal perforator instead of a proximal one or the sapheno-femoral junction. It should not be forgotten, that depending on the length of the segment affected by the shunt type 0, the hydrostatic pressure column increases and can condition the formation of refluxive tributaries to drain the volume, thus, a shunt type 0 could be a precursor of a shunt, as described in Sect. 3.8.2.

3.8 Closed Shunts

A closed shunt (see Sect. 3.7.1) is a recirculation with reflux point and re-entry point, where the blood returns to its origin. In shunt types 1 and 3, the saphenous veins are filled directly from the deep veins. Together they are the most frequent shunt types, accounting for about 60% of cases. Shunt types 4 and 5 filled by supra-inguinal reflux sources are the next frequent group (about 25% of cases), followed by shunt type 2 (about 15% of cases). Shunt 6 is seldom to be found.

3.8.1 Shunt Type 1

This recirculation always affects the **saphenous veins (N2)**. Its source is the deep system (N1 → N2). The saphenous vein is filled directly from the sapheno-femoral or sapheno-popliteal junction or through a perforating vein (Fig. 3.22). The recirculating blood drains back into the deep system directly from the saphenous vein through a perforating vein without being diverted through a tributary. The N3 network is not involved in the principal recirculation. The principal circuit is therefore deep vein (N1), saphenous vein (N2) and deep vein (N1).

Usually, **N3 tributaries** are also filled from the refluxive N2 vein which may themselves

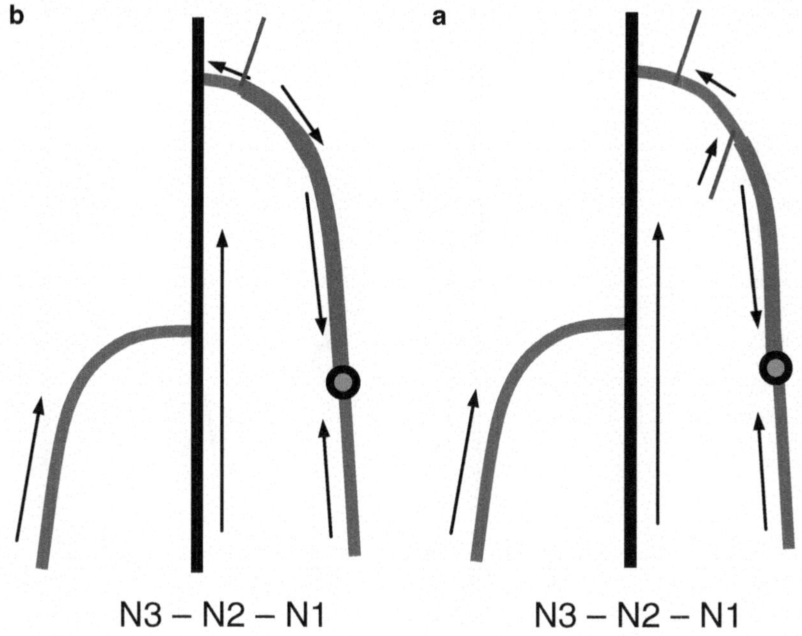

Fig. 3.21 Shunt type 0. (**a**) Physiologically draining tributaries (N3) feed the saphenous vein. The valves are not competent; the drained blood flows footwards and drains through a perforator into the deep vein. No compartment jumps visible, only backflow of longer than 0.5 s. (**b**) Evolution of the situation depicted in image (**a**). All the tributaries feed the saphenous vein retrogradely—the only competent valve is the terminal valve. Still there is no tributary with a retrograde flow lasting longer than 0.5 s (as would happen with a pelvic reflux, see Sects. 3.8.5, 3.8.6 and 3.8.7). With kind permission from [16]

become refluxive and varicose. An important point defining shunt type 1 is that the drainage from the saphenous vein occurs irrespective of additional tributary drainage (see also Sect. 3.8.3). Shunt type 1 with refluxive tributaries is called shunt type 1 + 2. A pure shunt type 1 with no refluxive tributaries is rare.

The most important criterion for the shunt type 1 is that blood is transported directly from the dilated saphenous vein by a dilated **perforating vein** back into the deep system: Deep vein (N1) – Junction/perforator to saphenous vein (N2) – Perforating vein to deep veins (N1).

In Summary Shunt Type 1

(1) Reflux source from the deep veins directly into the saphenous vein. (2) Reflux down the saphenous vein. (3) Re-entry through a perforating vein directly from the saphenous vein.

3.8.2 Shunt Type 2

The deep veins are not involved in the classical closed shunt type 2 (see Fig. 3.19a). The recirculation occurs only in the superficial veins. Consequently, a smaller volume of blood is involved in the recirculation. The general clinical appearance is of mildly dilated tributaries which are only cosmetically undesirable. The reflux source is from a N2 saphenous vein with normal antegrade flow. This fills an N3 tributary which then drains back into the saphenous vein (Fig. 3.19a). This closed type of shunt 2 is not often found. Mostly an open deviated shunt is found with drainage of the reflux into a perforating vein (Fig. 3.19b) or the other saphenous vein. This situation is termed as **open deviating shunt** because there is no recirculation. The blood does not flow back to its source (see Sect. 3.7.2).

In type 2 open shunts, the system is **not overloaded by volume** because of the absence of a recirculation circuit. However, the tributary may also be cosmetically bothering. This is because it

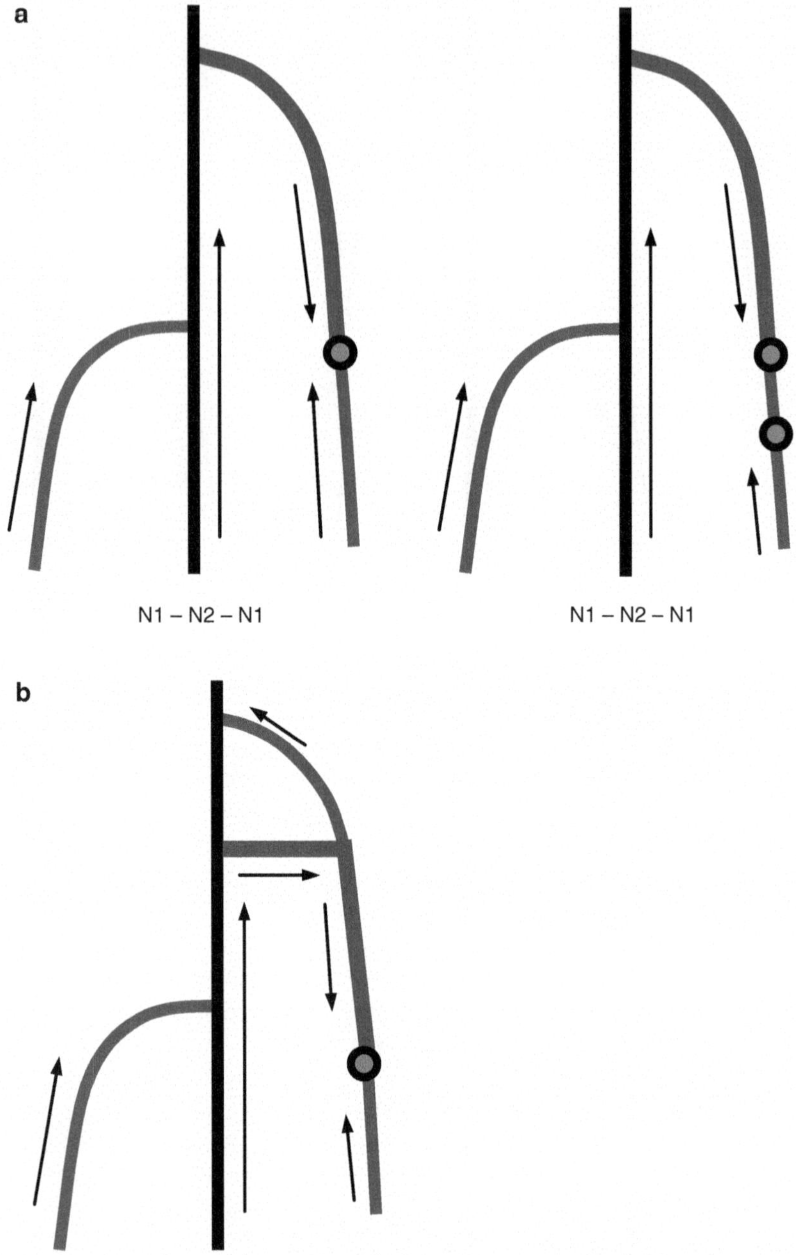

Fig. 3.22 Shunt type 1. (**a**) Refluxing great saphenous vein, escape point; sapheno-femoral junction, re-entry; direct perforator connecting the saphenous vein with the deep vein N1 → N2–N1 on the left; on the right we find two direct perforators. No refluxive tributaries are found. (**b**) Competent sapheno-femoral junction with reflux originating from the perforating vein in the adductor canal, re-entry like in (**a**). With kind permission from [16]

dilates to accommodate the blood from the relatively larger diameter saphenous vein.

Regardless of whether there is an open or closed type 2 shunt, a **reversal of saphenous flow** may occur above the outflow point of the incompetent tributary. This can be detected with duplex ultrasound as a weak signal over a variable distance upwards. The source of this reflux is not easily identified. It is not from a proximal reflux source arising from a junction with the deep veins. Instead, the blood leaking into the saphenous vein is from healthy tributaries further up (see also shunt type 0, Sect. 3.7.4). The flow direction in the saphenous vein between the healthy tributaries and the refluxive tributary is retrograde for a segment until it flows out into the refluxive tributary. One or two incompetent valves in the saphenous vein facilitate this process (see also Fig. 3.22). To identify these conditions, the shunt type 2 has been further subdivided into three groups [26]:

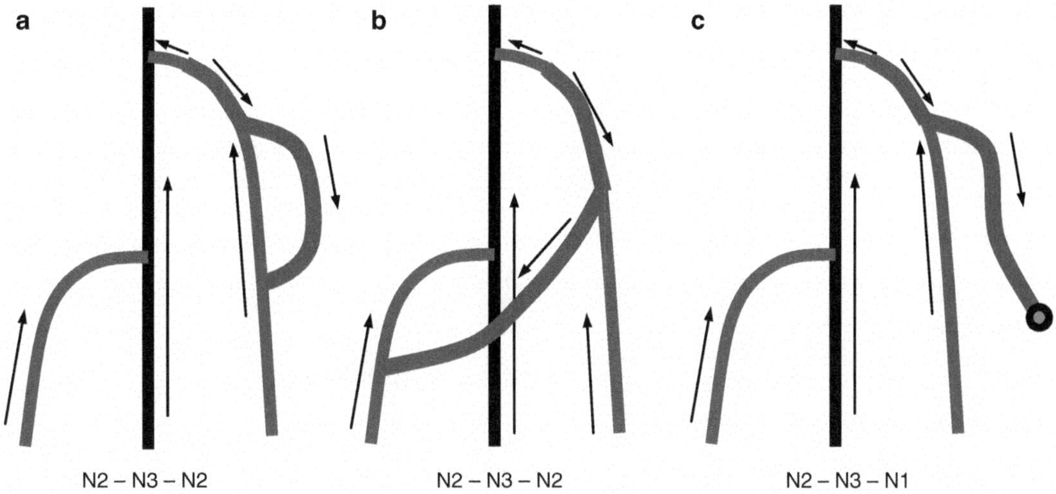

Fig. 3.23 Shunt type 2B. Reflux in the great saphenous vein without escape point, filling a refluxing tributary. This one drains: (**a**) Into the saphenous vein (closed shunt), (**b**) Into the other saphenous vein (open deviated shunt), (**c**) Into a perforating vein (open deviated shunt). With kind permission from [16]

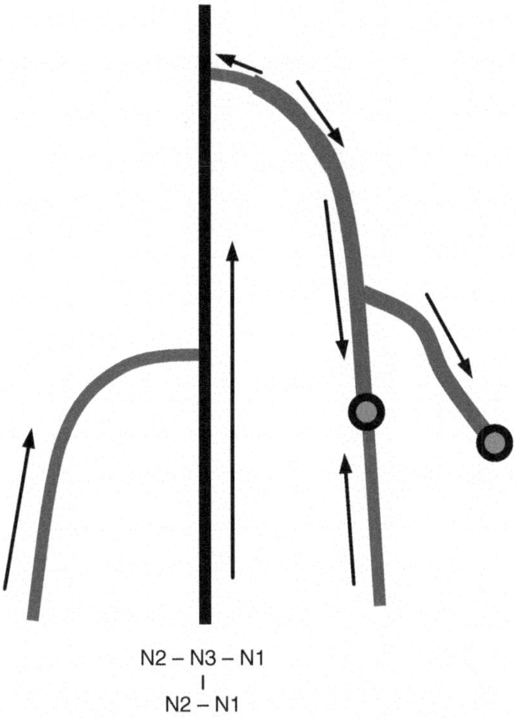

Fig. 3.24 Shunt type 2C. Reflux in the great saphenous vein without escape point, draining into a perforating vein on the saphenous vein itself and through a tributary, which also drains into a perforating vein (open deviated shunt). With kind permission from [16]

- A In case no reflux is found in the saphenous vein above the refluxive tributary (see Fig. 3.19).
- B In case reflux with no escape point is found in the saphenous vein above the refluxive tributary—but no draining perforator can be identified on the saphenous vein (see Fig. 3.23).
- C In case reflux with no escape point is found in the saphenous vein above the refluxive tributary and—in addition to the refluxive tributary—a draining perforator is found on the course of the saphenous vein (see Fig. 3.24).

In type 2A shunt, the escape point is from N2 to N3, without saphenous vein incompetence, so characterizing a mild N3 overload is easy to be treated by the interruption of the N3 flush at the confluence with N2.

In type 2B shunt, the escape point is also from N2 to N3, but the refluxing saphenous vein segment above the escape point is longer and without any focused re-entry point perforator. N3 is overloaded in proportion to this refluxing saphenous vein segment height. Its disconnection leaves behind a no more refluxing GSV segment but a heavy high blood column that could lead to more frequent recurrences.

The type 2C shunt is like 2B except for the presence of one or more re-entry perforators draining the saphenous vein high refluxing segment. These re-entry point could ease the drainage of the N2 remaining column after the N3 disconnection, leaving a shunt type 0 (see Sect. 3.7.4) and reducing the risk of recurrence.

In Summary Shunt Type 2
(1) Reflux source from a saphenous vein into a tributary. (2) Reflux in tributary. (3) Re-entry through the same saphenous vein (closed shunt) or a perforating vein or another saphenous vein (open deviated shunt).

3.8.3 Shunt Type 1 + 2

As described in shunt type 1, the "pure" form—without refluxive tributaries—is seldom. Most of the times, in addition to the recirculation affecting the saphenous vein and draining through a perforator, refluxive tributaries are fed from the recirculating blood. This condition is called shunt type 1 + 2, because both shunts are present see (Fig. 3.25).

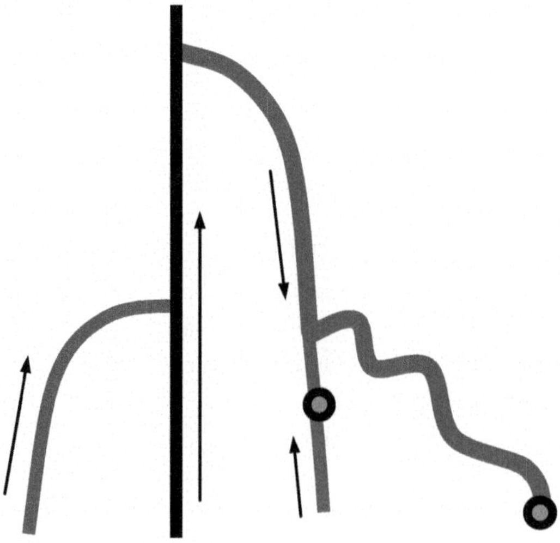

Fig. 3.25 Shunt type 1 + 2. Combination of a shunt 1 (N1 → N2–N1) with an open shunt 2 (N2 → N3–N1). With kind permission from [16]

Independently on the amount of refluxive tributaries present, a recirculation would persist, if all the tributaries would be removed, because it still would be a drainage on the saphenous vein through the re-entry perforator (see also Sect. 3.8.9).

3.8.4 Shunt Type 3

As with shunt type 1, the primary reflux source in shunt type 3 is a connection between the deep veins and the N2 network (N1 → N2). The saphenous vein is filled directly from the deep vein, either through a saphenous junction or a perforating vein. In contrast to shunt type 1, no efficient draining perforator is found in the refluxive segment of the saphenous vein. Even though perforators are present, they are not involved in the drainage of the shunt. Thus, the whole refluxive volume passes to one or more tributaries (N3). It is the N3 tributaries which return the blood to the deep veins. This may occur in different ways, either directly through a perforating vein (Fig. 3.26a) in which case the tributary may split and lead the blood to several perforating veins, alternatively, back into a saphenous vein (Fig. 3.26b and c). The small saphenous vein may also act as a drainage pathway and become incompetent as a result (Fig. 3.26d).

It is important to note that only those perforating veins which are dilated on ultrasound may be considered in shunt classification. A strategy to differentiate between shunt types 1 and 3 is described in Sect. 3.8.9.

In shunt type 3, the reflux begins in the saphenous vein having originated from the deep veins. Thereafter it does not flow from the saphenous vein into the deep system directly but through an intermediate tributary. This varicose tributary is a key player in the recirculation circuit. Without the tributary, there would be no recirculation.

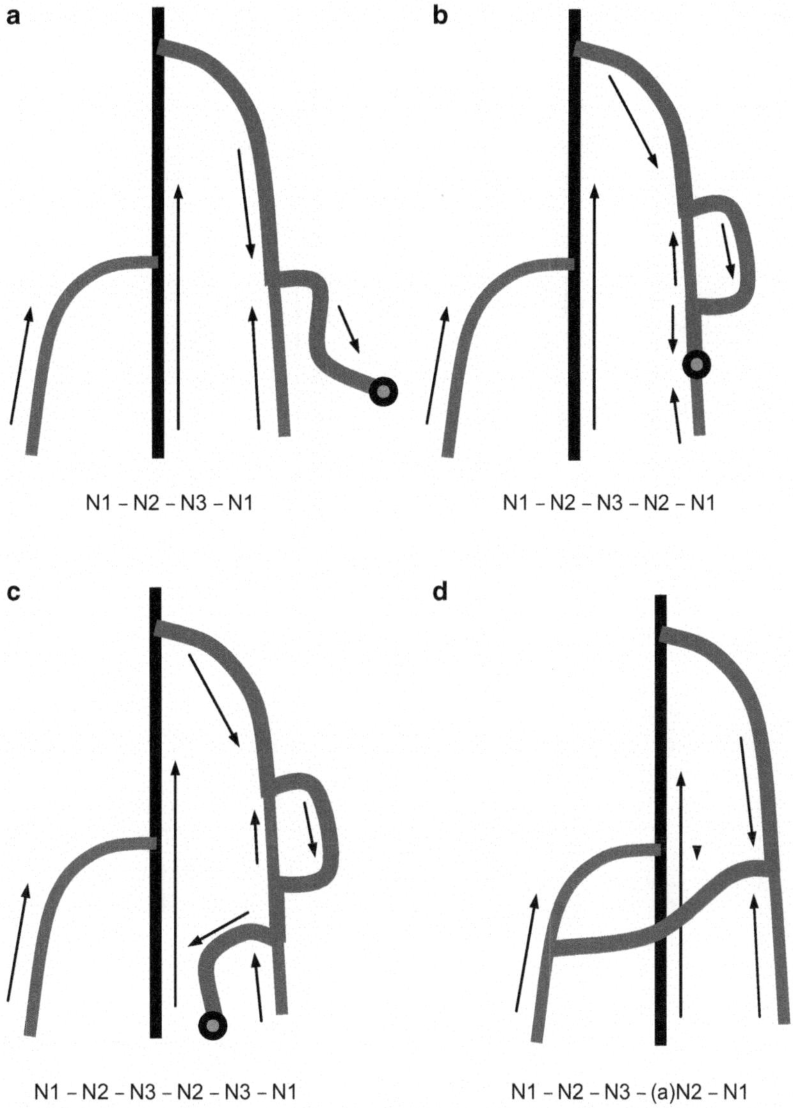

Fig. 3.26 Shunt type 3. Reflux from the deep vein fills the great saphenous vein and drains through a tributary. The segment of the great saphenous vein immediately distal to the offspring of the refluxive tributary is competent. The tributary might drain: (**a**) **Via a perforator** N1 → N2 → N3–N1, (**b**) Via the great saphenous vein and a direct perforator N1 → N2 → N3–N2–N1, (**c**) Via the great saphenous vein and a new tributary draining into a perforator (N1 → N2 → N3 → N3–N3–N1), (**d**) Via the small saphenous vein (N1 → N2 → N3–(another) N2–N1). With kind permission from [16]

> **In Summary Shunt Type 3**
> (1) Reflux source from a deep vein directly into the saphenous vein. (2) Reflux through the saphenous vein and a tributary. (3) Re-entry through a tributary into a perforating vein or saphenous vein.

3.8.5 Shunt Type 4

In shunt type 4, the recirculation involves the saphenous vein. However, the reflux source is not N1–N2. There is no reflux through the junction or a direct perforating vein. Instead the reflux source is from pelvic veins (pelvic shunt type 4, the commonest, Fig. 3.27a) or from a perforating vein, which fills the saphenous vein through a tributary (perforating shunt type 4, less common Fig. 3.27b). The re-entry point of the recirculation is through a perforating vein, directly from the saphenous vein, irrespective of whether there are further re-entry points from a distal varicose tributary. The shunt type 4 re-entry corresponds to the re-entry in shunt type 1.

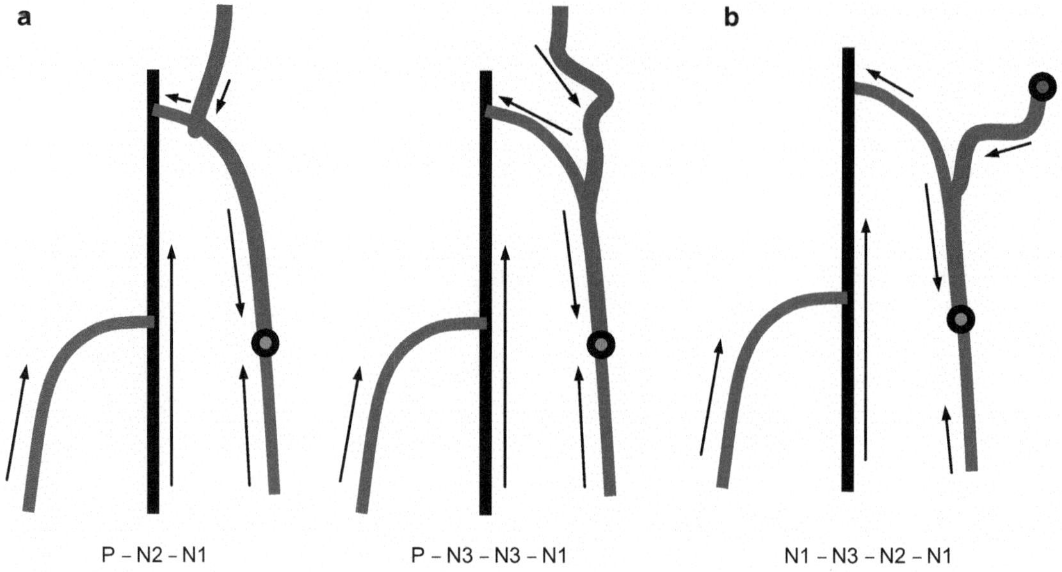

Fig. 3.27 Shunt type 4. (**a**) Pelvic type feeding the saphenous vein via a groin tributary (left): P → N2–N1 or via a subcutaneous tributary (right): P → N3–N2–N1, (**b**) Perforating type N1 → N3–N2–N1. With kind permission from [16]

In Summary Shunt Type 4

(1) Reflux source from a pelvic or perforating vein into the saphenous vein. (2) Reflux down the saphenous vein. (3) Re-entry through a perforating vein directly from the saphenous vein.

3.8.6 Shunt Type 4 + 2

The same as in the case of shunt type 1, most often we find in addition to the drainage through the perforator connected to the saphenous vein one or more refluxive tributaries fed by the refluxing saphenous vein. In analogy, this situation is called shunt type 4 + 2 (see Fig. 3.28).

3.8.7 Shunt Type 5

In the shunt type 5, the reflux source into the saphenous vein is the same as shunt type 4. There is also the pelvic shunt type 5, the commonest (Fig. 3.29a), or a perforating shunt type 5, less common (Fig. 3.29b). The pelvic shunt might feed the saphenous vein directly through a groin tributary or via a tributary, as described for shunt type 4.

However, re-entry is different. The re-entry volume flows into a tributary at the lower end of the refluxive segment of saphenous vein. In contrast to shunt type 4, there are no draining perforating veins on the saphenous vein.

In Summary Shunt Type 5

(1) Reflux source from the pelvic compartment or perforating vein into the saphenous vein. (2) Reflux down the saphenous vein and a tributary. (3) A tributary is interposed between the refluxing saphenous vein and the re-entry perforating vein.

There are many possible **reflux sources** in pelvic shunt types 4 and 5.

– The reflux enters the great saphenous vein through the junction tributaries. The reflux starts just below the sapheno-femoral confluence.

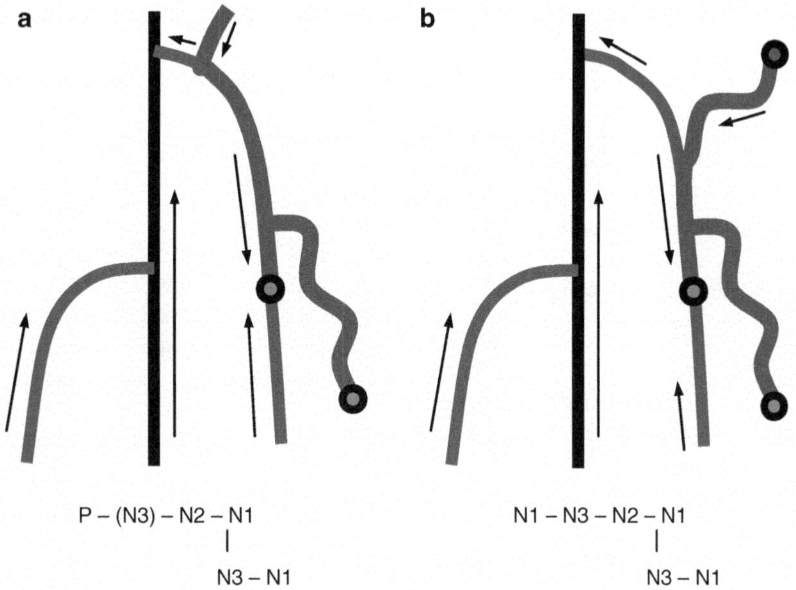

Fig. 3.28 Shunt type 4 + 2 reflux source as in Fig. 3.27, the principal drainage remains directly from the saphenous vein (N2–N1) irrespective of other refluxive tributary drainage points. (**a**) Pelvic type feeding the saphenous vein via a groin tributary P → N2–N1 (the option with an interposed tributary has been left out), (**b**) Perforating type N1 → N3–N2–N1. With kind permission from [16]

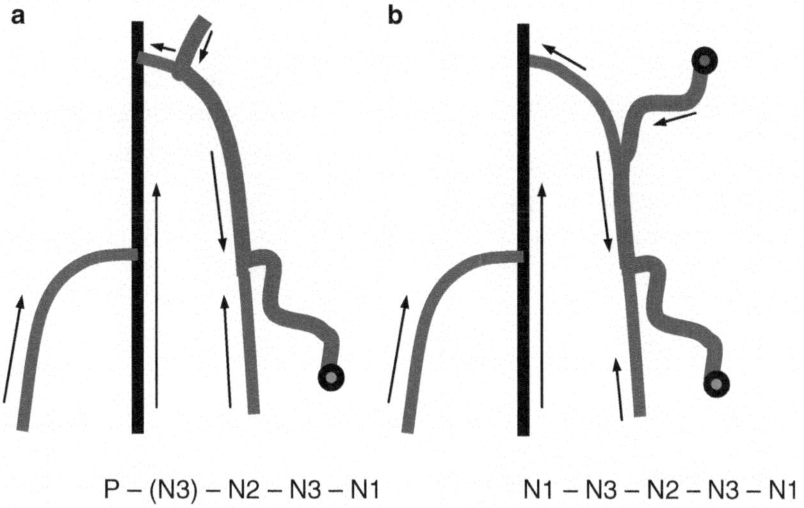

Fig. 3.29 Shunt type 5. (**a**) Pelvic type with reflux from the supra-inguinal networks: P → (N3)–N2 → N3–N1. (**b**) Perforating type N1 → N3–N2 → N3–N1. Note that there is no draining perforator on the saphenous vein. With kind permission from [16]

- Recirculation through the labia into a reticular network in the inner thigh which leads into the posterior accessory saphenous vein and then the great saphenous vein. This may result in a varicose reticular network on the inner and posterior thigh.
- The reflux from a junction tributary fills the anterior or posterior accessory saphenous veins which derive the reflux via a tributary into one of the two saphenous trunks. The great saphenous vein is the commonest trunk involved.

3.8.8 Shunt Type 6

All other possibilities of a recirculation circuit without refluxing pathways through the saphenous veins can be defined as a shunt type 6 (see Fig. 3.30).

In Summary Shunt Type 6
(1) Reflux source from a pelvic or perforating vein. (2) Reflux through tributaries. (3) Re-entry into a perforating vein or healthy saphenous vein.

3.8.9 Differentiation Between Shunt Type 1 and 3 or Type 4 and 5

Differentiating between the two commonest shunt types (1 and 3) and the less common shunt types 4 and 5 has clear therapeutic implications. This is because of the importance of the tributary (shunt types 3 and 5) as a re-entry point. For the design of the strategy, the differentiation between a refluxive saphenous vein drained by a perforator and drained by a tributary is of high importance (see Sect. 6.4.1). The differentiation is performed using duplex ultrasound. The test is called the reflux elimination test = RET (Fig. 3.31) [11, 16, 39].

3.9 Combination of Shunts

3.9.1 Combination of Open deviated and Closed Shunts

Most of the time, two different shunt types coexist in the different anatomical compartments.

A closed shunt with an escape point from N1 to N2 and a re-entry point from N2 to N1 can be overlapped to an open deviating shunt with an escape point from N2 to N3 and a re-entry point from N3 to N1 (see Shunt Type 1 + 2, Sect. 3.8.3, Fig. 3.25).

Suppressing one single pressure gradient from N1 to N2 or from N2 to N3 would maintain the driving force feeding the reflux, so leading to a strategy failure. Thus, both shunts must be identified and interrupted, at the N2–N1 and N3–N2 junctions.

3.9.2 Combined Deep and Superficial Venous Incompetence

The "competitive reflux"

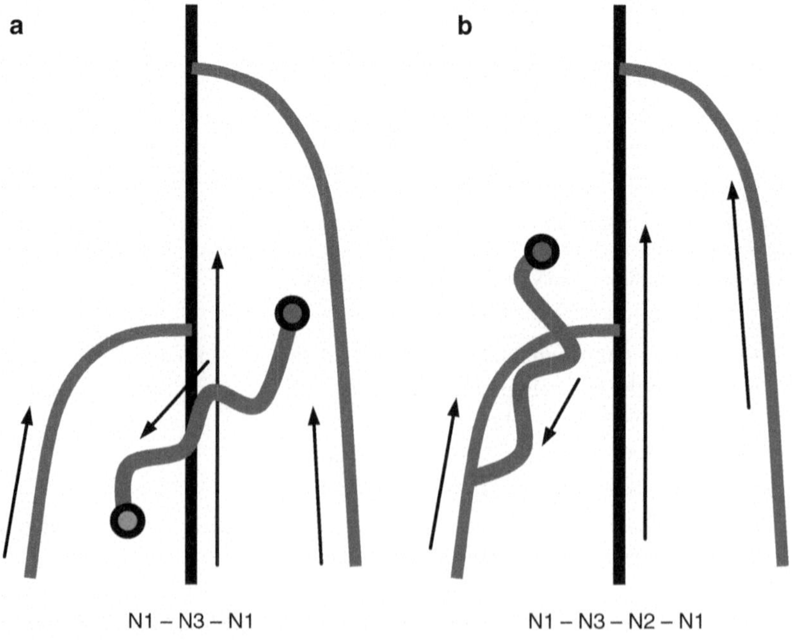

Fig. 3.30 Shunt type 6. Reflux from the deep vein via a perforator into a tributary. The draining pathway can be via another perforator (**a**) *or via a competent saphenous vein* (**b**). With kind permission from [16]

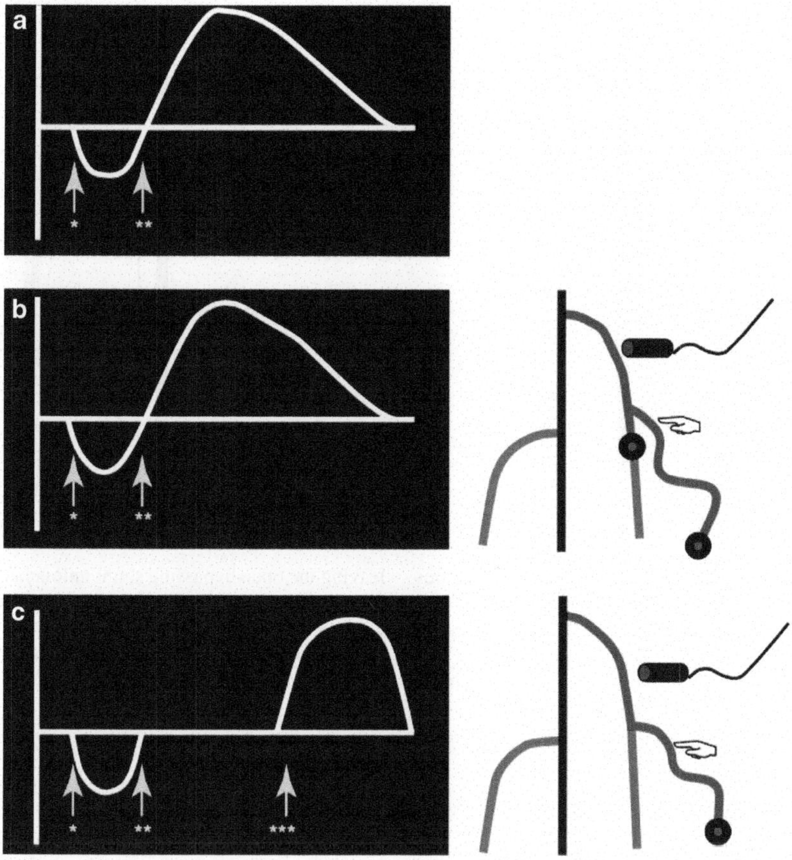

Fig. 3.31 Reflux elimination test, differentiating between shunt types with and without drainage via a direct perforator (1 and 3, as well as 4 and 5) using duplex ultrasound. (**a**) Flow profile in the proximal refluxive segment of the saphenous vein in both shunt types demonstrating antegrade flow (under the line) and reflux (above the line). * Manual compression of the calf, or toe elevation manoeuvre; ** decompression of the calf, or relaxing the toes. (**b**) Flow profile at the same point as in (**a**) with digital compression of the tributary in shunt type 1. The reflux profile remains unchanged starting at the beginning of muscular diastole. (**c**) Flow profile at the same point as in (**a**) with digital compression of the tributary in shunt type 3. Reflux is eliminated by digital compression until *** the moment of digital release. With kind permission from [16]

Deep venous obstruction can lead to open bypassing shunts (see Fig. 3.20). After some time, the superficial vein gets dilated and, in case of a tributary, also varicose. Another scenario could be when a patient with an existing closed shunt in the saphenous vein suffers a deep vein thrombosis. The untreated superficial incompetence will take over as the draining path for the deep insufficiency.

Whenever deep venous insufficiency coexists with a large but in diastole non-refluxing superficial varicose vein, the re-entry point diastolic aspiration into the deeper compartment is hampered. The venous muscle pump fails in creating the pressure gradient forcing the shunted blood to come back into the deep system. The superficial reflux decreases proportionally to the increase of the deep incompetence. It can be tested also by a simple Perthes manoeuvre: placing a tourniquet at the varicose vein root won't make it collapse at the muscle pump activation, because of the high-pressure values affecting the same deep system.

In this scenario CHIVA strategy doesn't give indication to open deviating shunt and closed shunt disconnection when no reflux is evoked in the superficial varicose veins by the dynamic manoeuvres and Perthes test doesn't collapse them.

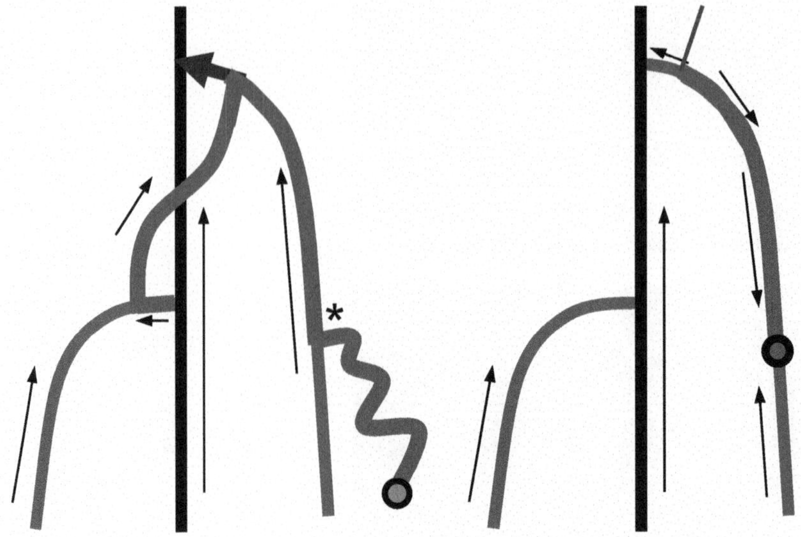

Fig. 3.32 Mixed shunt, open bypassing or vicarious shunt, N1 → N2 (SSV) → N2 (Giacomini) → N2 (GSV)–N1 combined with a closed shunt type 3: N1 → N2 (SSV-Giacomini-GSV) → N3–N1. The disconnection of the tributary at the level of the * would treat the closed shunt leaving the open bypassing shunt untouched. The draining part of the open bypassing shunt is shown with a dark red arrow to differentiate it from the refluxive distal great saphenous vein (GSV). With kind permission from [16]

3.9.3 Mixed Systolic and Diastolic Shunts

Mixed Shunts are constituted by one or more consecutive veins, competent or not, that play the role of open bypassing shunt during the muscular systole and the role of a closed shunt during the diastole. They are possible in all the networks, assuming that they share the escape point, but the re-entry points are different one from the other.

In a mixed shunt, the escape point and the initial part of the venous path are common to both, the open bypassing shunt and the closed shunt, while the terminal paths and re-entry point are different and divergent.

Anatomic example: Taking into consideration the previously described Giacomini vein involvement in an open bypassing shunt from a femoral obstruction (see Sect. 3.7.3), a great saphenous vein incompetence can coexist. The distal great saphenous vein is fed during diastole by the reflux coming from the small saphenous vein junction, via the Giacomini vein, and draining at the calf—at a point below the knee to close the shunt and following the pressure gradients (see Fig. 3.31).

Similarly, considering the previously described spontaneous Palma open bypassing or vicarious shunt, in case of a homo- and/or contralateral great saphenous vein incompetence, a closed shunt will be overlapped to the open bypassing shunt.

In both examples, the open bypassing shunt will be active during muscular systole, while closed shunt during the diastole.

When planning the treatment strategy, the open bypassing shunt has to be preserved, so the common escape point and the common initial path as well as open bypassing shunt terminal path have to be kept untouched. Conversely, the path corresponding isolately to the closed shunt is treated according to the CHIVA strategy; in the case of Fig. 3.31, a flush ligation and disconnection of the tributary at the distal great saphenous vein would interrupt the closed shunt (Fig. 3.32).

Literature

1. Dodd H, Cockett FB. The pathology and surgery of the veins of the lower limb. Edinburgh: Churchill Livingstone; 1976.
2. Lattimer CR, et al. Saphenous pulsation on duplex may be a marker of severe chronic superficial venous insufficiency. J Vasc Surg. 2012;56(5):1338–43.
3. Katz A. Flow through a collapsible tube. Biophys J. 1969;9(10):1261–79.
4. Baird RN, Abbott WM. Elasticity and compliance of canine femoral and jugular vein segments. Am J Physiol. 1977;233(1):H15–21.
5. Norgren L, Thulesius O. Pressure-volume characteristics of foot veins in normal cases and patients with venous insufficiency. Blood Vessels. 1975;12(1):1–12.
6. Davies AH, Magee TR, Baird RN, Sheffield E, Horrocks M. Vein compliance: a preoperative indicator of vein morphology and of veins at risk of vascular graft stenosis. Br J Surg. 1992;79(10):1019–21.
7. Davies AH. Vein factors that affect the outcome of femorodistal bypass. Ann R Coll Surg Engl. 1995;77(1):63–6.
8. Zamboni P, Marcellino MG, Cappelli M, Feo CV, Bresadola V, Vasquez G, Liboni A. Saphenous vein sparing surgery: principles, techniques and results. J Cardiovasc Surg (Torino). 1998;1998(39):151–62.
9. Zamboni P, Marcellino MG, Portaluppi F, Manfredini R, Feo CV, Quaglio D, Liboni A. The relationship between in vitro and in vivo venous compliance measurement. Int Angiol. 1996;15(2):149–52.
10. Zamboni P, Portaluppi F, Marcellino MG, Quaglio D, Manfredini R, Feo CV, Stoney RJ. In vitro versus in vivo assessment of vein wall properties. Ann Vasc Surg. 1998;12(4):324–9. PubMed PMID: 9676928.
11. Zamboni P. Physical principles of venous haemodynamics. In: Franceschi C, Zamboni P, editors. Principles of venous haemodynamics. New York: Nova Science; 2010. p. 13–21.
12. Kamm RD, Pedley TJ. Flow in collapsible tubes: a brief review. J Biomech Eng. 1989;111(3):177–9.
13. Mendoza E, Lattimer CR, Morrison N. Duplexultrasound of superficial leg veins. New York: Springer; 2014.
14. Labropoulos N, Tiongson J, Pryor L, Tassiopoulos AK, Kang SS, Mansour A, Baker WH. Definition of venous reflux in lower-extremity veins. J Vasc Surg. 2003;38:793–8.
15. Habenicht M, Rabe E, Amsler F, Mendoza E. Toe elevation manoeuvre to assess venous rflux in comparison to manual calf compression and release. Vasa. 2016;45(4):299–304.
16. Mendoza E. Handbuch CHIVA, Arrien GmbH; 2002.
17. Chiu JJ, Chien S. Effects of disturbed flow on vascular endothelium: pathophysiological basis and clinical perspectives. Physiol Rev. 2011;91(1):327–87. https://doi.org/10.1152/physrev.00047.2009.
18. Tisato V, Zamboni P, Menegatti E, et al. Endothelial PDGF-BB produced ex vivo correlates with relevant hemodynamic parameters in patients affected by chronic venous disease. Cytokine. 2013;63(2):92–6.
19. Tisato V, Zauli G, Voltan R, et al. Endothelial cells obtained from patients affected by chronic venous disease exhibit a pro-inflammatory phenotype. PLoS ONE. 2012;7(6):e39543.
20. Tisato V, Zauli G, Gianesini S, Menegatti E, Brunelli L, Manfredini R, Zamboni P, Secchiero P. Modulation of circulating cytokine-chemokine profile in patients affected by chronic venous insufficiency undergoing surgical hemodynamic correction. J Immunol Res. 2014;2014:473765.
21. Zamboni P, Spath P, Tisato V, Tessari M, Dalla Caneva P, Menegatti E, Occhionorelli S, Gianesini S, Secchiero P. Oscillatory flow suppression improves inflammation in chronic venous disease. J Surg Res. 2016;205(1):238–45.
22. Franceschi C, Cappelli M, Ermini S, Gianesini S, Mendoza E, Passariello F, Zamboni P. CHIVA hemodynamic concept, strategy and results. Int Angiol. 2016;35(1):8–30. Epub 2015 Jun 5.
23. Gianesini S, Occhionorelli S, Menegatti E, Zuolo M, Tessari M, Spath P, Ascanelli S, Zamboni P. CHIVA strategy in chronic venous disease treatment: instructions for users. Phlebology. 2015;30:157–71.
24. Trendelenburg F. Ueber die Unterbindung der Vena saphena magna bei Unterschenkelvaricen. Beiträge zur Klinischen Chirurgie (Tübingen) 1891;7:195–210. Translation to English to be found on www.chiva.info/Informationen für ärzte.
25. Hach W, Girth E, Lechner W. Classification of saphenous vein reflux in 4 grades (German: Einteilung der Stammvarikose in 4 Stadien). Phlebol Proktol. 1977;6:116–23.
26. Franceschi C, Zamboni P. Principles of venous haemodynamics. New York: Nova Science; 2010.
27. Franceschi C. Théorie et pratique de la cure Conservatrice et Hémodynamique de l'Insuffisance Veineuse en Ambulatoire. Precy-sous-Thil: Editions de l'Armançon; 1988.
28. Franceschi C. Theory and practice of the conservative haemodynamic cure of incompetent and varicose veins in ambulatory patients. Translated by Evans J. Precy-sous-Thil: Editions de l'Armançon; 1988.
29. Labropoulos N, Giannoukas AD, Delis K, Mansour MA, Kang SS, Nicolaides AN, et al. Where does venous reflux start? J Vasc Surg. 1997;26(5):736–42.
30. Bernardini E, et al. Development of primary superficial venous insufficiency: the ascending theory. Observational and hemodynamic data from a 9 year experience. Ann Vasc Surg. 2002;24:709–20.
31. Pittaluga P, Chastanet S, Locret T, Barbe R. The effect of isolated phlebectomy on reflux and diameter of the great saphenous vein: a prospective study. Eur J Vasc Endovasc Surg. 2010;40(1):122–8.
32. Pittaluga P, Chastanet S. Treatment of varicose veins by ASVAL: results at 10 years. Ann Vasc Surg. 2017;38:e10. https://doi.org/10.1016/j.avsg.2016.07.021; Epub 2016 Oct 11.

33. Ramelet AA, Crebassa V, Carlos D'Alotto C, Buero G, Gillet JL, Grenot-Mercier A, Kuepfer S, Mendoza E, Monsallier JM, Obermayer A, Pacheco K, Pros N, Rastel D, Soulie D. Anomalous intraosseous venous drainage: bone perforators? Phlebology. 2017;32(4):241–8.
34. Mendoza E. Duplex ultrasound investigation of perforating veins. Phlebologie. 2014;43:206–9.
35. Mendoza E. Topographical anatomy of the great saphenous vein: duplex-ultrasound study. (German: Zur topographischen Anatomie der Vena saphena magna: Eine duplex-sonographische Studie im Hinblick auf chirurgisch relevante Aspekte). Phlebologie. 2001;30:140–4.
36. Franceschi C. La Cure Hemodynamique de l'Insuffisance Veineuse en Ambulatoire. J Mal Vasc. 1992;22(2):91–5.
37. Hammarsten J, Pedersen P, Cederlund CG, Campanello M. Long saphenous vein saving surgery for varicose veins. A long-term follow-up. Eur J Vasc Surg. 1990;4(4):361–4.
38. Carandina S, Mari C, De Palma M, Marcellino MG, Cisno C, Legnaro A, Liboni A, Zamboni P. Varicose vein stripping vs haemodynamic correction (CHIVA): a long term randomised trial. Eur J Vasc Endovasc Surg. 2008;35(2):230–7.
39. Zamboni P, Cisno C, Marchetti F, Quaglio D, Mazza P, Liboni A. Reflux elimination without any ablation or disconnection of the saphenous vein. A haemodynamic model for venous surgery. Eur J Vasc Endovasc Surg. 2001;21:361–9.

Duplex Ultrasound of Superficial Leg Veins in the Context of Saphenous Vein Sparing Surgery

4

Erika Mendoza and Erica Menegatti

4.1 General Information on Duplex Ultrasound

The advent of duplex ultrasound revolutionised the treatment of superficial leg veins. Previous methods to investigate veins like phlebography and continuous wave Doppler (CW Doppler) have become almost obsolete. The various duplex modes have allowed a deeper comprehension of the physiology of the venous system—this has led to new techniques in the ablation strategy and completely new approaches in the treatment of varicose veins. Saphenous vein sparing surgery would not have been possible without these new insights. If Trendelenburg [1] had the possibility to perform duplex ultrasound prior to his selective interruptions of the varicose recirculation, it could be argued that the current popular methods would never have arisen.

The physics behind the generation of ultrasound, the application possibilities and the technical details of an ultrasound device are explained in many books. Furthermore, the general investigation of superficial leg veins has been extensively published [2–5].

E. Mendoza, M.D., Ph.D. (✉)
Venenpraxis, Wunstorf, Germany
e-mail: erika.mendoza@t-online.de

E. Menegatti, Ph.D.
Vascular Diseases Center, University of Ferrara, Ferrara, Italy
e-mail: mngrce@unife.it

Details like optimising the examination environment, selection and the systematic process of performing the investigation are assumed as known. They have been covered extensively in an earlier book [5]. This chapter gives a comprehensive explanation of the many situations where it is possible to spare the saphenous vein and deliver a minimally invasive treatment to improve leg haemodynamics. It cannot be stressed enough that the knowledge of duplex ultrasound of superficial leg veins is the basis for the comprehension of CHIVA.

To be able to perform a preoperative mapping, the ultrasound machine must be fitted with a probe which detects flow in superficial and deep veins with colour and especially also with PW mode. Usually a linear probe with a frequency of 7–12 MHz is appropriate. In addition, an abdominal probe (curved array, 3–8 MHz) is required for the examination of the supra-inguinal veins and is helpful also in obese patients.

The patient will spend some time standing on an elevated platform. Elevation is important to protect the back of the investigator, as bending down to reach the leg in a person standing on the floor is uncomfortable. An additional display monitor positioned behind the leg of the patient is also helpful as this will limit neck strain. To avoid dizziness, the patient should stand on a large platform (on small areas people tend to feel they are falling). There should be the provision to hold onto a rail, with the examination table behind to give the feeling that they can sit or lie down any time.

P. Zamboni et al. (eds.), *Saphenous Vein-Sparing Strategies in Chronic Venous Disease*,
https://doi.org/10.1007/978-3-319-70638-2_4

Confusion that seems to exist between B-mode and B-flow is common. The differences are explained below:

The plain ultrasound image without any Doppler effects is termed B-mode. It just reflects off the tissue as an image. The newer generation of ultrasound devices can detect erythrocyte aggregates moving through the veins. Slow movement and stationary regions can be seen as slightly different echogenic patterns (see Fig. 3.6). This is termed erythrocyte sludge [6, 7]. After a fast emptying of veins with a calf compression or contraction, the lumen appears black. After a few seconds, the aggregates appear again. Flushing manoeuvres aid in the identification of small veins which would otherwise be obscured by the is-dense surroundings. Colour-coded duplex can be applied to B-mode where flow is seen as red or blue, depending on the direction of flow.

The highly sensitive image of blood flow which applies Doppler and different enhancing techniques is termed B-flow. Only high-end devices are fitted with this option. It does not suffer with blooming which is the overpainting of the vessel edges with colour artefact. Further information can be found in basic ultrasound duplex books [8].

4.2 Flow Patterns in Superficial Leg Veins

The basis to recognise physiologic or pathologic flow in the superficial venous system is the flow curve in PW mode. In the standing position, only a little spontaneous flow is detectable. Different provocation manoeuvres have been described to augment the flow. They will be discussed in Sect. 4.3.

A physiological flow, as described in Chap. 3, is directed from superficial to deep and from the periphery towards to the heart. It is produced mainly by vis-a-tergo forces which include the heart, and this is augmented by muscle contraction of the venous leg pumps. This is called leg muscle pump systole. In standing position, it is often followed by a short flow in the opposite direction due to gravitational forces. This is called muscle pump diastole. Diastolic flow is impeded by valve closure in healthy veins. This is shown in Fig. 4.1 (see also Sect. 2.3.1).

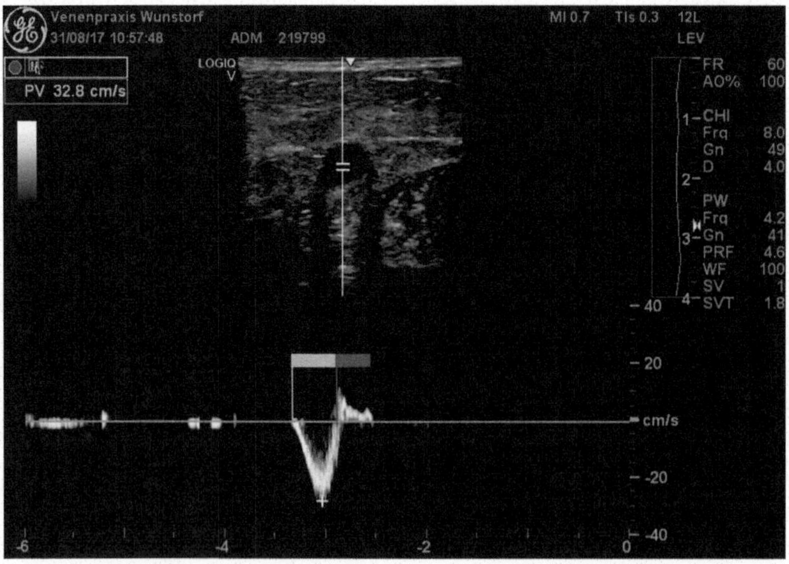

Fig. 4.1 Flow after a provocation manoeuvre in a competent leg vein. The flow in pulsed wave (PW) mode is defined as negative (below the "zero" line) when the flow is away from the probe and as positive when the flow is directed towards the probe. Antegrade physiological flow will be directed towards the heart or from superficial to deep. Here, the PW curve will be "under" zero, as shown in the image; this is the flow during muscular systole (green line), followed by a short flow in the opposite direction during the muscular diastole, caused by gravitational forces. This flow is very short, because closing valves are impeding a further flow in the false direction (red line)

If the valves do not close during diastole, in standing position there will be a retrograde flow (reflux) lasting longer than 0.5 s. Labropoulos studied healthy legs and found out that all veins with competent valves had a retrograde flow below 0.5 s [9]. This was taken as cut-off value between competent and incompetent superficial leg veins. In a recent study, it was shown that patients with reflux have mostly reflux curves lasting longer than 1 s following at least one provocation manoeuvre [10].

The PW Doppler mode measures the **velocities** of the erythrocytes per unit of time within the measurement window set by the investigator. The PW curve records these velocities as white points along the time axis. If the velocities of the individual erythrocytes are similar (laminar flow), a curve will be formed with a white contour and a black space under the curve. If different velocities are recorded (turbulent flow), the space under the curve will be filled in with white points.

Reflux may be assessed by its duration velocity. In veins these are not measured as accurately as in arteries, because of the lack of laminar flow. Besides, the vein runs parallel to the skin. This makes it difficult to achieve an angle of 45°–60° between the vein and the probe to improve the curve quality and the accuracy of the velocity measurement. Nevertheless, the shape of the curve provides useful information about the venous drainage pathways. A large vein, like a dilated saphenous vein, fed by another large vein, like the femoral vein, which then drains back into the deep veins via a large perforating vein, will have a rapid retrograde flow (see Fig. 4.2a). Long-lasting retrograde flow with slow velocity (see Fig. 4.2b) is typical in one of the following cases:

- Small blood reservoir as a source of reflux. For example, reflux from a healthy saphenous vein into a refluxing tributary.
- Small calibre link between a reflux source and refluxing vessel. For example, reflux from the pelvis through the pudendal or epigastric veins.
- Re-entry path into the deep veins that has less diameter than the refluxing segment. In this case, the drainage will be slower and more prolonged.
- Lack of compliance in the refluxing vein so that it cannot receive large blood volumes. This may occur with fibrosis after a thrombosis episode or after radiation.
- Reflux path is partially obstructed, for example, by a superficial vein thrombosis or extraluminal compression of the reflux path.

So, the shape of the reflux curve can already give us an information about some of the physiological aspects playing a role in the reflux

4.3 Provocation Manoeuvres

To examine the recirculation circuits of the superficial venous system, venous flow is an essential requirement. In the standing position, there is little spontaneous flow for assessment. Therefore, in most cases, a provocation manoeuvre is required. Competent superficial veins have little flow and will not respond well to a provocation manoeuvre. However, incompetent superficial veins will answer with a reflux in the standing position in the following situations:

- Under pressure in the abdomen, provoking reflux from above (Valsalva) (see Sect. 4.3.1)
- After having challenged the valves with an antegrade flow from below with manual compression and release of the calf or with dynamic manoeuvres like Paraná or Wunstorf (see Sect. 4.3.2)
- After the venous reservoir have been completely emptied, challenging the valves with gravitational forces like after the orthostatic manoeuvre (see Sect. 4.3.3)

Overviews about provocation manoeuvres can be found at the following links: https://www.youtube.com/watch?v=e76GcnWB7gg (German video with clear demonstration of manoeuvres)

https://phlebo.schattauer.de/inhalt/archiv/issue/1812/issue/special/manuscript/20571/show.html (download of English version)

4.3.1 Manoeuvres Using Pressure

These manoeuvres work by elevating the pressure in the thoraco-abdominal compartment, in order

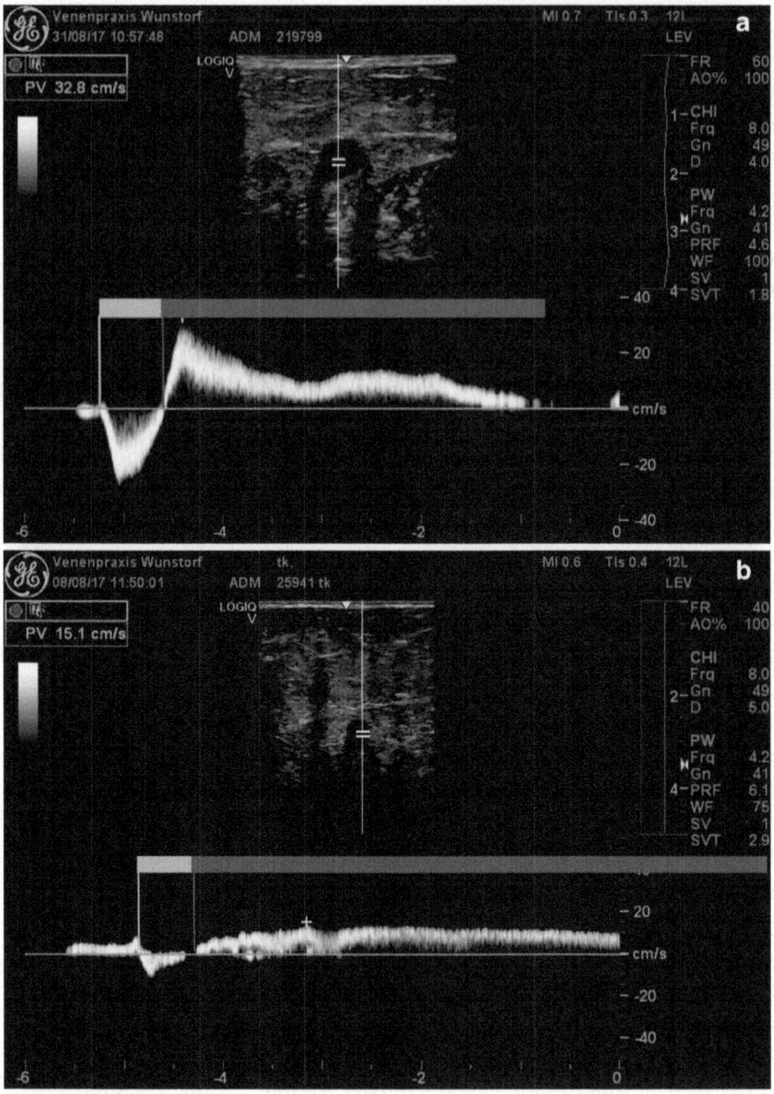

Fig. 4.2 (**a**) Well-drained refluxing vein with a high peak velocity and duration of approximately 3.5 s. Systole (green) followed by reflux (red). This image was found in a shunt type 1 with additional drainage via a tributary. (**b**) Long-lasting reflux, longer than the display of the ultrasound screen (red line). This velocity is slow which is typical for a non-drained system. This reflux was found in a pelvic shunt type 5. Typically, the antegrade flow in systole in these cases is also very slow (green)

to force venous blood back down into the legs. When the valves are competent, the flow will stop and an anterograde flow will reappear after finishing the pressure. When the valves are incompetent, the retrograde flow will be prolonged whilst the pressure is applied. These manoeuvres are independent of gravitational forces and thus can be used lying as well as standing.

These manoeuvres were the first applied in a time, when patients used to be investigated in recumbent position. Today, in standing position, the value of these manoeuvres is less—as the gravitational manoeuvres are optimal in standing position. Nevertheless, the pressure manoeuvres are especially sensitive to demonstrate pelvic reflux and should always play a role when exploring the groin.

4.3.1.1 Standard Valsalva Manoeuvre

The Valsalva manoeuvre is a blocked expiration (closed glottis) similar to defecation, delivery or weight bearing. Valsalva provokes a retrograde flow if valves are incompetent due to the transmission of a hyper-pressure gradient along the wall [11]. The reappearance of the anterograde flow when the manoeuvre stops confirms that it was properly performed. Standardised variations with devices have been developed, most of them too complicated for a daily office situation.

4.3.1.2 Cremona Manoeuvre

The Cremona manoeuvre, developed by Claude Franceschi and Roberto Delfrate, is easier to apply than the standard Valsalva manoeuvre. The patient blows air through a straw when asked. This induces a pressure increase in the thorax and abdomen, thereby forcing the venous blood back into the legs, and allows a dosage of pressure during the exploration.

4.3.2 Manoeuvres Provoking Antegrade Flow

In the standing position and with competent veins, blood flow will be antegrade, with a little backflow until the valves have closed (see Fig. 4.1). To discriminate competent from incompetent vein segments, manoeuvres need to be applied which first expel blood upwards (muscular systole) and then wait for the flow situation on muscle relaxation (muscular diastole) (see Sect. 2.3.1). Compression manoeuvres, with the hand squeezing the calf or external pneumatic cuffs, include the superficial veins and are not physiological. They should be distinguished from the physiological muscle contraction manoeuvres which involve only the venous blood within the pumping chamber [6, 7].

4.3.2.1 Manual Compression and Release of the Calf

The manual calf compression and release manoeuvre is the most common provocation test used in the evaluation of the leg veins. The calf is squeezed with one hand (systole) and then released (diastole). The manoeuvre can also be done by compressing the foot or thigh with the hand. It can be performed with standardised cuffs applying the pressure for study situations. This is not usable in daily clinical setting.

Calf compression causes antegrade flow in the superficial and deep veins. If venous incompetence is present, there will be retrograde flow when the pressure is relaxed. This manoeuvre can be performed any time without the assistance of the patient, and it always causes blood flow in open veins. The response depends on the size, force and speed of the operator's hand. It may cause pain and it provokes not a blood flow to be found in physiological conditions.

4.3.2.2 Automated Compression and Release of the Calf

Pneumatic pumps can be wrapped around the calf which can be inflated to a predetermined pressure and then deflated suddenly to induce reflux. They can be manually operated by a foot pedal leaving the examiners hands-free. Alternatively, an automated pump can be applied delivering a cycle of compression, relaxation and time for refilling to occur before the next compression cycle. The advantage of these methods is that it standardises the compression test and refilling time. Standardisation is a requirement if reflux is being quantified [12].

4.3.2.3 Paraná Manoeuvre

The Paraná manoeuvre is a physiologic manoeuvre and consists of a gentle forward push of the patient's lower back, thus provoking a calf reflex contraction to avoid falling down. This contraction causes an upstream blood flow (systole), followed by a reflux in cases of valvular incompetence [13].

4.3.2.4 Wunstorf or Toe Elevation Manoeuvre

The Wunstorf manoeuvre is a physiologic manoeuvre. It was inspired in the Paraná manoeuvre and proposed as a simple test that is easy to perform and is not demanding for the patient. Furthermore, it does not require the participation of the examiner. A big advantage of this manoeuvre is that the leg itself is not moved whilst remaining a physiological test. It is performed with the patient standing and flexing or extending the forefoot followed by a relaxation. Dorsal flexion involves hyperextension of the toes and raising them off the floor (systole) followed by a relaxation phase (diastole). Plantar flexion involves flexing the toes so that they curl under raising up the metatarsal heads and foot arch (see Fig. 4.3). These forefoot contraction and relaxation manoeuvres activate the foot muscle pump [14, 15].

In almost all patients, hyperextension of the toes causes an antegrade flow impulse,

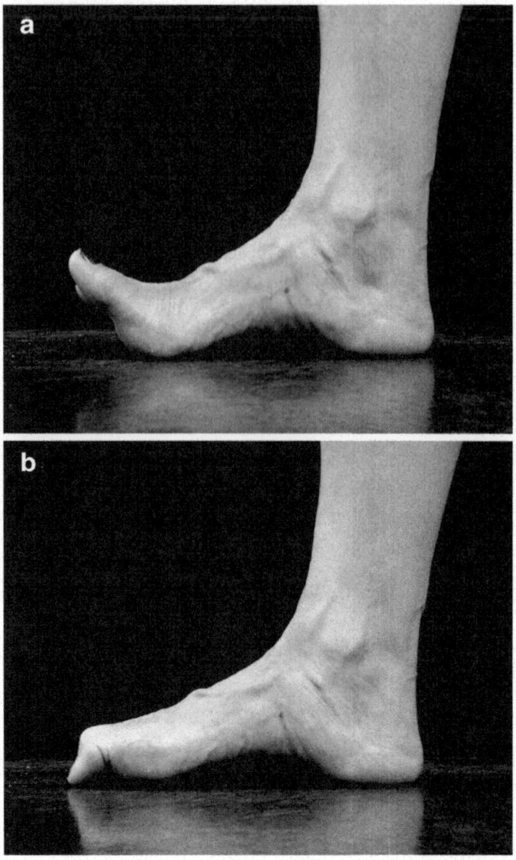

Fig. 4.3 (**a**) Wunstorf or toe elevation manoeuvre. (**b**) Alternatively, the toes can be flexed to provoke a flow in superficial leg veins. With permission by [5]

which can be measured up to the common femoral vein. Antegrade flow is generally also found in the saphenous trunk veins after the Wunstorf manoeuvre. In patients with deep or superficial vein incompetence, retrograde flow (reflux) follows the antegrade flow on relaxation.

In a recent study, these manoeuvres demonstrated to be as efficient as calf compression and release [10].

4.3.3 Manoeuvres Using Gravitation and Gravitational Volume Changes

Most manoeuvres have the inconvenience that their result depends on how the manoeuvre is performed. Inability to breathe as expected in Valsalva, small hands in compression manoeuvres and muscular contraction variations whilst maintaining stability can all influence the results. Thus, all studies which compare manoeuvres lack the security of a standardised provocation test possibly leading to interpretation errors.

4.3.3.1 Elevation-Dependency Manoeuvre

The elevation-dependency manoeuvre may close this gap: Here, the patient lies down on his or her back, with the leg to be investigated elevated straight up for half a minute. Then the patient stands up whilst the duplex ultrasound probe is simultaneously applied over the vein to be assessed. Alternatively, the emptying and filling can be performed on a tilt table.

In case of competent leg veins, no reflux will be found. In case of valve incompetence, a continuous retrograde flow is seen until venous reservoir filling. This retrograde flow will last between 20 s up to minutes, thereby giving the examiner time to look for incompetent veins [16]. The reflux ends only when the venous reservoir is full to capacity and there is no more space to accommodate further reflux [17]. This is independent of the patient or the examination factors, which leads to less bias in the results. In some patients, with visible varicose veins and lack of flow after classical provocation manoeuvres, this manoeuvre will uncover valvular incompetency that would otherwise remain undetected. This is especially true in case of non-drained systems (see Fig. 4.4).

4.4 Sapheno-femoral Junction

4.4.1 Anatomy of the Sapheno-femoral Junction

Under the groin crease, the great saphenous vein (GSV) pierces the fascia (ostium) to drain into the common femoral vein. In its last few centimetres, the GSV has two valves, the terminal valve next to the common femoral vein, at the ostial

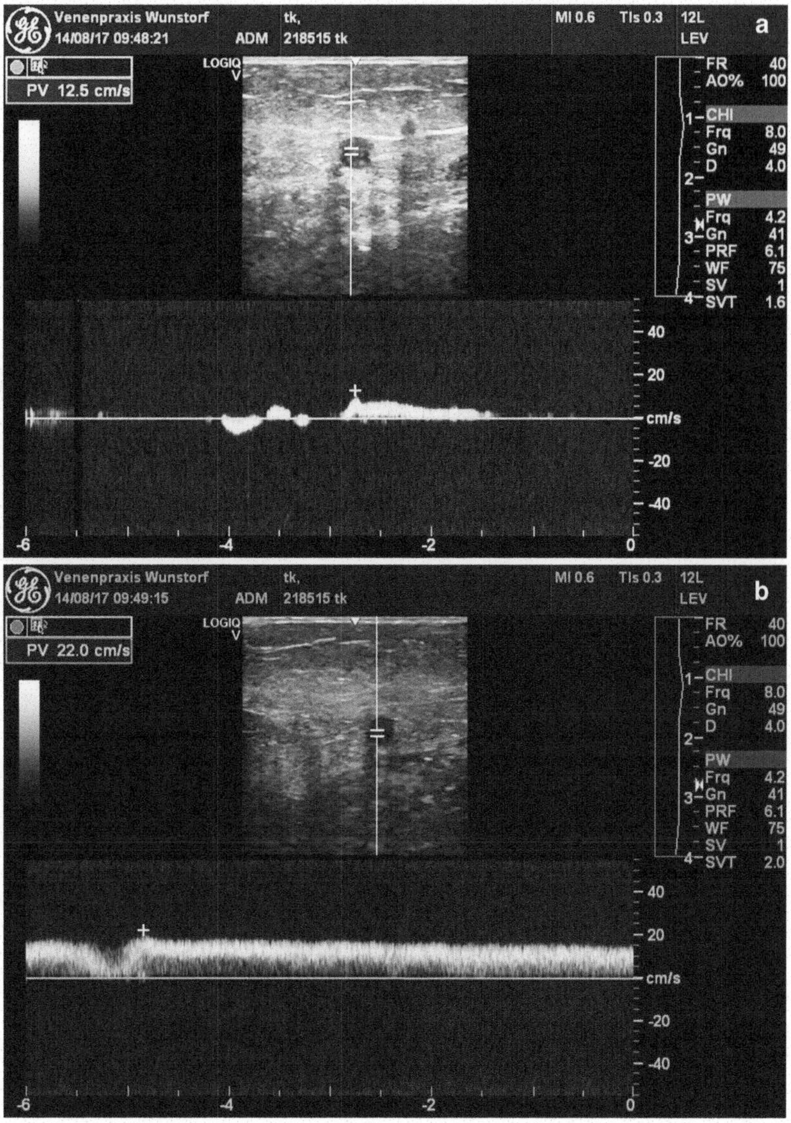

Fig. 4.4 (**a**) Little flow is observed in a patient with obvious varicose tributaries after manual compression of the vein immediately below the measuring point to improve the outcome, after finding nearly no flow with physiologic muscle contraction manoeuvres. (**b**) Flow in the same vein after lying down, lifting the leg for 30 s and then standing up again. The reflux is prolonged and lasts until the venous reservoir is full to capacity

level which is where the GSV pierces the fascia, and the preterminal valve at some centimetres further down and below the confluence of those tributaries which join in at the groin level (see Fig. 4.5).

There are many tributaries joining in the GSV at the SFJ (see Figs. 4.6 and 4.7):

- Pudendal vein from the medial side
- Posterior accessory saphenous vein (PASV), also from medial, but usually some cm further down
- Anterior accessory saphenous vein (AASV) coming from the lateral side after running on the anterior aspect of the thigh
- Epigastric and circumflex veins from lateral and coming down from the abdomen

AASV and epigastric or circumflex veins can join independently (Fig. 4.6f) or alternatively form a common vein that drains at one into the GSV (see Fig. 4.6a, b, e). These mentioned veins may be absent. And the relation between these veins and the valves is highly variable.

4.4.2 Flow in the Sapheno-femoral Junction

The sapheno-femoral junction is involved in the vast majority of patients with varicose veins. Thus, the investigation of this point of the recirculation circle is of highest importance. A recent study investigating the frequency of incidence and distribution of reflux sources in 2019 patients with venous incompetence involving the GSV at the groin is represented in Table 4.1 [19].

Of all legs, 53% had a reflux with an incompetent terminal and preterminal valve, two thirds of all patients had a reflux from the common femoral vein. Exclusive periosteal reflux was identified in 21%, and 8% had reflux from both sources

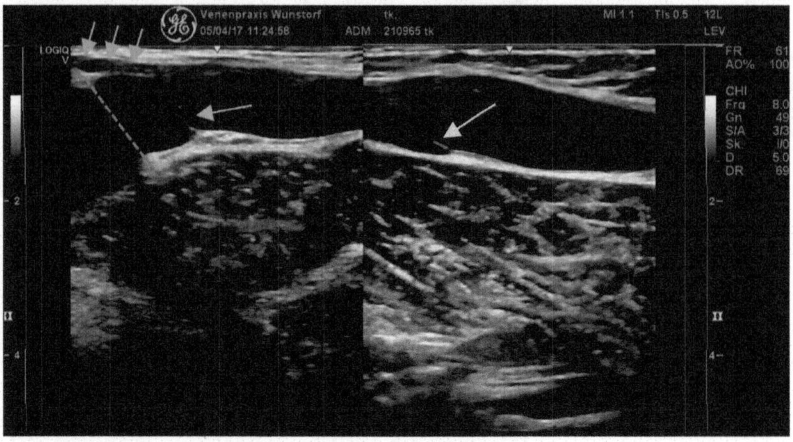

Fig. 4.5 Longitudinal view of the GSV next to the junction (composed image). At the left margin: common femoral vein, the ostium level (dotted line), the terminal valve (blue arrow) and the preterminal valve (yellow arrow) in the GSV. Joining into the GSV, we find the epigastric vein (green arrows)

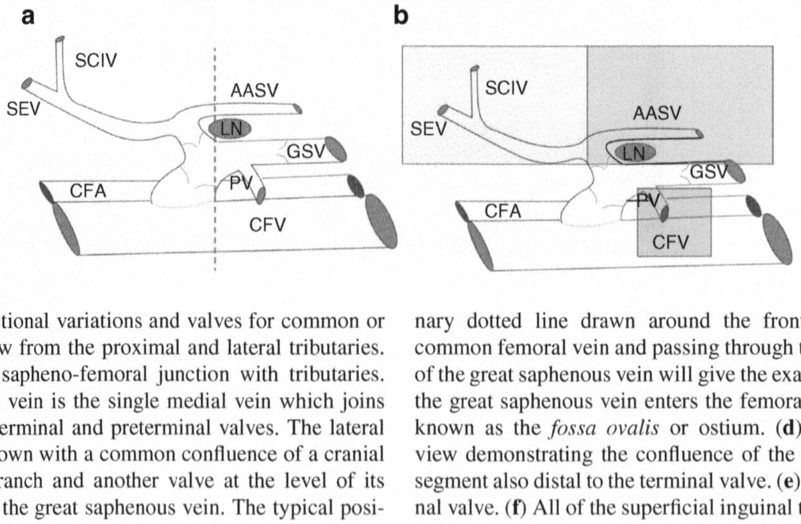

Fig. 4.6 Junctional variations and valves for common or separate inflow from the proximal and lateral tributaries. (**a**) Standard sapheno-femoral junction with tributaries. The pudendal vein is the single medial vein which joins between the terminal and preterminal valves. The lateral segment is shown with a common confluence of a cranial and caudal branch and another valve at the level of its junction with the great saphenous vein. The typical position of a lymph node (LN) lateral to the great saphenous vein is shown. The perpendicular red-dotted line marks the caudal edge of the ostium (dotted line on the CFV). (**b**) Additional information defining the lateral segment (*light green/light purple*) and the medial segment (*light brown*). The lateral segment is divided into cranial (*green*) and caudal (*light purple*) parts. (**c**) Transverse view of the lateral segment distal to the terminal valve (TV). An imaginary dotted line drawn around the front wall of the common femoral vein and passing through the confluence of the great saphenous vein will give the exact point where the great saphenous vein enters the femoral vein. This is known as the *fossa ovalis* or ostium. (**d**) Longitudinal view demonstrating the confluence of the lateral cranial segment also distal to the terminal valve. (**e**) Absent terminal valve. (**f**) All of the superficial inguinal tributaries join independently between the terminal and the preterminal valves (*CFA* common femoral artery, *LN* lymph node, *TV* terminal valve, *CIV* circumflex iliac vein, *SEV* superficial epigastric vein, *PV* pudendal vein, *AASV* anterior accessory saphenous vein, *GSV* great saphenous vein) (Drawings Dr. Andreas Hildebrandt. Berlin; by kind permission. Ultrasound images Erika Mendoza). With permission by [5]

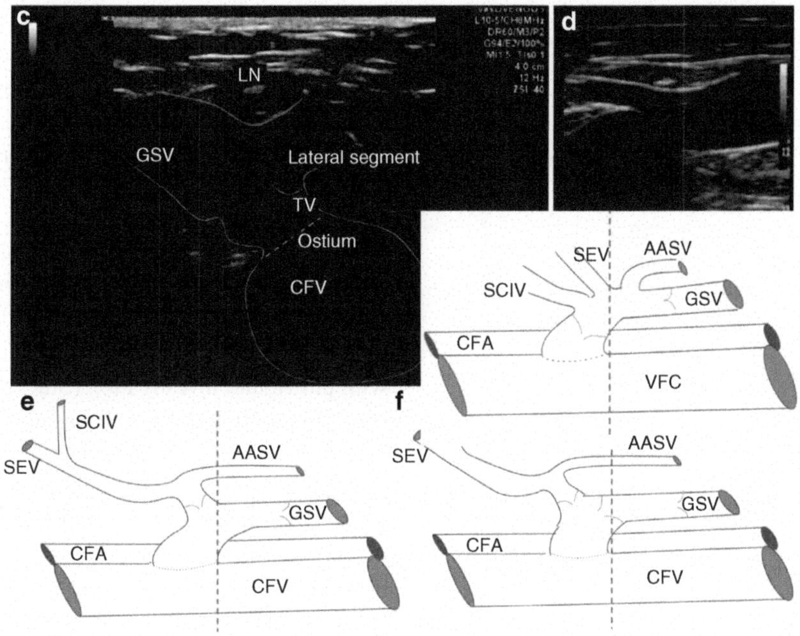

Fig. 4.6 (continued)

(periosteal and ostial). Four percent of the study population had neither a reflux from the common femoral nor the cranial tributaries (shunt type 0; see Sect. 3.7.4).

4.4.2.1 Competent Valves

When the valves are competent, there is no reflux through the valves and no backflow from the deep to the superficial vein at the SFJ. In muscular systole, the PW curve will show an inflexion "downwards" followed by a short retrograde flow (inflexion "upwards") to close the valve (curve; see Fig. 4.1).

The tributaries of the groin behave the same with a short flow towards the SFJ in diastole. Occasionally a pelvic leak point is present draining through the SFJ without provoking a reflux into the GSV. This is identified as a prolonged draining flow through the junction lasting longer than 0.5–1 s, which is fed by a refluxing pudendal, circumflex or epigastric vein. This is seen easily during a Valsalva manoeuvre: the draining flow through the junction fed by the reflux in the groin tributary will last as long as the manoeuvre. This situation is not a pathological condition for the GSV, but a drainage through the SFJ of pathologic reflux from the pelvic network. It could develop to a situation of venous insufficiency of the legs to be re-evaluated at a later stage.

4.4.2.2 Incompetent Terminal Valve and Competent Preterminal Valve

If only the terminal valve is incompetent and the preterminal is not, then there will be a reflux emerging from the deep vein through the SFJ, and it will escape into the anterior accessory saphenous vein (AASV) (see Sect. 6.5.2). This condition has been described by Stücker as Stücker type 1 (see Fig. 4.7) [20].

A schematic representation of this reflux is found in Fig. 4.7. As there is the possibility of connections between the refluxing AASV and the GSV along the leg, it is important to follow the GSV downwards the leg to make sure no calibre changes and further refluxing segments are present.

On ultrasound, the AASV is situated between the skin and the CFV in the groin, called the "alignment sign". The GSV is situated medial to the CFV (see Fig. 4.8). Therefore, a large calibre AASV

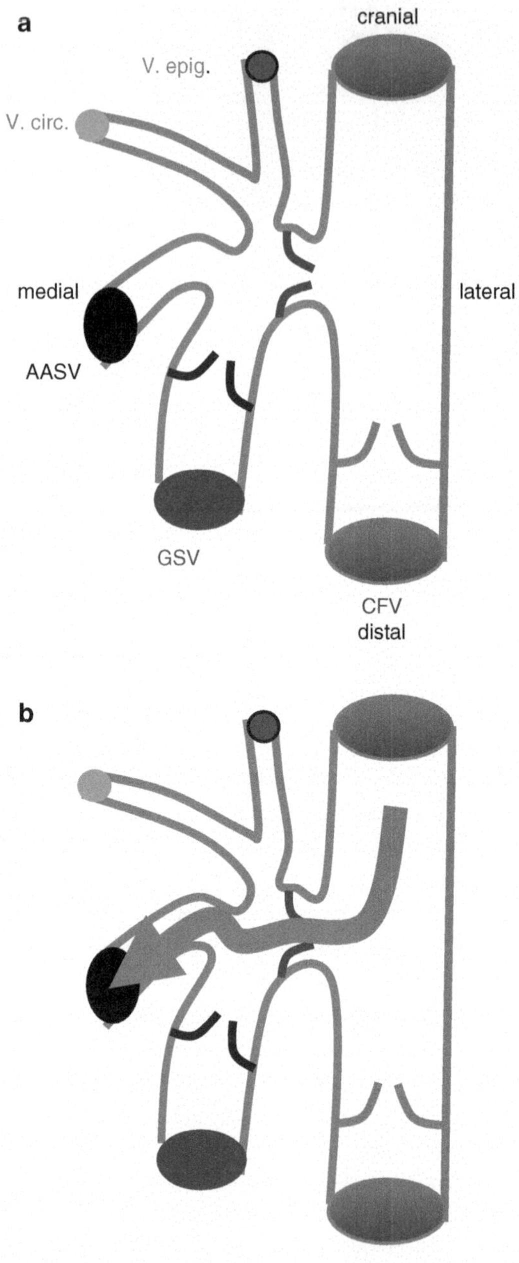

Fig. 4.7 (**a**) Schematic representation of the SFJ with terminal valve (green) and preterminal valve (violet) with legend for (**b**), Figs. 4.9 and 4.13. (**b**) Reflux path in case of incompetent terminal valve and competent preterminal valve (orange arrow) (Stücker type 1). With permission from [18]

directly over the CFV may be confused with an incompetent GSV. During systole in colour-coded duplex ultrasound, both veins are seen with antegrade blue flow (Fig. 4.8a). During diastole, the red colour represents an incompetent terminal valve with reflux escaping into the AASV (Fig. 4.8b).

4.4.2.3 Competent Terminal Valve and Incompetent Preterminal Valve

This condition is one of the most difficult to detect with ultrasound investigation (Stücker type 2, see Figs. 4.9, 4.10 and 4.11). It has also been called "para-ostial reflux", as this reflux does not emerge through the ostium. This configuration needs a confident diagnosis for saphenous sparing techniques. However, with saphenous ablation it makes no difference, whether the reflux in the GSV emerges from the deep vein or from the pelvic network. This is because in any case the reflux path will be destroyed. Recognition that the reflux source may be exclusively from a groin tributary will influence the saphenous sparing tactic and the follow-up.

The reflux might emerge from the pudendal vein (see Fig. 4.10) or the epigastric vein (see Fig. 4.11). It is important to show the competence of the terminal valve with a PW curve at this site (see Fig. 4.12) and a reflux beyond that goes into the GSV at the preterminal valve level. A Valsalva manoeuvre is essential in these cases for confirmation and to exclude a pelvic reflux source. Occasionally concurrent reflux occurs from a tributary vein as well as the junction thereby combining ostial and para-ostial reflux in one situation (see Fig. 4.11).

4.4.2.4 Incompetent Terminal and Preterminal Valve

The most frequent reflux condition in the groin is the incompetence of the terminal and pretermi-

Table 4.1 Possible combinations of reflux sources at the sapheno-femoral junction in 2.019 legs

N (%)	GSV	AASV	PASV	GSV + AASV	GSV + PASV	GSV + AASV + PASV	Sum
Type AFemoral reflux	106752.8%	1226.0%	20.1%	1547.6%	20.1%	1<0.1%	134866.8%
Type B"Both" femoral and cranial reflux	1175.8%	221.1%	0–	311.5%	0–	0–	1708.4%
Type CCranial reflux	31415.6%	743.7%	20.1%	391.9%	1<0.1%	0–	43021.3%
Type 0	633.1%	30.1%	0–	50.2%	0–	0–	713.5%
Sum	156177.3%	22110.9%	40.2%	22911.3%	30.1%	1<0.1%	2019100%

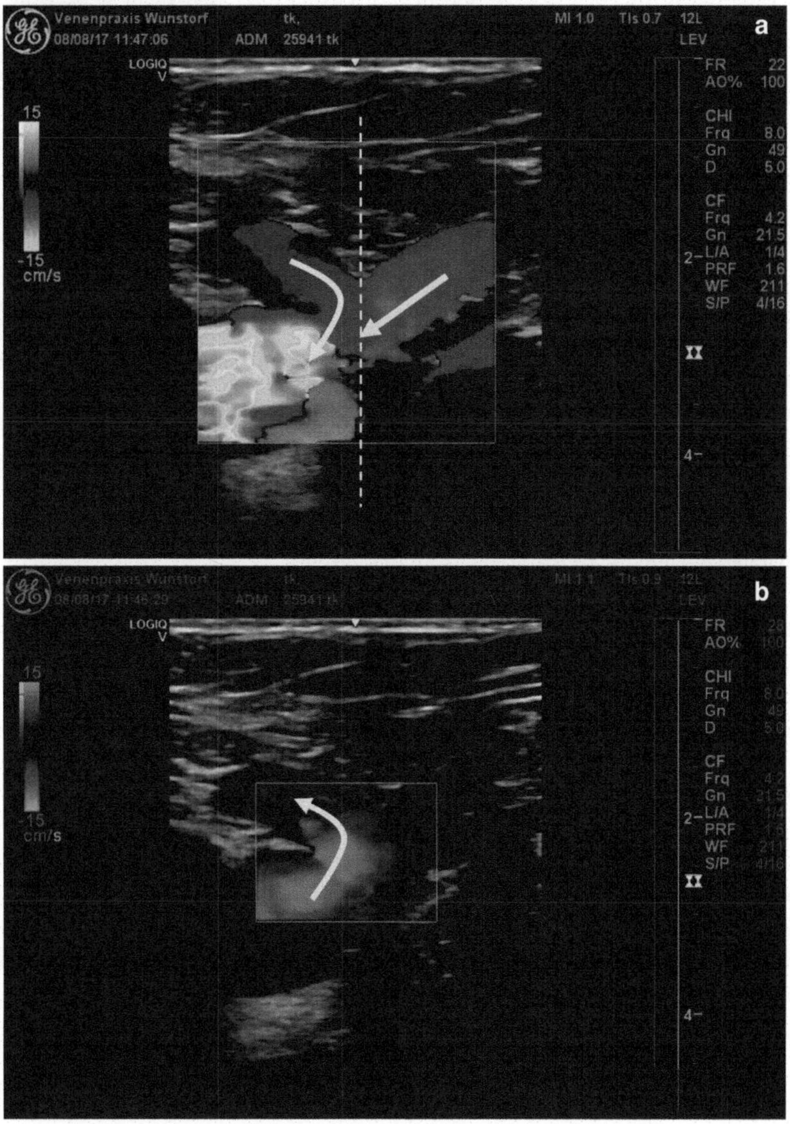

Fig. 4.8 (**a**) Cross-section through the groin during muscular systole. Both the AASV (yellow arrow) and the GSV (blue arrow) represent blue flow in colour-coded duplex ultrasound. This is because the flow is away from the probe and towards the deep vein. In the deep vein the flow has to change direction, provoking turbulences. This is represented with blue, yellow and red flow signals. The dotted line at the medial margin of the CFV explains the "alignment sign": Medial to this line the GSV is found, lateral, between the CFV and the skin, the AASV. (**b**) Muscular diastole with reflux from the CFV through the incompetent terminal valve into the AASV (yellow arrow). The GSV does not receive any reflux

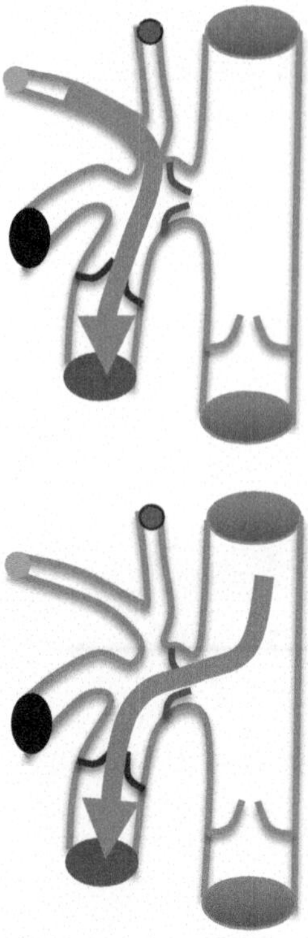

Fig. 4.9 Schematic representation of a para-ostial reflux (Stücker type 2) with an incompetent terminal valve and competent preterminal valve. Reflux into the GSV is via an incompetent circumflex vein. Note that the reflux could also emerge from the epigastric or pudendal vein. With permission from [18]

nal valve. Here the reflux arises from the femoral vein through the junction into the GSV and down the thigh (Stücker type 3; see Fig. 4.13). It is important to demonstrate using ultrasound the origin of the reflux in the femoral vein and passing through the terminal valve (see Fig. 4.14).

4.4.2.5 Summary: Reflux Sources at the Sapheno-femoral Junction

At the sapheno-femoral junction (SFJ), there are many different reflux source possibilities, alone or in combination (see Table 4.2). It is important in the context of saphenous vein sparing surgery to differentiate these diverse reflux situations properly prior to deciding the strategy.

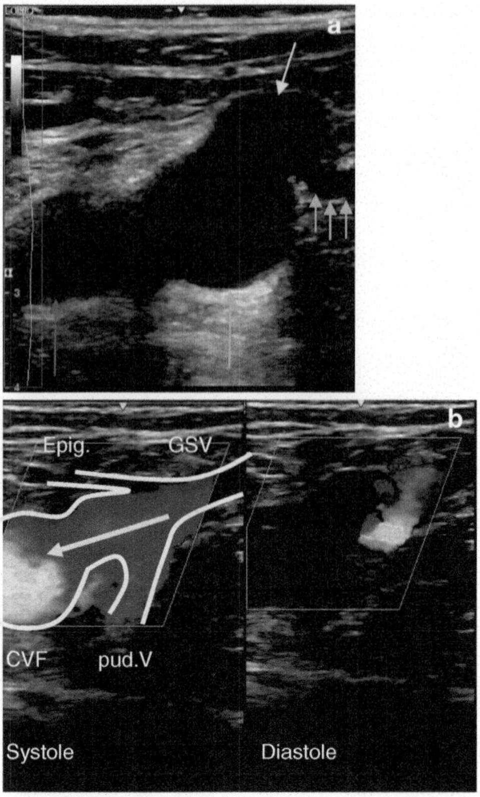

Fig. 4.10 (**a**) Cross-section through the right groin demonstrating the common femoral artery (left, red arrow), the common femoral vein (middle, single blue arrow), the SFJ and the GSV (yellow arrow). The pudendal vein (blue arrows) is shown draining into the GSV. (**b**) Flow in colour-coded duplex ultrasound with a diagonal representation of the SFJ (another patient than **a**). The anatomic structure is painted as "overlay" to the left image. A pudendal and an epigastric vein is present. Left image in systole: antegrade flow draining into the CFV (yellow arrow) and filling the last centimetre of the pudendal vein, which is not the physiologic situation. Right image in diastole: reflux from the pudendal vein into the GSV (pudendal vein with red flow). There is no reflux from the deep vein into the GSV

Summarising the different reflux sources or finding out which of these is the one present in each patient, a flow chart can be applied (see Fig. 4.15) or a table (see Table 4.2).

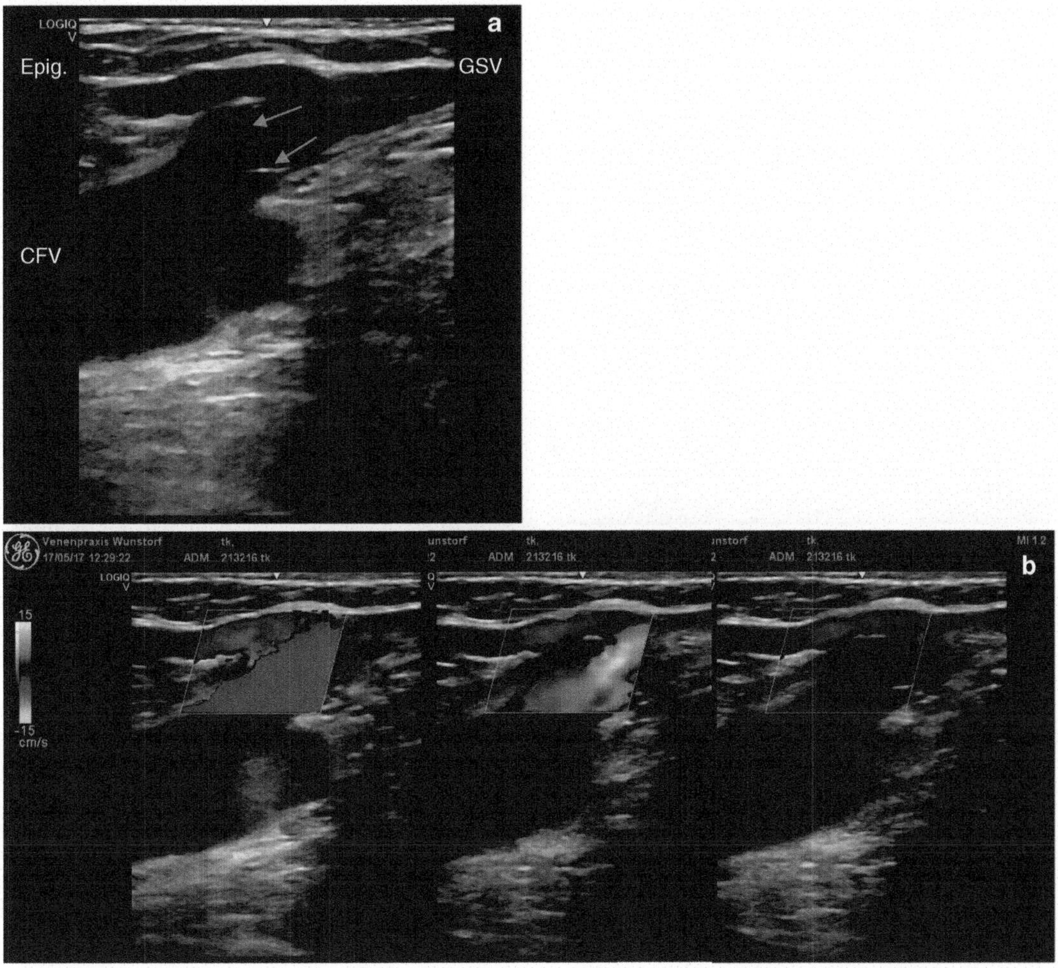

Fig. 4.11 (**a**) Longitudinal section through the common femoral vein (CFV) and the sapheno-femoral junction with visible terminal valves (blue arrows). (**b**) Same patient in colour duplex examination: left, systole with antegrade flow (blue) from the GSV through the SFJ into the CFV. The epigastric vein drains into the GSV (red flow). Middle: early diastole with reflux from the deep vein and the epigastric vein into the GSV. Right: later diastole; the reflux through the terminal valve is finished; only a long-lasting reflux through the epigastric vein feeds the GSV. This is a case of combined Stücker types 2 and 3. If only the reflux situation depicted on the right image was present, it would be an isolated epigastric reflux or para-ostial reflux, Stücker type 2

4.5 Great Saphenous Vein

The vein involved in the majority of situations with superficial vein insufficiency is the great saphenous vein (GSV). It is also the vein mostly taken as a graft for femoral or cardiac bypass interventions.

4.5.1 Anatomy

The GSV runs from the inner part of the foot anteriorly to the medial malleolus up to the groin, as shown in Fig. 4.16. As described in Sect. 2.2.3, it is wrapped between the muscle and the saphe-

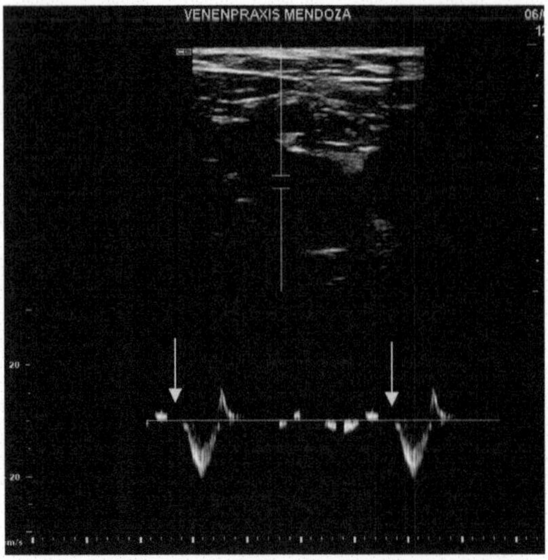

Fig. 4.12 Examination of the competence of the terminal valve using PW: the competence or incompetence of the terminal valve is assessed with PW inside the femoral vein at the ostium level; the competence or incompetence of the terminal valve is identified. This can be performed in cross-section as shown or in longitudinal section (see Fig. 4.14d). Yellow arrows: antegrade flow in systole. Short backflow in diastole until the terminal valve closes. No reflux is present

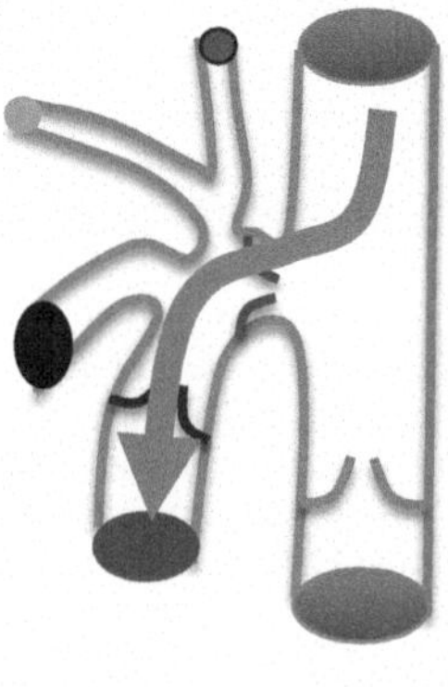

Fig. 4.13 Schematic representation of Stücker type 3: incompetent terminal and preterminal valve. Reflux from the common femoral vein trespasses the incompetent terminal and preterminal valve and fills the GSV. With permission from [18]

nous fasciae. Sometimes its course is aplastic or hypoplastic, with continuing superficial tributaries acting as a bypass for these segments. There are three typical possibilities (depicted in Figs. 4.17, 4.18 and 4.19: type I, Fig. 4.17; type h, Fig. 4.18; type s, Fig. 4.19). Very seldom a double GSV is found in the fascial compartment (1%). The GSV has to be examined in B-mode from the groin to the ankle to see calibre variations, mayor tributaries, perforating veins and aplastic segments. These are all relevant for the treatment plan. Diameters at the junction and 15 cm below should be measured in cross-section, as they will help in decision-making. It is easier to follow the GSV in cross-section, though sometimes a longitudinal scan will show more details. The GSV is easy to find at the mid-thigh by positioning the probe in cross-section. The GSV runs between the fasciae with the typical image of the Egyptian eye (see Fig. 4.17).

4.5.2 Flow and Reflux in the Saphenous Vein and Tributaries

In combination with the B-mode examination, the flow in the examined segments will be measured. Although this is easier to do in colour-coded duplex, the documentation should be performed in PW modus. If these measurements are taken in cross-section, the probe will have to be positioned slightly angulated, allowing an angle between the flow and the probe. In perpendicular position over the skin, no flow may be detected with misleading results. The top of the probe should always be angulated upwards (see Fig. 4.20).

Also in PW mode, possible supplemental reflux sources can be assessed. At the end of the

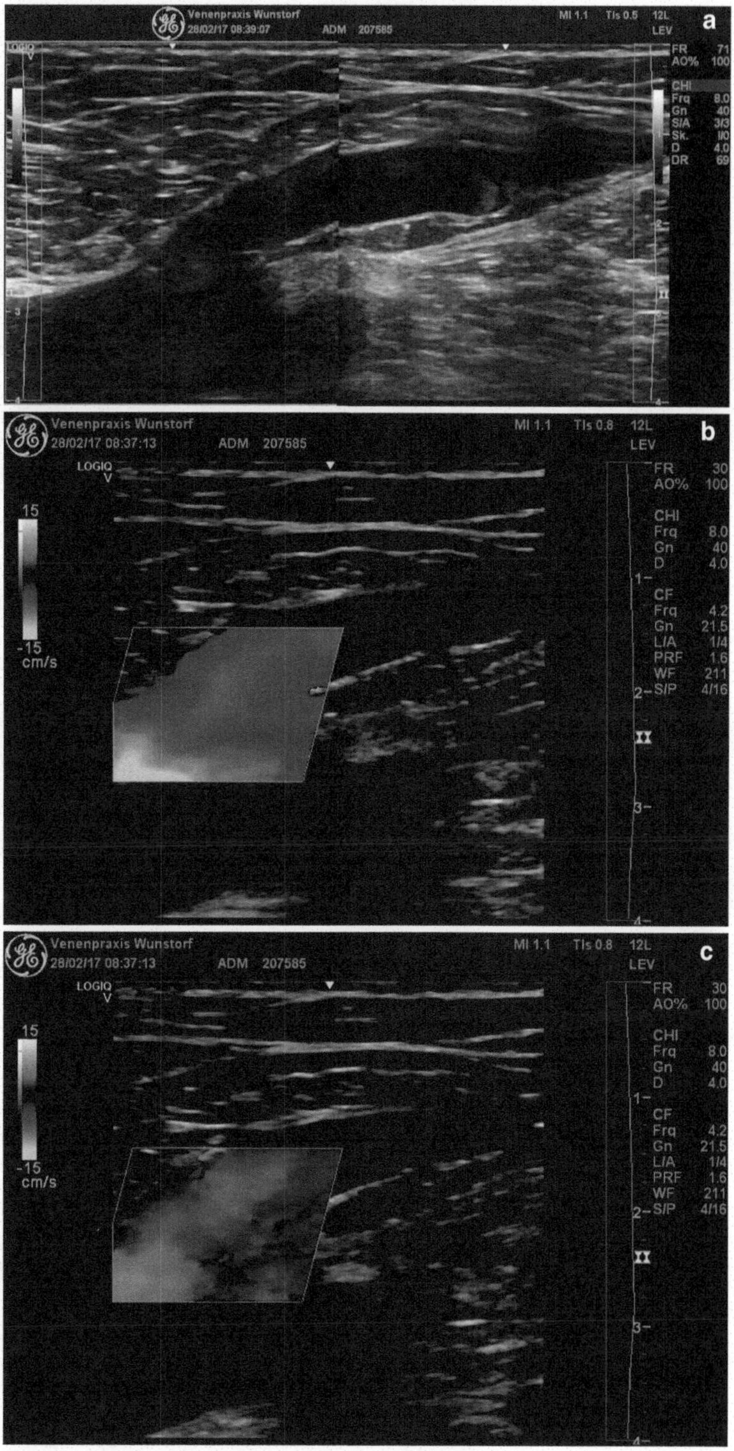

Fig. 4.14 (**a**) Longitudinal representation of the sapheno-femoral junction with terminal and preterminal valve. (**b**) Muscular systole in colour-coded duplex with antegrade flow from GSV into CFV. (**c**) Muscular diastole with retrograde flow from CFV into the GSV through an incompetent terminal valve. (**d**) Measurement in PW mode in longitudinal section at the level of the terminal valve with reflux. (**e**) Measurement in PW mode at the level of the preterminal valve with reflux. (**f**) Measurement in PW mode at the ostium in cross-section demonstrating reflux—compare with Fig. 4.12

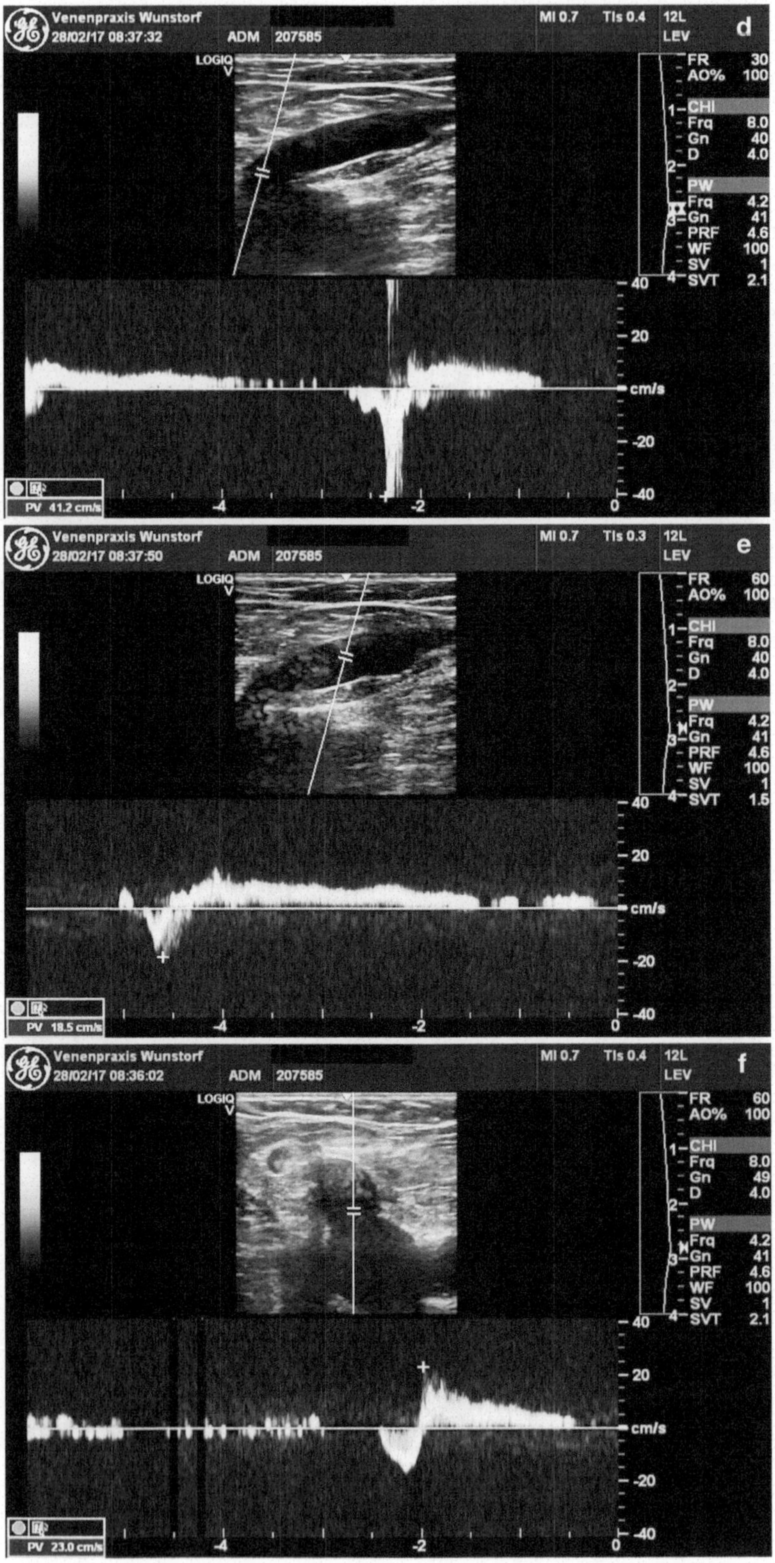

Fig. 4.14 (continued)

Table 4.2 Paths for different flow patterns in the groin region, including the Stücker type and the shunt type (explanation: see Sect. 3.8)

Path	Description	Clinics	Stücker type	Shunt type
CFV–TV–GSV–AASV	Incompetent terminal valve. Competent preterminal valve. GSV is only affected for a short distance. "Ostial reflux"	Visible tributaries on the anterior thigh	1	3
CFV–TV–GSV–PTV	Ostial reflux, GSV reflux above and below knee	Tributaries along the medial aspect of thigh and calf	3	1 or 3
PV–GSV–PTV	Para-ostial reflux feeding the GSV, competent TV	Tributaries along the anterior thigh and calf	2	4 or 5
PV–AASV	Reflux from pelvic venous network directly into AASV, without involving the GSV or flowing "through" it between the TV and PTV but without incompetence of any of both	Tributaries on the anterior thigh	4[a]	6
GSV (sufficient)–AASV	Antegrade flow in GSV feeding the AASV	Small tributaries at the ventral aspect of the thigh	–	2
SSV–PASV–GSV	GSV filled via a Giacomini anastomosis (origin SSV). The TV is competent and in most cases the PTV also	Tributaries at the medial aspect of the calf, possibly veins at the dorsal thigh	–	Combined 3 (SSV) and 4 or 5 (GSV)
PV–PASV–GSV	GSV filled from pelvic reflux via PASV. The TV is competent and in most cases the PTV also	Tributaries at the medial aspect of the calf or distal thigh, possibly veins at the dorsal thigh	–	4 or 5

CFV common femoral vein, *TV* terminal valve, *PTV* preterminal valve, *GSV* great saphenous vein, *SSV* small saphenous vein, *AASV* anterior accessory saphenous vein, *PASV* posterior accessory saphenous vein, *PV* pelvic veins
[a]Lit: Mendoza and Stücker [21]

examination of a refluxing GSV, the following points need answers:

- The source of the reflux.
- A possible second source, like a perforating vein.
- Is there only one segment refluxing or is there multisegmental reflux in the GSV?
- The length of the refluxing segment.
- The drainage path of the reflux load into a perforating vein or a tributary.

4.5.2.1 Reflux Source

The most frequent reflux source for the GSV is the groin region (see Sect. 4.4). Other options are:

- Refluxing tributaries, possibly fed by:
  - Pelvic vein reflux
  - Refluxing small saphenous vein via the Giacomini vein at the thigh
  - Refluxing small saphenous vein via communicating vein at the calf
  - Tributaries fed by perforating veins and draining into the GSV
  - Healthy tributaries draining into the GSV
- Perforating veins feeding the GSV directly at the mid-thigh or from paratibial perforating veins below the knee

After examining the sapheno-femoral junction, the probe will be held transversally, and the GSV will be followed down the thigh, passing

Fig. 4.15 Flow chart to determine the possibility of reflux in pelvic or inguinal tributaries as reflux source for great saphenous vein (GSV) or accessory anterior saphenous vein (AASV). Abbreviations (see legend Table 4.2). Adapted from [5]

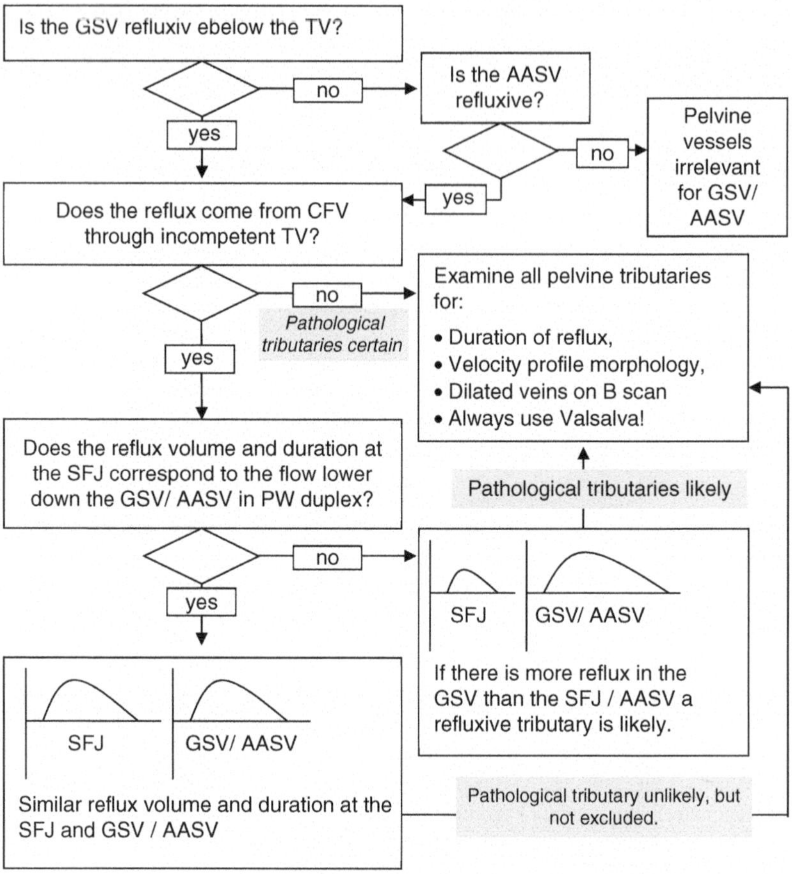

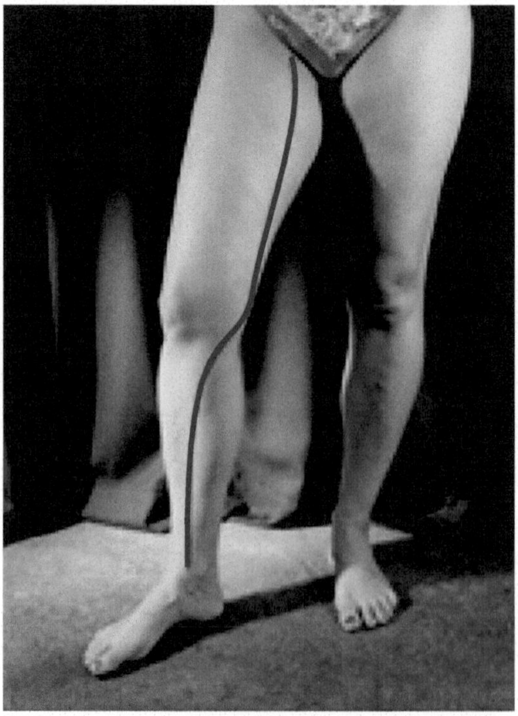

Fig. 4.16 Course of the great saphenous vein along the right leg. With permission by [5]

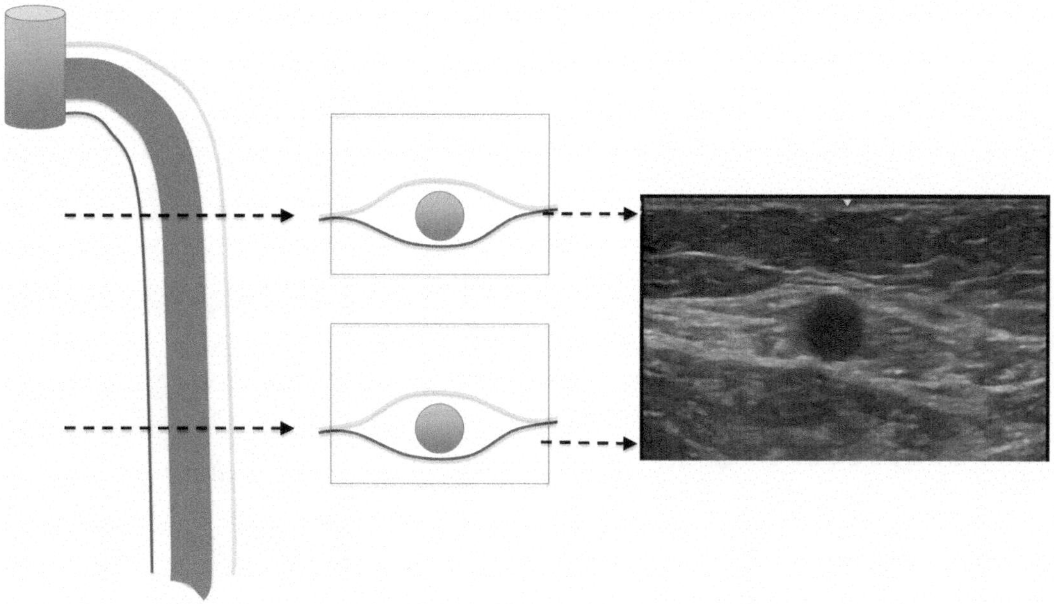

Fig. 4.17 Course of the GSV type “I”. The vein has a straight course within the saphenous fascia which is confirmed at both ultrasound points in the thigh; on the right side is a typical image, visible on ultrasound at both points (Course of GSV at the thigh and knee. Schematic representation of a typical ultrasound image in B-mode in cross-section. Red, muscle fascia; yellow, saphenous fascia; blue, saphenous vein). With permission by [5]

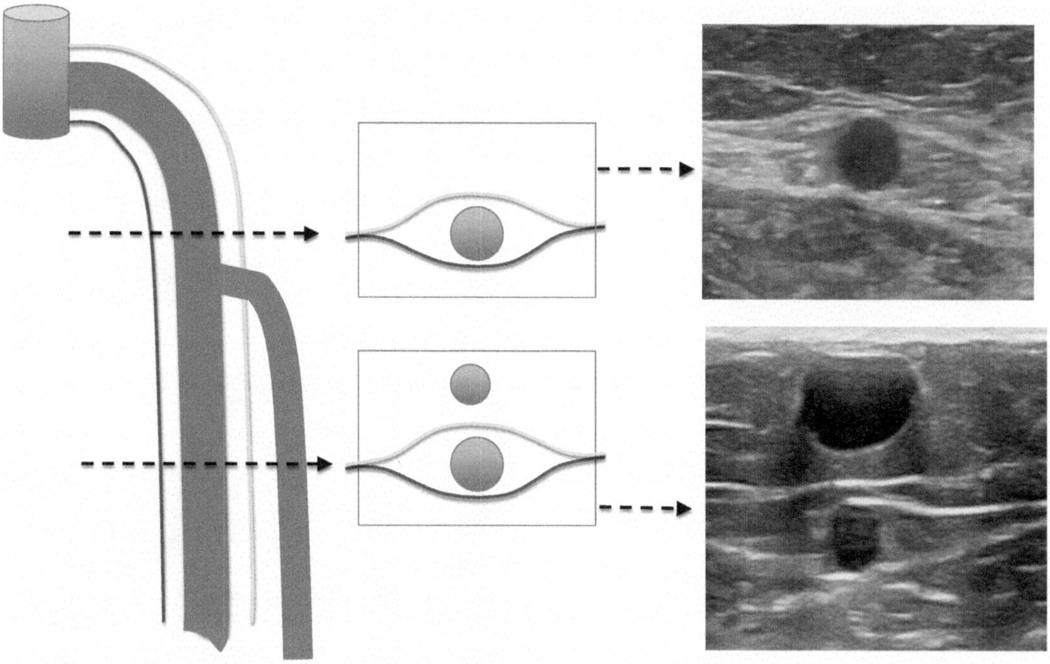

Fig. 4.18 Course of GSV type “h”. The GSV has a straight course within the saphenous fascia. There is a parallel extrafascial tributary, joining the GSV at the mid-thigh. At the proximal point, the saphenous vein is seen in the compartment, and at the distal ultrasound point, there are two veins, one in the compartment and the other in the extrafascial tributary (Course of GSV at the thigh and knee. Schematic representation of a typical ultrasound image in B-mode in cross-section. Red, muscle fascia; yellow, saphenous fascia; blue, saphenous vein). With permission by [5]

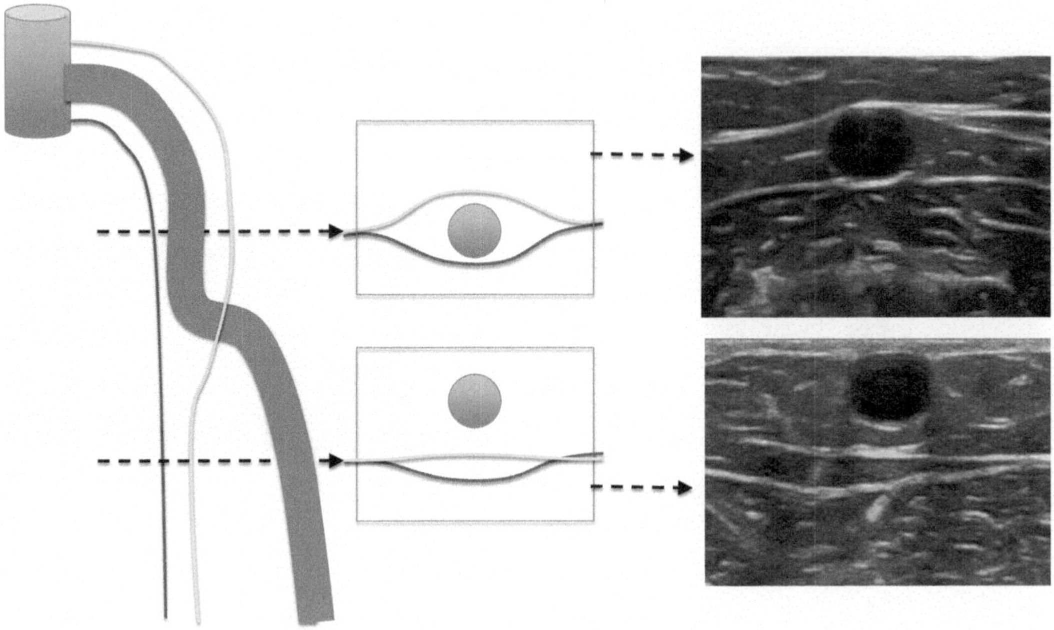

Fig. 4.19 Course of GSV type "s". The vein runs in the fascial compartment at the proximal point and leaves the fascia so that at the distal point there is no vein seen inside the fascial compartment. However, an aplastic or hypoplastic rudiment is present on histology, but not visible by ultrasound. The main continuing tributary takes over the blood flow of the GSV as a superficial natural bypass (Course of GSV at the thigh and knee. Schematic representation of a typical ultrasound image in B-mode in cross-section. Red, muscle fascia; yellow, saphenous fascia; blue, saphenous vein). With permission by [5]

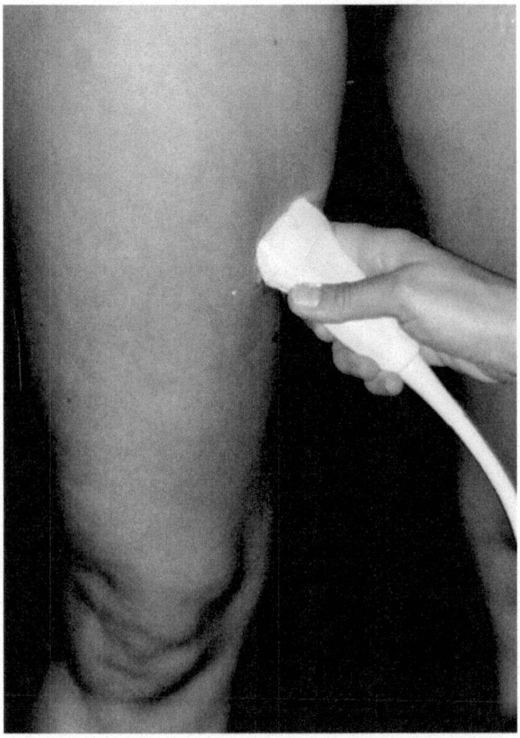

Fig. 4.20 Probe position to measure a flow in the superficial leg veins when exploring with the probe in transversal position. The tip of the probe is angulated upwards

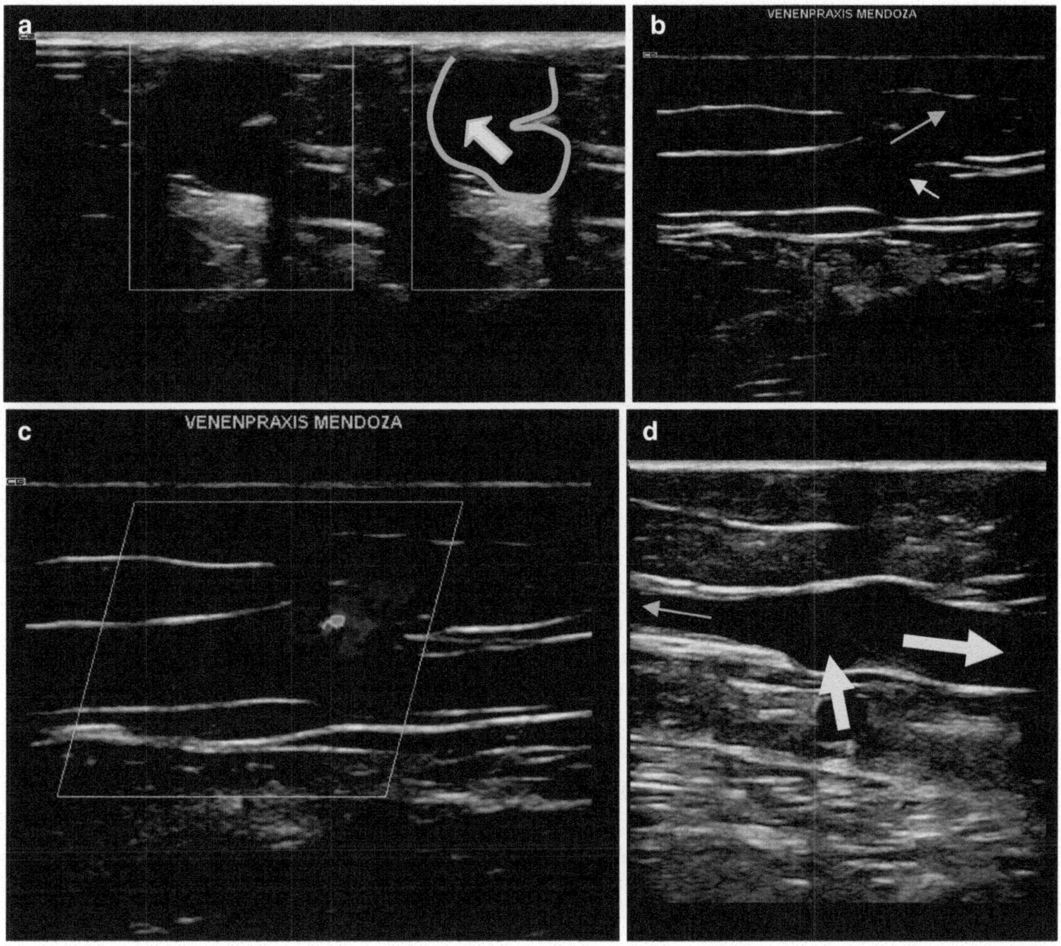

Fig. 4.21 Calibre changes in the GSV. (**a**) Cross-section at the medial thigh in colour-coded duplex during diastole: a tributary is refluxing and the reflux emerges from the saphenous vein to feed the tributary. On the right side, the shape of the GSV and the emerging tributary is depicted in blue; the direction of the flow from the GSV to the tributary is shown with a yellow arrow. During systole (not shown), the flow in the tributary and the GSV is antegrade, "blue" (Image with kind permission of Viavital from: Mendoza E. Duplexsonographie der oberflächlichen Beinvenen in Rabe E. Stücker M Phlebologischer Bildatlas. Viavital. 2015). (**b**) Longitudinal representation of the GSV at the mid-thigh in B-mode. Proximal (left part of the image) the GSV is larger; after a tributary joins the GSV (blue arrow), the distal GSV is smaller. A valve can be seen in the GSV (yellow arrow). Distally to the valve, the GSV is competent. (**c**) Same patient than in (**b**) in muscular diastole in colour-coded duplex. The reflux from the proximal GSV fills the tributary. (**d**) Longitudinal representation in another patient. Proximal GSV is competent (blue arrow). At the mid-thigh, a calibre change is seen, where a refluxing perforating vein feeds the distal GSV with reflux (yellow arrows)

the knee and then down to the ankle. Any variation of the calibre of the vein and any branching vein—perforating vein or tributary—with more than approximately 2 mm diameter must be analysed with duplex in PW mode (see Fig. 4.21). Keep in mind, that there are possibly more than one reflux sources or drainage pathways present. Awareness to this possibility will lead to less error and encourage to a better, more informative, examination.

Sometimes a reflux in the GSV is found with apparently no reflux source. This situation is called "reflux without source" and is based on the physiological feeding of the GSV by tributaries.

Here the valves in the GSV are not competent, and this physiological blood volume is drained retrogradely and demonstrated as reflux in the GSV (see Fig. 4.22).

4.5.2.2 Refluxive Segments

The most common configuration is that the GSV has one segment of reflux, fed by the SFJ and is drained via one or more tributaries or one or more perforating veins or both. Occasionally, GSV reflux feeds a tributary, the distal GSV is competent for a segment and further down will be fed again by the same tributary or another reflux source. After the exploration, it has to be clear, which segment or segments of the GSV is refluxing (Fig. 4.23).

4.5.2.3 Drainage Pathways

Identification of the drainage pathways is crucial if saphenous vein sparing surgery is performed. In the GSV the drainage of the reflux is only possible via one or more perforating veins or tributaries or both. They will be found exploring the complete GSV and analysing the flow behaviour inside the vein above and below any visible tributary or perforating vein. The reflux elimination test is useful to determine whether a segment is drained by a tributary (described in Sect. 3.8.9).

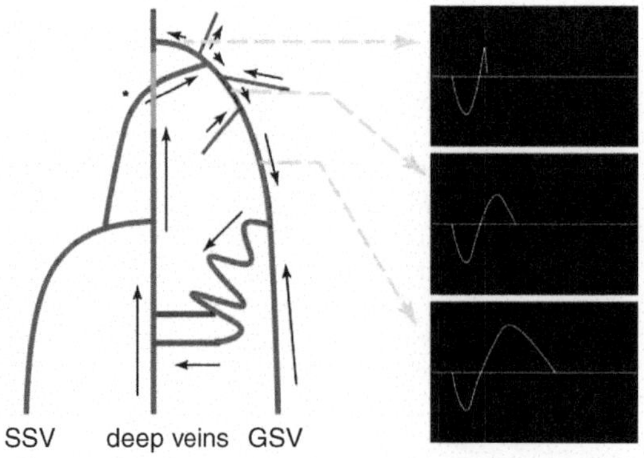

Fig. 4.22 Reflux without source according to Cappelli and Franceschi. The terminal valve of the great saphenous vein (*GSV*) remains competent. Antegrade blood from healthy tributaries, including the posterior (*) and anterior accessory saphenous veins, drain progressively into the great saphenous vein, causing retrograde flow within an incompetent segment of the GSV. There is no pathological connection with the deep system. The reflux curves are of small volume but progressively increase down the great saphenous vein. These are shown on the right at three different stages. *SSV* small saphenous vein. With permission by [5]

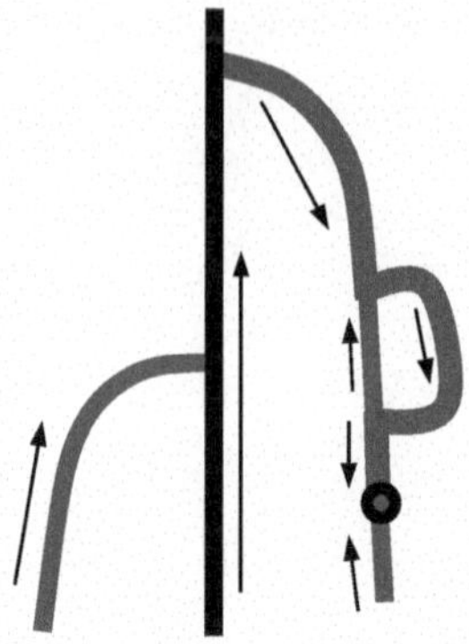

Fig. 4.23 GSV with two refluxing segments: One from the groin to the distal thigh, where the reflux drains into a tributary, which further down again joins the GSV and fills it with reflux. This second, distal segment drains into a paratibial perforating vein. The segment of GSV at the knee level is competent, as it is being bypassed by the refluxing tributary. The segment of the GSV between the ankle and the draining perforating vein is also competent, because the reflux path is diverted away by the re-entry perforating vein. With permission by [22]

4.6 Small Saphenous Vein

The small saphenous vein is the shorter, interfascial vein in the leg, running at the back of the calf (see Fig. 4.24). It is less commonly affected by a reflux.

4.6.1 Anatomy

The SSV runs from the lateral malleolus at the back of the calf, usually ending at the knee level. In 60% of cases, it has a thigh extension, which often meets the posterior accessory saphenous vein forming the Giacomini anastomosis, which connects both saphenous veins at the thigh (see Figs. 4.24 and 4.25c, f). Unlike the GSV, which always drains into the deep vein at the saphenofemoral junction below the groin crease, the drainage of the small saphenous vein is variable (see Fig. 4.25). Rarely, it drains into muscle veins below the knee or via a communicating vein into the GSV, also below the knee. In these cases, the SSV will be absent in the popliteal fossa (see Fig. 4.25g). Usually, the SSV drains into the popliteal vein in the popliteal fossa or into the first segment of the femoral vein, where it may pierce or not a muscle at the back of the lower thigh (see

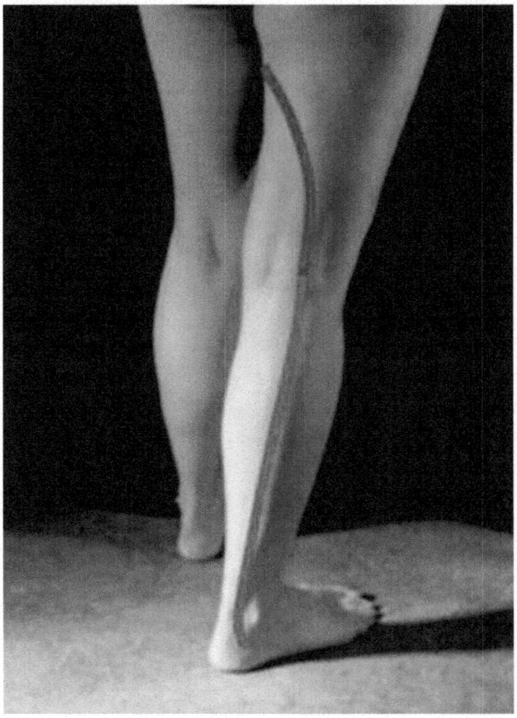

Fig. 4.24 Posterior view of the leg demonstrating the course of the small saphenous vein (SSV) as a green line and the course of its thigh extension or Giacomini anastomosis as a red line. With permission by [5]

Fig. 4.25a, d, e). In addition, it may give a connecting vein into a muscle vein before draining into the deep vein (see Fig. 4.25b).

Prior to any treatment decision, it is crucial to identify, which of the described conditions are present and which of these paths have reflux (see Sect. 6.7).

The SSV runs between two fasciae, like the GSV. It is possible to confuse the SSV with a muscle vein, especially when the muscle vein has reflux (see Fig. 4.31).

4.6.2 Flow and Reflux in the Small Saphenous Vein

The small saphenous vein has to be examined from the popliteal fossa to the ankle in cross-section with close attention to flow, calibre changes, joining tributaries and perforating veins. As in the GSV, the SSV can have one or more reflux sources and one or more refluxing segments (see Sect. 4.5.2).

Many different reflux sources may feed the SSV with reflux:

- Popliteal vein via sapheno-popliteal junction (see Figs. 4.26, 4.27, 4.28 and 4.29)
- Muscle vein connecting to the SSV (see Fig. 4.30)
- Refluxing Giacomini vein, fed by the GSV (see Sect. 6.11.6.1), a posterior thigh perforating vein or by pelvic reflux
- Refluxing tributaries, fed by the GSV or occasionally a perforating vein
- Refluxing perforating vein (see Fig. 4.31)

Reflux in the SSV may be systolic, diastolic or both. A systolic reflux at the sapheno-popliteal junction is a sign of an antegrade thigh drainage obstruction to the venous flow of the deep veins (see Sect. 3.9.3). In these cases, the SSV is often only affected for a very short segment, between the deep vein and the origin of the Giacomini vein.

4.7 Perforating Veins

Perforating veins usually drain blood from superficial veins to the deep venous system during diastole. This flow is with the orientation of the venous valves which face inwards. Only dilated perforating veins or perforating veins involved as reflux source or drainage pathway for a varicose vein have to be investigated with flow measurement.

4.7.1 Anatomy

There are lots of perforating veins in the leg. Some of them concentrate along the GSV, others along the SSV and some independent veins can be also important for venous pathology. This includes the perforating vein on the back or lateral part of the mid-thigh ("Hach" perforating vein), often feeding an isolated refluxing tributary.

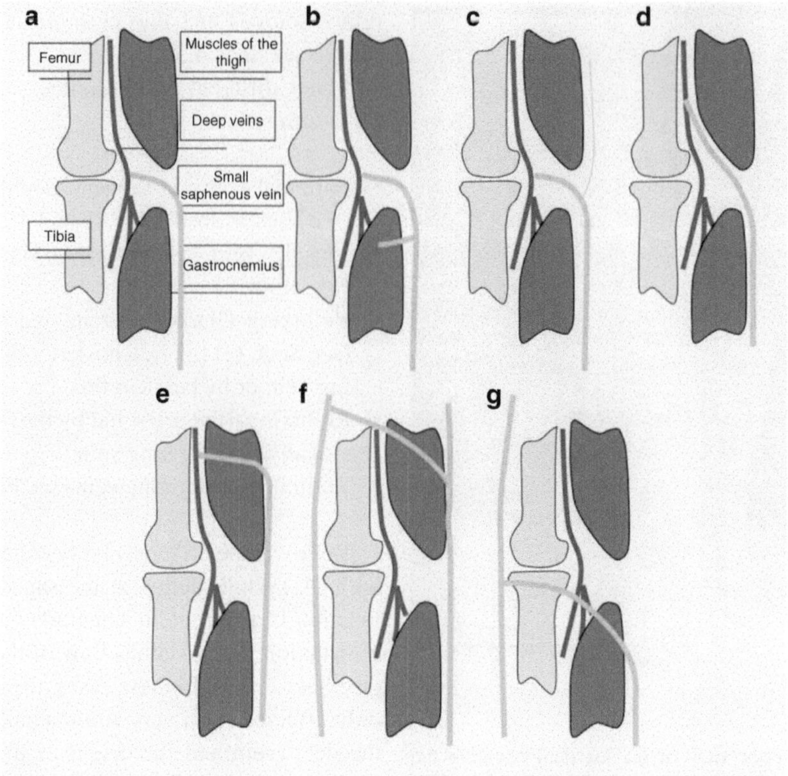

Fig. 4.25 Variations of the termination of the small saphenous vein: (**a**) Termination of the small saphenous vein (SSV) in the popliteal fossa draining into the popliteal vein (see Fig. 4.26). (**b**) Termination of the SSV in the popliteal fossa with an additional connection to the deep vein through the muscle veins (see Fig. 4.30). Sometimes the SSV only drains via a muscle vein and not directly into the popliteal vein (see Fig. 4.27). (**c**) Termination of the SSV in the popliteal fossa. The SSV has a "thigh extension" running cranially to drain via a perforating vein or meet the posterior accessory saphenous vein with an additional connection to the GSV. This intersaphenous connection is called Giacomini anastomosis (Fig. 4.26). (**d**) Termination of the SSV above the popliteal fossa without piercing the muscle fascia (Fig. 4.28). (**e**) Termination of the SSV above the popliteal fossa where it pierces the muscle fascia and the muscles of the back of the thigh. (**f**) No junction at the knee level. Termination of the SSV draining into the vein of Giacomini or femoropopliteal vein with drainage into the great saphenous vein or the gluteal veins (see Fig. 4.29). (**g**) Termination of the SSV via a connecting branch vein into the great saphenous vein below the knee. The true terminal segment of the SSV is absent, and there is no sapheno-popliteal junction present in the popliteal fossa. With permission by [22]

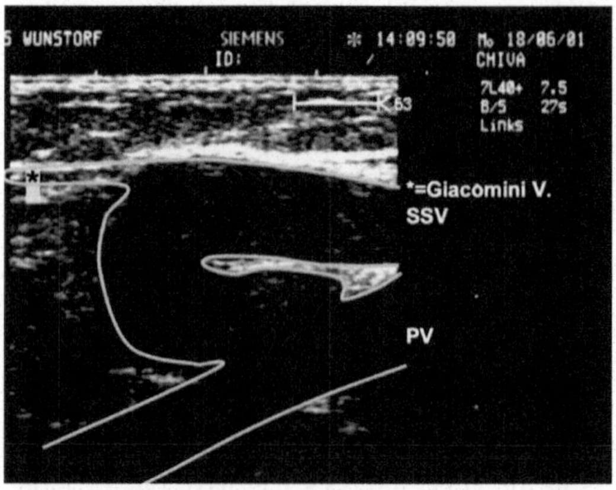

Fig. 4.26 Longitudinal scan through the popliteal fossa showing a very enlarged and refluxing SSV draining into the popliteal vein (PV). A small Giacomini vein (*) drains into the SSV (treatment: see Fig. 6.22c). With permission by [5]

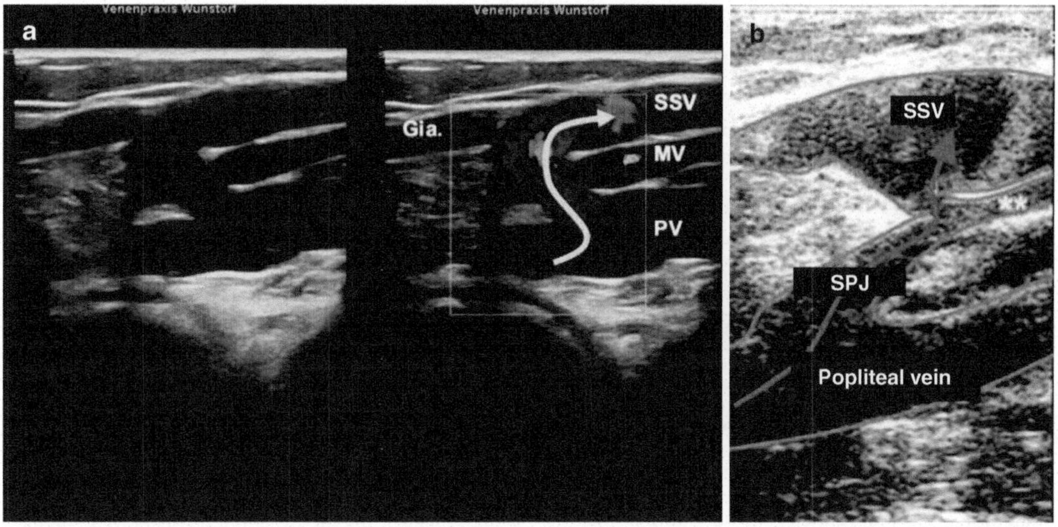

Fig. 4.27 (a) Longitudinal scan through the popliteal fossa showing the drainage of the SSV into a muscle vein. Both together drain into the popliteal vein. Reflux from the popliteal vein into the SSV is shown during the muscular diastole in colour-coded duplex ultrasound. (**b**) Longitudinal scan through the popliteal fossa demonstrating a venous aneurysm at the termination of the small saphenous vein (*SSV*). This joins the popliteal vein together with a competent muscle vein (**). The aneurysm has partially thrombosed. The arrow indicates the direction of flow of the refluxing blood. *SPJ* sapheno-popliteal junction (treatment: see Fig. 6.22b). With permission by [5]

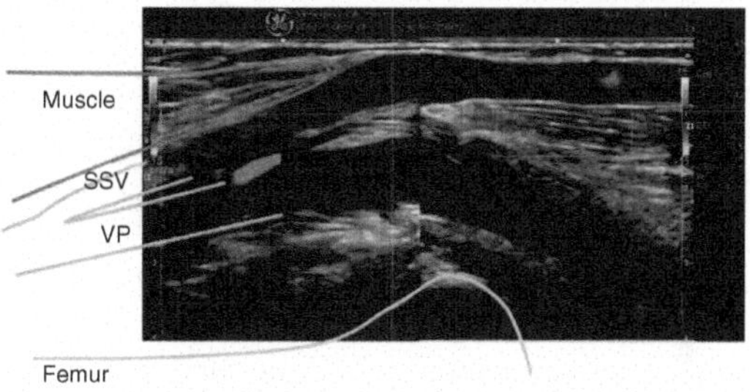

Fig. 4.28 Longitudinal image of the popliteal fossa with a SSV draining into the deep vein below the thigh posterior muscle, above the knee crease

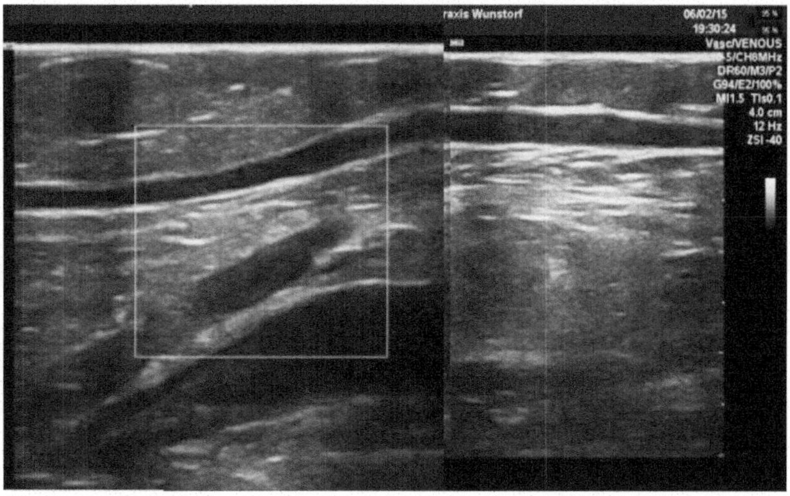

Fig. 4.29 Longitudinal composite image of the popliteal fossa with a SSV passing through the fossa without connection to the deep vein. Usually in this configuration, there is no reflux in the SSV

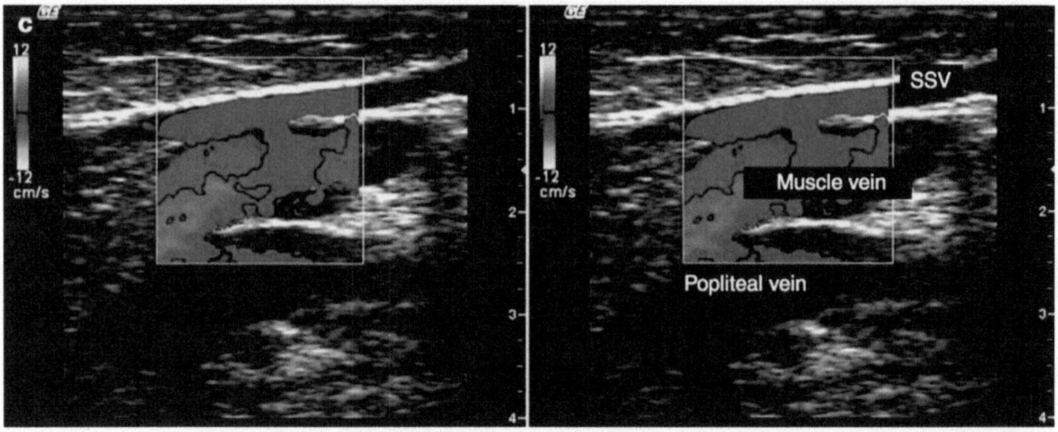

Fig. 4.30 Longitudinal view through the lower part of the popliteal fossa. The small saphenous vein (*SSV*) has reflux at the junction (not shown). In addition, there is reflux via a muscle vein. There is often a connection with the muscle veins in this region. If only the junction of the small saphenous vein is interrupted because this distal connection was not discovered in preoperative scan, then distal SSV reflux may persist. With permission by [5]

Figure 4.32 shows the most important perforating veins as a schematic representation. Perforating veins have been renamed in an international consensus. However, many people still use the former names. In these figures both names will be mentioned.

4.7.2 Flow in Perforating Veins

Dilated perforating veins have been thought to be pathologic in the sense of them being "responsible for varicose veins" for a long time. It was the ultrasound that identified the truth. Most of the perforating veins are dilated, because they drain the blood from the varicose veins back into the deep veins (see Sect. 2.4.2 and Fig. 4.35). Only those perforating veins with outward flow in systole and/or diastole are pathological (see Table 3.2 and Sect. 3.5.3 and Figs. 4.33 and 4.34).

Usually those perforating veins, which exhibit reflux in diastole, are the reflux source of a varicose vein. They are mostly found at the thigh and very seldom at the calf (see Fig. 4.33). A perforating vein can also be the second reflux source along an incompetent vein. Occasionally an incompetent saphenous vein can be fed through the sapheno-femoral junction and fed again by reflux via a perforating vein of the medial thigh. Rarely a refluxing perforating vein is identified in systole. If they are seen, they are usually part of an open bypassing shunt after deep vein thrombosis (see Fig. 4.34 and Sect. 3.7.3).

Draining perforating veins will have flow in diastole from superficial to deep and can be found at the end of the refluxing segment of a vein (terminalising perforating vein) or on the way of a refluxing segment (non-terminalising perforating vein) (Fig. 4.35).

4.8 Tributaries

Tributaries are veins running in the subcutaneous tissue superficial to the saphenous fascia. The most important tributaries are:

- Tributaries from the GSV (see Fig. 4.35)
  - Anterior accessory saphenous vein (AASV)
  - Posterior accessory saphenous vein (PASV)
  - Accessory vein at the calf (anterior and posterior)

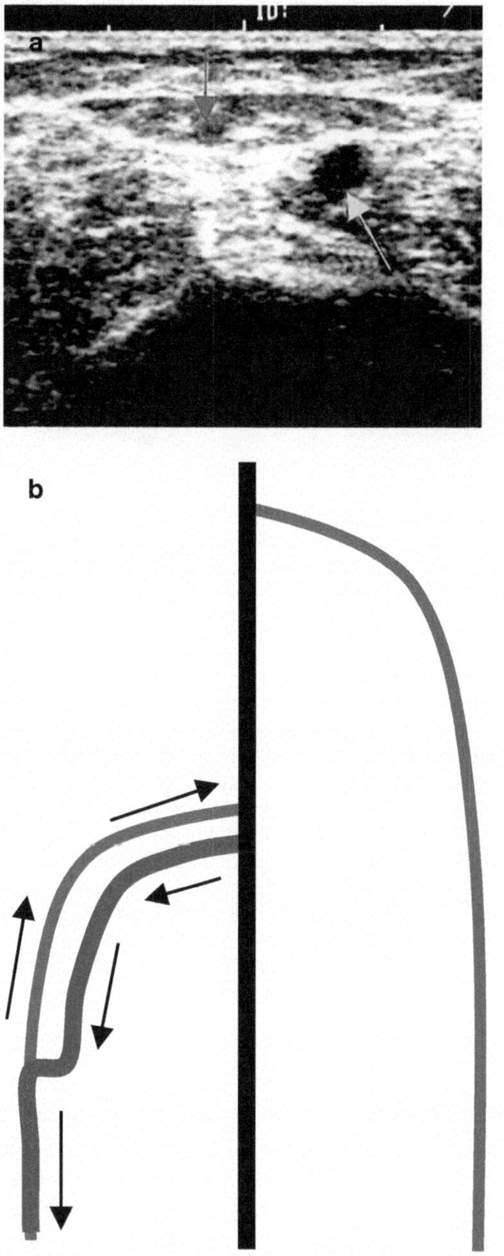

Fig. 4.31 (**a**) Transverse view through the back of the calf showing a competent small saphenous vein (*blue arrow*) and a refluxing muscle vein (*yellow arrow*). (**b**) Diagram of the recirculation circuit with incompetence of a muscle vein (red) arising from the popliteal fossa. This fills the lower part of the small saphenous vein which is also refluxing the proximal part of the SSV remains competent (blue). (**a**) With permission by [5]. (**b**) With permission by [22]

  - Communicating vein between AASV and GSV
  - Communicating vein between GSV and SSV at the calf
  - Giacomini vein
- Tributaries from the SSV (usually at the knee crease or mid-calf)

These tributaries are present, but are not always visible. If pathological they are dilated and much more likely to be visible clinically and when examining the GSV or SSV with ultrasound.

Every dilated vein connecting with a saphenous vein has to be examined with duplex ultrasound.

- Blue flow will be present:
  - If they drain into the GSV with normal physiologic blood flow less than 1 s in diastole
  - If they fill the GSV with reflux excessive blood flow lasting longer than 1 s in diastole, like in case of reflux from pelvic venous network draining into the GSV or multisegmental reflux in GSV
- Red flow will be present if the tributary is filled with reflux from the saphenous vein being dilated by the volume overload (Fig. 4.21)

The special flow behaviour of the AASV and PASV has been explained in Sect. 4.4.

Apart from the veins connected to the saphenous vein, every visible dilated and meandering superficial vein has to be examined making sure the source and the termination point of the reflux. The reflux source can be a perforating vein, the pelvic network, a saphenous vein or another tributary that branches into several other tributaries. Drainage pathways usually are perforating veins, but saphenous veins can also serve as a draining pathway for tributaries.

To detect if there are one or several draining or branching points along a very meandering tributary, the technique explained in Fig. 4.36 can be

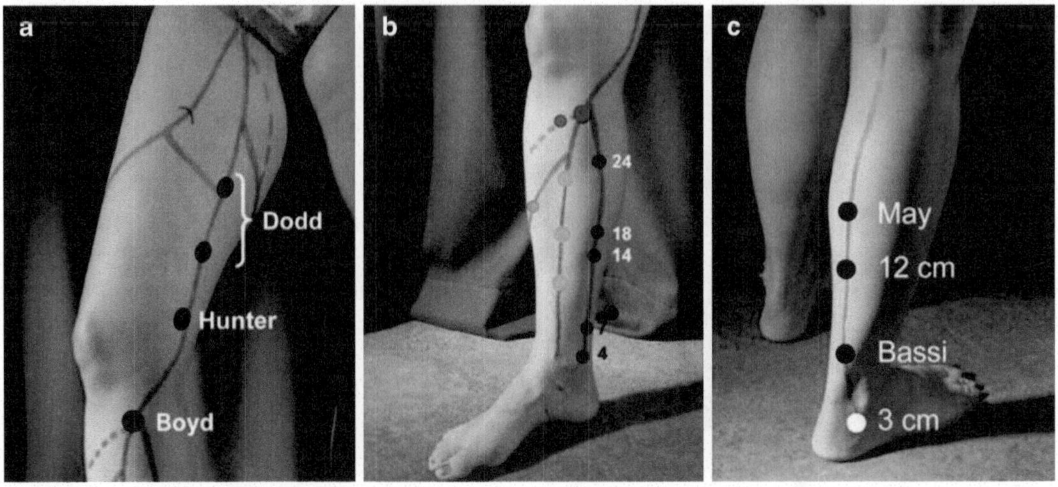

Fig. 4.32 (**a**) Location of the perforating veins of the adductor canal (formerly Dodd and Hunter) in the above knee great saphenous vein and location of the highest and most important paratibial perforating vein (formerly Boyd) in the below knee great saphenous vein. (**b**) Location of the perforating veins on the front and inner sides of the calf. *Blue*, perforating veins of the anterior arch vein; *green*, paratibial perforating veins of the great saphenous vein; *dark green*, formerly Boyd perforating vein; *light green*, paratibial perforating veins with drainage into the posterior tibial veins; *black*, posterior tibial perforating veins. These are perforating veins draining the posterior arch vein, formerly known as Cockett I–III, depending on the distance in cm between the floor and the vein. The posterior ankle perforating veins were formerly known as Kuster veins, starting at 4 cm. (**c**) Location of the perforating veins of the SSV from proximal to distal: The soleal perforating vein (formerly May) connects the SSV with the muscle veins in the middle of the calf at the so-called gastrocnemius point, a perforating vein at a height of 12 cm, a para-Achillean perforating veins (formerly Bassi). Both these connect the small saphenous vein with the fibular veins. Below the lateral malleolus, there is a direct connection between the small saphenous vein and the fibular (peroneal) veins at a height of 3 cm (lateral ankle perforating vein). With permission by [5]

applied: First, the probe is placed at the upper end of the vein to be examined. Next, the subject is told to raise and lower his toes (Wunstorf manoeuvre). In this way reflux can be confirmed in this vein segment. Then the segment below the varicose vein is compressed with one finger, and the subject is again asked to activate the muscle pump. If there is no drainage point between the probe and the point of digital compression, there will be no reflux in the first phase of muscular diastole. However, after the digital compression is released (top two curves in Fig. 4.36), reflux will resume. If a refluxing tributary branches off between the middle and lowest compression point, the waveform changes. With digital compression at the lowest point of the varicose vein in the figure, the reflux begins at the onset of muscular diastole which is independent of digital compression. This is because the refluxing volume is now drained by another tributary (bottom curve).

4.9 Deep Veins

Blood flow in the deep veins should be directed to the heart, just like in the superficial veins during systole with a short retrograde flow until the valves close. This should be no longer than 1 second to define competency of valves. The normal vein wall is represented as a thin line without thickenings or bulges.

The pathology and exploration of the deep leg veins are explained in Chap. 8. Nevertheless, during the exploration of the superficial veins, deep veins at the groin (common femoral vein) and the knee (popliteal vein) are automatically in the focus of the probe. In the groin, the com-

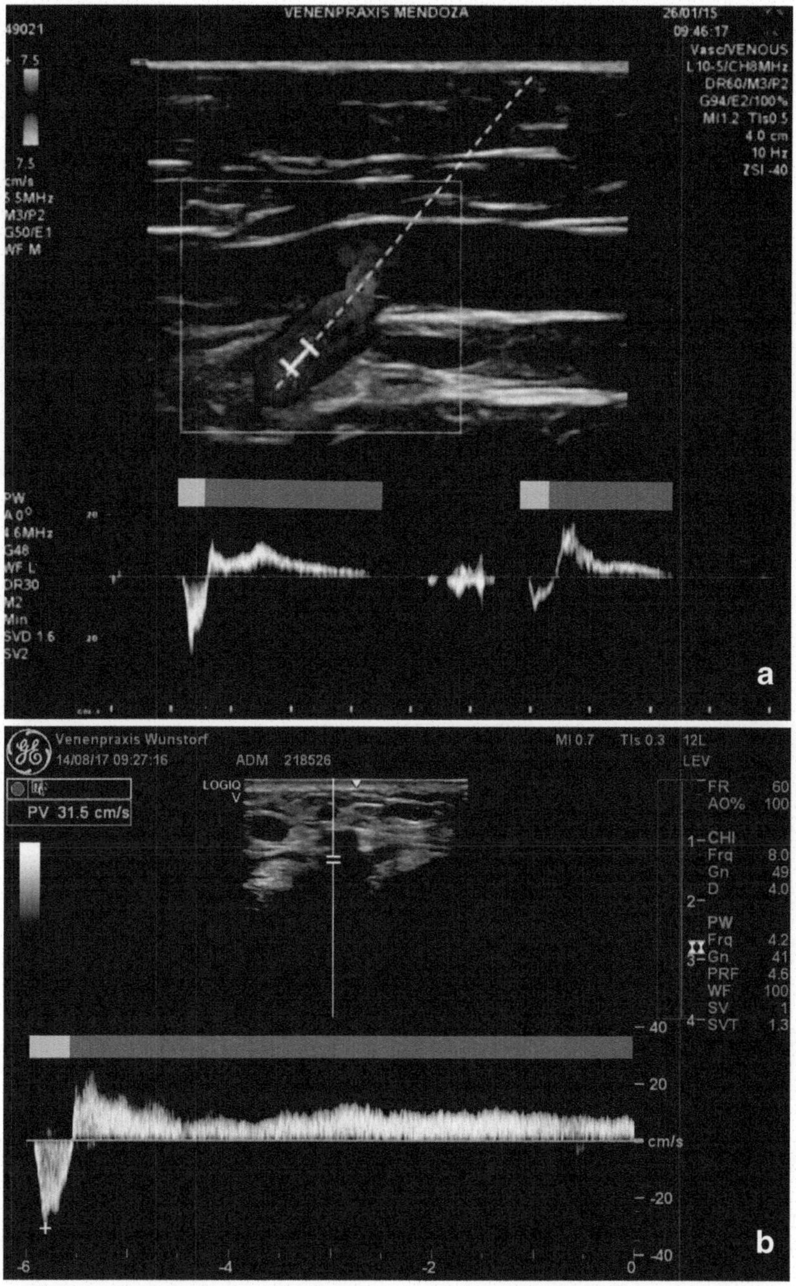

Fig. 4.33 Perforating vein as a reflux source: (**a**) Longitudinal representation of the GSV at the inner thigh. The proximal GSV (to the left of the image) is competent; the distal GSV (at the right of the image) has reflux. In colour the perforating vein and the distal GSV are shown to be refluxing (red) in diastole. On the bottom, the PW measurement in the perforating vein is added. Note that during systole the flow is antegrade (inwards) and during diastole a reflux is seen outwards and then downwards. (**b**) Refluxive perforating vein at the calf: the cross-section at the medial calf shows a paratibial perforating vein with antegrade (inward) flow in systole and long-lasting, retrograde flow in diastole. This is not a common finding in the calf

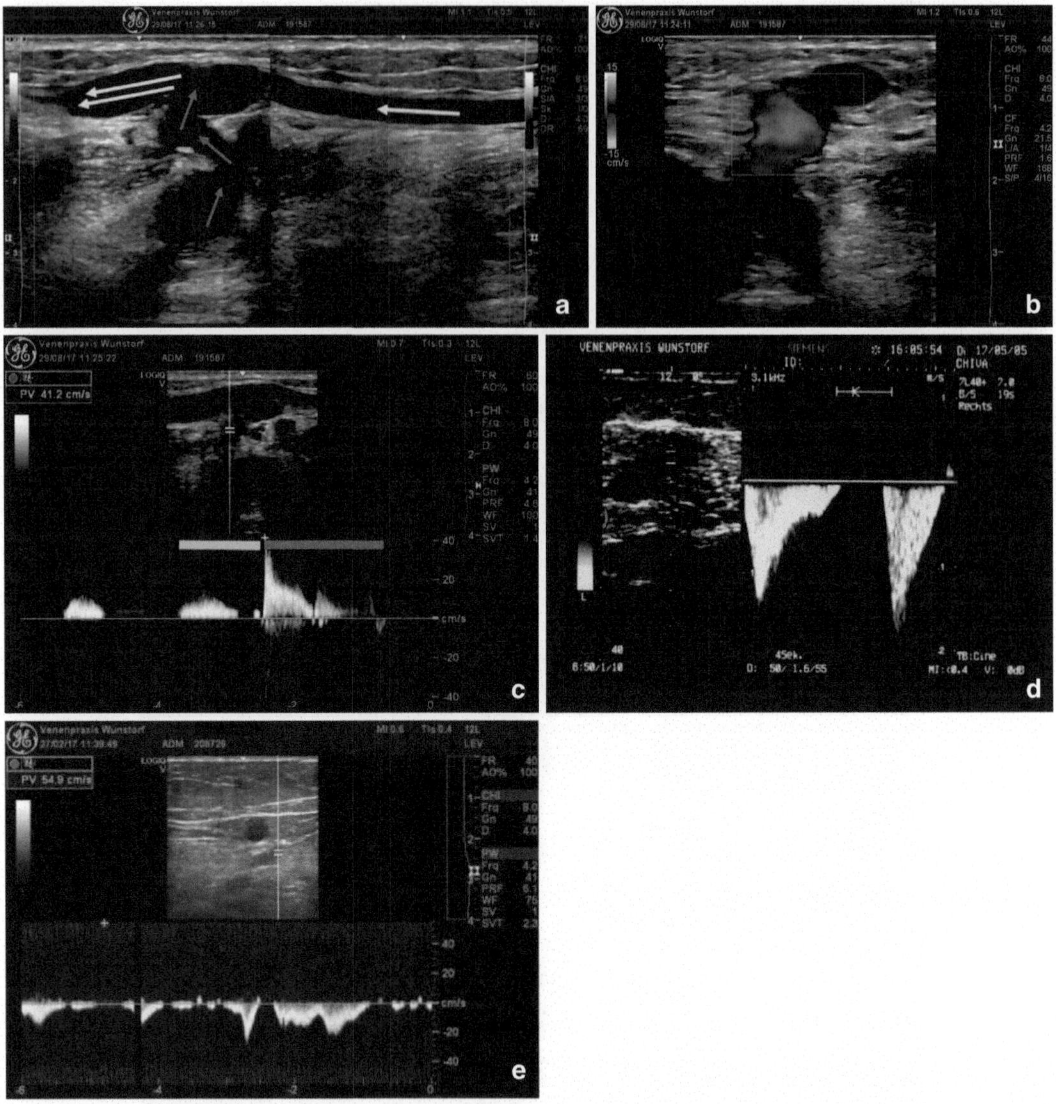

Fig. 4.34 Perforator as part of a bypass for the deep venous system after thrombosis (open vicarious or bypass shunt). (**a**) Longitudinal image or the proximal inner part of the calf with GSV. On the right part of the image, the distal GSV is draining physiologically upwards (one blue arrow). On the left part of the image, red arrows show the blood flow through the paratibial perforating vein. The GSV on the left part of the image is dilated segment, also with antegrade flow. This is required to transport the additional blood entering the GSV from the perforating vein as part of a deep venous bypass. (**b**) Cross-section of the proximal calf of the same patient with the tibia at the left border of the image. The GSV is to the right and is being filled with red (refluxing) blood from the paratibial perforating vein during muscular systole. (**c**) Measurement using PW mode in the perforating vein in systole and diastole. In both phases, incompetent flow is observed from deep vein to superficial, filling the proximal GSV (same patient as **a** and **b**). (**d**) Draining perforating veins. Non-terminalising perforating vein at the mid-thigh with draining (inwards) flow in systole and diastole. (**e**) Terminalising perforating vein at the calf with draining (inwards) flow in systole and diastole. With manual compression of the calf over lax muscles during "systole", an outward flow can be seen, which can cause confusion. (**d**) With permission by [5]

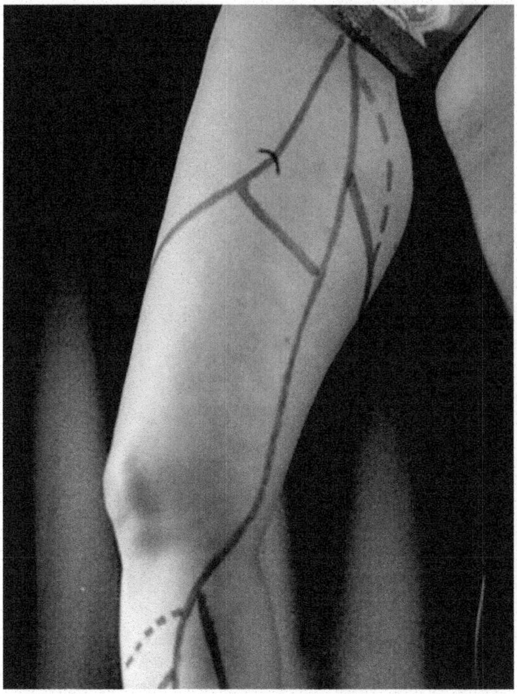

Fig. 4.35 Major tributaries of the GSV, at the thigh: anterior and posterior accessory saphenous veins (red) demonstrating variations in their termination with the great saphenous vein (green). The dotted line marks the alternative course of the posterior accessory saphenous vein into the confluence of superficial inguinal veins. The black mark indicates where the anterior accessory saphenous vein leaves the fascial compartment of the great saphenous vein and becomes epifascial. Distal of this point, there is very often a connecting vein between the anterior accessory saphenous vein and the great saphenous vein. At the calf, the posterior accessory arch vein plays an important role in the drainage of refluxing veins towards the calf perforating veins (red dorsal line). From this vein a communicating vein towards the SSV is possible. With permission by [5]

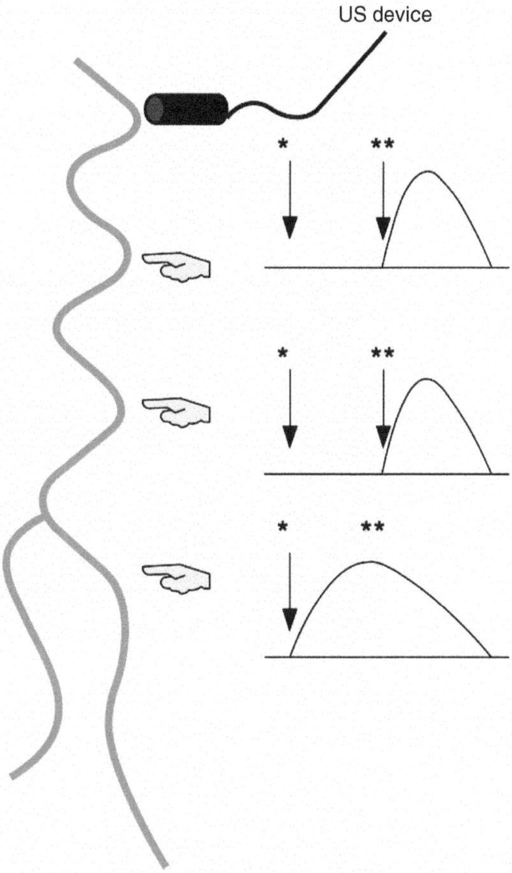

Fig. 4.36 Diagram of the examination technique used to determine the site of important drainage points. The probe is placed at the upper end, and the hands indicate the points at which the vein is compressed with the finger. The curve on the right shows the velocity profile in each case after muscle contraction (rising the toes). One star (*) shows the beginning of the muscular diastole (lowering the toes); two stars (**) show the moment of the release of the digital compression. For further explanations please see the text. With permission by [5]

mon femoral vein is examined together with the SFJ. It can be seen in cross-section and in longitudinal view. In the popliteal fossa, the popliteal vein structure and flow pattern is best seen in longitudinal view. However, a cross-section is best to rule out a thrombosis (see Fig. 4.37). In order for reflux to arise from the deep vein into a superficial vein, the reflux must start in the deep vein. This can lead to the incorrect interpretation, that also the deep vein has also reflux (see Fig. 4.38) [14, 15]. Thrombosis or post-thrombotic changes are visualised as hyperechoic structures inside the vein (see Fig. 4.39).

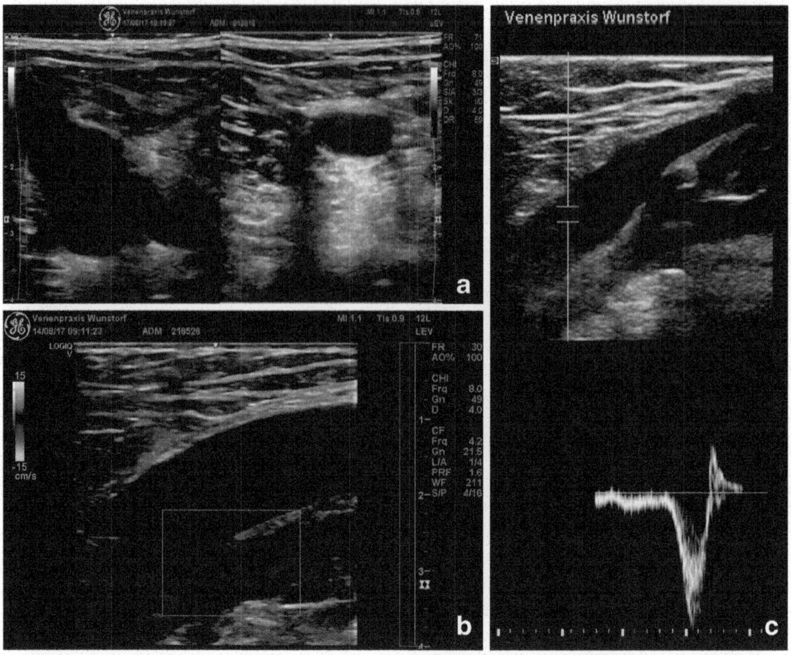

Fig. 4.37 Normal deep veins. (**a**) Compression ultrasound to rule out the presence or absence of a thrombus. This should be done and documented before any treatment of the superficial vein is performed. On the left part of the image is cross-section without compression, where the common femoral vein and sapheno-femoral junction, as well as tributary (blue arrows) and common femoral artery (red arrows) are seen. On the right part is a cross-section at the same place with compression. Only the artery lumen remains (red arrows). The veins have been completely compressed, demonstrating absence of thrombotic material. (**b**) Longitudinal representation of a normal popliteal vein and artery (artery with red blood flow). The vein has smooth walls without bulges or thickenings. (**c**) Flow curve in a normal popliteal vein, measured slightly ahead of the knee crease

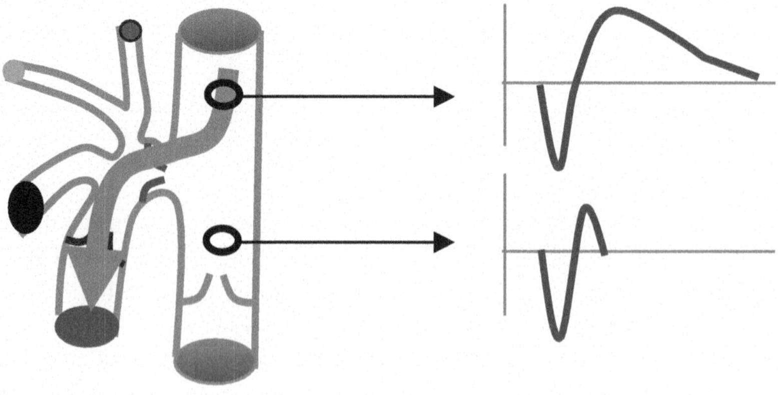

Fig. 4.38 Flow in the deep vein (CFV) above and below the sapheno-femoral junction in a patient with terminal valve incompetence (Compare Fig. 4.13). In the CFV the flow curve shows a reflux in diastole. This is the flow from the deep vein draining pathologically into the GSV when there is superficial vein incompetence. After treating the superficial vein incompetence, the reflux in the deep vein will stop, because there will be nowhere for the blood to go. Distal to the junction, the flow is normal in the deep vein. With permission by [18]

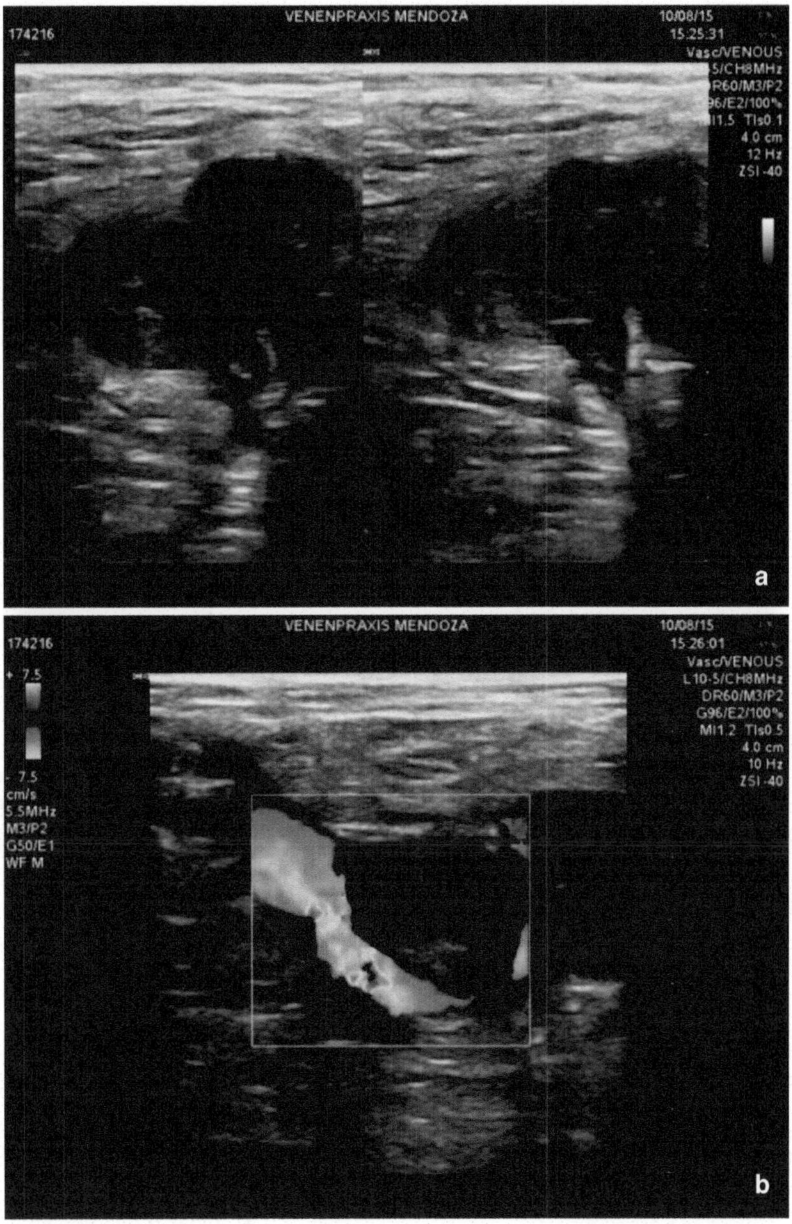

Fig. 4.39 (**a**) Cross-section of the left groin without compression (left) and with compression (right). (Superficial) femoral artery, red arrows; profound femoral artery, orange arrows; CFV, blue arrows. With the compression, the deep vein is not compressed, demonstrating the presence of a thrombus. (**b**) Colour-coded ultrasound of the same site without any manoeuvre. Permanent blood flow from the GSV into the CFV, around the thrombus

4.10 A Routine Exploration

Deep veins can be examined in the lying, sitting or standing position.

A routine examination of the superficial veins should be performed in the standing position. Every specialist is free to develop his standards, but the routine should be always the same to avoid forgetting a part of the exploration.

The following routine is an example:

- Start in the right groin with in B-mode, colour and PW flow:
  - The common femoral vein (also with compression)
  - The artery
  - Sapheno-femoral junction with all its branches

- Follow the GSV down to the ankle, measuring:
  - The diameter at the proximal thigh
  - Blood flow at proximal thigh
  - The site of any calibre changes
  - Exploring flow in visible tributaries and perforating veins
- Turn the patient with the back to the examiner and explore the knee crease in B-mode and Duplex:
  - Popliteal vein (also with compression)
  - Popliteal artery
  - Sapheno-popliteal junction and Giacomini vein, if present, follow it up to the thigh
- Follow the SSV down to the ankle, measuring:
  - The diameter and blood flow below the knee
  - The site of any calibre changes
  - Flow in visible tributaries and perforating veins
- Look at any additional visible varicose veins and examine their origin and draining pathways

4.10.1 Questions to Be Answered at the End of the Examination: Great Saphenous Vein

Morphology

- Is there any anomaly of the sapheno-femoral junction?
- Is an aneurysm present?
- Is the great saphenous vein visible in the fascial compartment throughout its length?
- What is its diameter at the standardised point 10–15 cm below the junction?
- Are there any changes in saphenous calibre?
- Is its course typical in relation to topographical anatomy?
- Is there a duplication or aplastic segments present over part of its course?
- Is there evidence of thrombosis or post-thrombotic changes?
- Are any dilated tributaries or perforating veins apparent in the course of the great saphenous vein?
- Are there any pathological soft-tissue changes surrounding the great saphenous vein?
- Has all or part of the saphenous vein been treated before?

Function

- Is there reflux through the sapheno-femoral junction?
- Is the terminal valve competent?
- Is the preterminal valve competent?
- Are the superficial inguinal tributary veins competent (including AASV)?
- Is there reflux in the great saphenous vein?
- Where is the proximal reflux source?
- Are tributaries or perforating veins involved in the recirculation circuit?
- Does the reflux leave the great saphenous vein by a tributary or a perforating vein?
- Are one or more segments of the vein refluxing?
- How is the draining pathway of the saphenous vein?

4.10.2 Questions to Be Answered at the End of the Exploration: Small Saphenous Vein

Morphology

- Does the small saphenous vein join the popliteal vein?
- Is an aneurysm present?
- At which level is the sapheno-popliteal junction in relation to the posterior knee crease?
- Is the small saphenous vein connected to muscle veins in the region of the junction?
- Does a thigh extension of the small saphenous vein exist?
- Does it become a Giacomini vein?
- Is there any anomaly in the junction of the small saphenous vein?
- What is its diameter at a standardised point, 5 cm below its junction?
- Are there any sudden changes in calibre?
- Is its course typical or does it deviate or duplicate?
- Does any segment have superficial vein thrombosis or post-thrombotic alteration?

- Are any dilated tributaries or perforating veins along the small saphenous vein's course?
- Are there any remarkable findings in the tissues surrounding the small saphenous vein?

Functional

- Is there reflux in the junction of the small saphenous vein refluxing?
- Is the thigh extension or the vein of Giacomini competent?
- Are the muscle veins competent?
- Does the small saphenous vein have reflux?
- Where does the proximal reflux source arise from?
- Does the reflux leave the small saphenous vein by a tributary or a perforating vein?
- Have one or more segments demonstrated reflux?

4.10.3 Questions to Be Answered at the End of the Exploration: Perforating Veins

Morphology

- Are there any dilated perforating veins in the course of the great and small saphenous veins?
- Are there any visible perforating veins in other typical locations, such as the posterior arch vein and the back or lateral side of the thigh or calf?
- If so, is it a muscle perforating vein (connection between deep vein, muscle vein via perforating vein to a superficial vein), and is there a posttraumatic cause in the case of dilation?
- Have the perforating veins suffered post-thrombotic damage?
- What is their diameter?

Functional in perforating veins of large diameter (>3 mm):

- Is the perforating vein incompetent and which is the reflux source?
- Is the perforating vein a re-entry point with draining flow?
- Is the reflux in the perforating vein systolic (bypassing shunt) or diastolic (filling varicose veins)?

4.11 Investigation After Treatment of Veins

Duplex ultrasound not only provides an evaluation of the patient prior to intervention but also a follow-up after the treatment. This is important to monitor the success of the intervention, recognise side effects or complications and determine the pathogenesis behind possible recurrences. Historically, phlebography was only applied when there were visible recurrences, but this test is invasive. Ultrasound does not harm the patient yet provides a comprehensive quality control instrument for the physician.

A basic issue when performing a follow-up is a good preoperative documentation of the findings. This is the only way to evaluate technical or tactical errors if the expected result is not achieved.

This chapter focusses on the duplex findings of the veins after saphenous sparing surgery is commented.

The hallmark of effect in all saphenous sparing intervention is the reduction in calibre of the saphenous veins in the follow-up [14, 15, 23].

4.11.1 Flow Patterns After CHIVA

In case of CHIVA 2 after surgery there are two possibilities:

- Competent saphenous vein (complete success of the strategy in one step)
- Same or less reflux in saphenous vein with drainage either through a perforating vein or a new tributary

When the reflux point has been interrupted, a distinction must be made between incompetent perforating veins or junctions.

After interruption of a perforating vein: If the perforating vein was the only reflux source, after its interruption the expected flow in the GSV or SSV will be antegrade in its whole length.

After **interruption of a junction**: Here the flow in the saphenous vein will be less than before the intervention but still footwards ("deflusso" or a deflux) (see Sects. 6.3.4.1 and 6.14.3 and Fig. 4.40). This blood flow originates from the physiologic blood flow from the tributaries. When the proximal exit point of the saphenous vein is closed, this tributary blood has to flow downwards to meet the next perforating vein and drain into the deep vein. The amount and velocity of this flow is very small. Often it appears after some delay following a provocation manoeuvre.

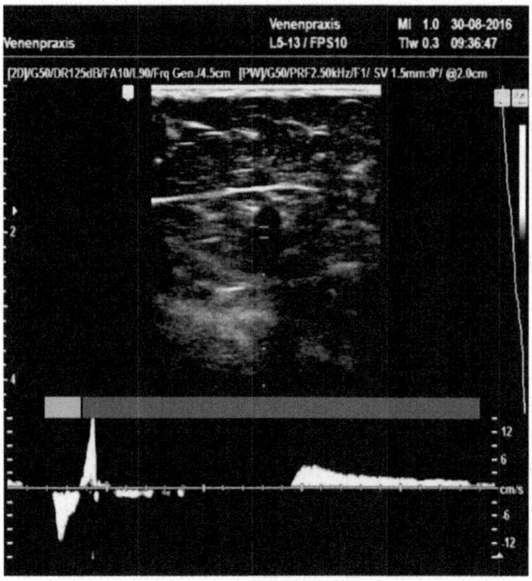

Fig. 4.40 Cross-section of the GSV at the mid-thigh after a crossotomy. Muscular systole (green line) with antegrade flow, followed by a short retrograde flow in diastole representing valve closure. A few seconds later, a very slow downwards flow is seen. It represents the drainage of the tributaries through the saphenous vein

This downwards flow is often confused with a persistent or new reflux when comparing crossectomy alone with crossectomy and stripping [24]. If a patent GSV is left in situ and connected with tributaries and perforating veins, the only possible flow direction is down, towards the lower perforating vein, as upwards flow is not possible, when this exit has been closed. Without this drainage pathway, the complete GSV would close by thrombosis after the intervention.

4.11.2 Flow Patterns in GSV After ASVAL

After the mini-phlebectomy of the varicose reservoir, the reflux in the great saphenous vein will automatically be lesser or even abolished. Depending on the preoperative situation of the saphenous vein reflux, we will find one of the following flow possibilities (see Table 4.3).

Table 4.3 Postoperative flow in GSV depending on the preoperative flow pattern

Preoperative	Postoperative after ASVAL
Segmental reflux in GSV without incompetence of the junction	The GSV will be competent
Competent terminal valve, incompetent preterminal valve, no draining perforating vein on GSV	The GSV will be competent in about 95% of cases (compare Fig. 6.43)
Competent terminal valve, incompetent preterminal valve, draining perforating vein on GSV	The GSV will have little reflux, draining through the perforating vein on the GSV. This situation can remain stable for years without clinics or cosmetic complaints (compare Fig. 6.41)
Incompetent terminal and preterminal valve and no draining perforating vein on GSV	The GSV can be competent or a tributary or draining perforating vein can develop a recurrent reflux in the GSV (compare Fig. 6.17b)
Incompetent terminal and preterminal valve and draining perforating vein on GSV	The GSV will have little reflux draining through the perforating vein on the GSV. This situation can remain stable for years without clinics or cosmetic complaints

4.11.3 Flow Patterns After Extraluminal Valvuloplasty

After the extraluminal valvuloplasty, the GSV is expected to be competent (see Chap. 13). The refluxing tributaries, if left in situ, will no longer be fed retrogradely by refluxing blood from the deep vein and will reduce their calibre. Alternatively, they will be fed with blood from the distal, antegrade flowing GSV (forming a shunt type 2 in this case).

If the valvuloplasty fails, two possible findings can be expected:

- Thrombosis of the proximal GSV causing a complete or partial obstruction of the saphenous vein till the next large perforating vein
- Reduced reflux in the GSV through a smaller SFJ

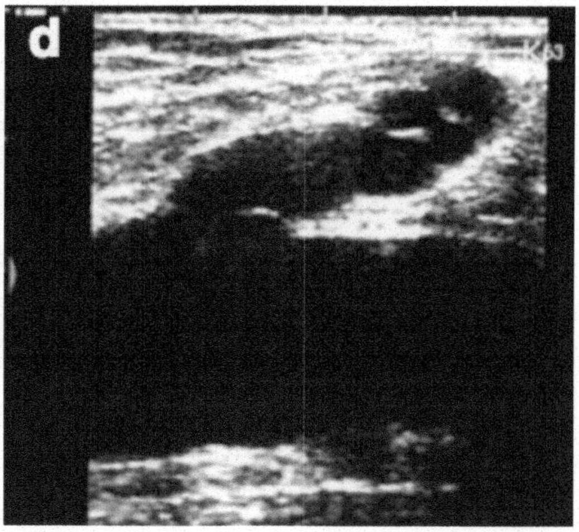

Fig. 4.41 Longitudinal representation of the SFJ: after ligation of the great saphenous vein approximately 2 cm distal to the SFJ in the context of a stripping procedure. The valve can be seen at the sapheno-femoral junction demonstrating that the vein has been left in situ. Typically, the formation of large convoluted venous tributaries arising from the distal end of the stump can be observed. With permission by [5]

4.11.4 Analysing Technical Errors

Technical errors refer to the operating technique. There are lots of possible errors if a crossotomy is not performed correctly, like the errors also known from the classical crossectomy. Leaving a stump is always a technical error leading to recidives (see Fig. 4.41).

At the popliteal junction, surgery is much more complex than in the groin region. If a Giacomini vein is present, the "stump" of the SSV is washed by this vein and therefore the stump may act as a beneficial draining pathway. Nevertheless, a reflux can still arise from this proximal segment of the SSV if a tactical error occurred, like the interruption of the junction when there is systolic reflux (see Sect. 4.11.5).

After performing CHIVA 2, a recurrence can arise at the site of the interruption if a non-flush ligation of the tributary is performed at the level of the saphenous vein (see Fig. 4.42). The consequence is either a matting or a new tributary with reflux. The same can happen after ASVAL, in case the reflux load after ablation of the reservoir in the GSV is large.

4.11.5 Analysing Tactical Errors

A tactical error occurs when the preoperative flow pattern is not properly analysed. This can happen in every strategy, but in CHIVA it will be noticed immediately, as the pathways are left in situ and not obliterated or removed. If the reflux source is not eliminated, the reflux path will persist and it will look like no change after intervention. Alternatively, if the system is interrupted without leaving a good drainage pathway, a non-drained situation will provoke early matting through little reticular veins. On ultrasound, the calibre of the GSV will not decrease.

The classical tactical error in CHIVA is to perform a crossotomy, which is a ligation of the GSV between the tributaries and the deep vein at the ostial level, in patients with pelvic reflux, also called para-ostial reflux. The reflux source will remain untouched and continue to fill the GSV (see Fig. 4.43). Not being aware of the fact that about 30% of patients have an isolated or combined para-ostial reflux (see Table 4.1) and applying a crossotomy without interruption of the refluxive tributary to all patients with SFJ reflux

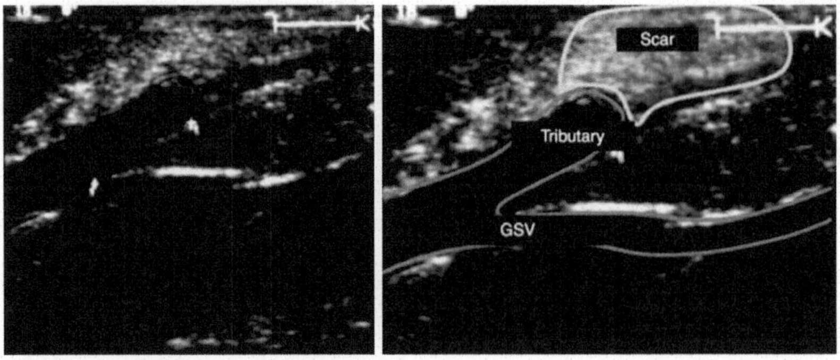

Fig. 4.42 Longitudinal representation of the inner aspect of the proximal thigh after surgery (CHIVA 2: Interruption of a tributary at the GSV). Left native image. Right annotated image: the scar (yellow) was not at the level of the junction between the tributary and the GSV, but distally. This was not a flush ligation but left a stump of proximal tributary. This resulted in a clinical recidive, with a visible tributary on the skin and persistence of reflux in GSV. With permission by [5]

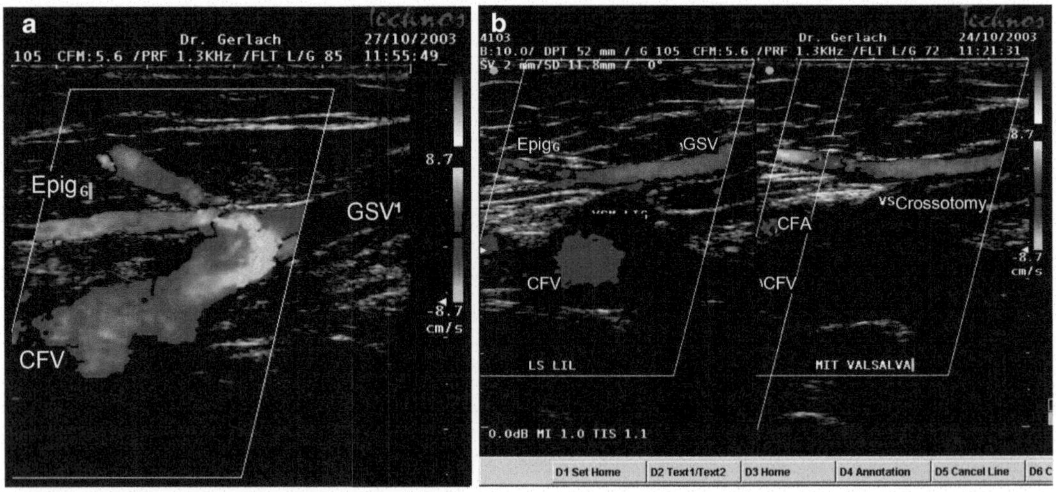

Fig. 4.43 (**a**) Preoperative image in longitudinal view of the SFJ in a patient with a refluxing epigastric vein. (**b**) Postoperative image of the same SFJ after crossotomy with persistent reflux from the epigastric vein into the GSV. Tactical error. From Dr. Horst Gerlach, Mannheim, with kind permission

would lead to reflux persistence due to tactical error in 30% of all treated patients!

Another tactical error is to close an open bypassing shunt. This will induce recurrences at the site of the ligation, like in the open bypassing shunt described in Sect. 3.9.3, if the Giacomini vein or the SSV is interrupted in the knee crease. The recurrence will appear soon after intervention with lots of new vessels through the scar.

4.11.6 Assessment After Endoluminal Treatment of the Junction

After endoluminal closure of the GSV or the SSV in the context of CHIVA, the first follow-up should be at 1 week to rule out a deep vein thrombosis and also to make sure the superficial vein has been closed.

In cross-section, the deep vein at the level of the SFJ is visualised and a compression ultrasound performed to make sure in the deep vein there is no thrombus. The SFJ is examined looking for the proximal end of the heat-induced closure of the vein. This should look like a superficial vein thrombus. This usually ends at the confluence of a tributary, which acts to wash out the SFJ. An "EHIT" (endoluminal heat-induced thrombus) occurs when thrombotic material from the heat closure is encroaching into the deep vein lumen. This has to be excluded. Although the natural history is usually benign, anticoagulation for 6 weeks is often recommended.

The flow in the proximal GSV is assessed with colour-coded duplex. No flow is expected beyond the SFJ in the proximal part of the GSV. This part of the GSV has to be uncompressible in cross-section.

One possible failure of endoluminal CHIVA is that the reflux from the deep vein continues through the terminal valve and into the anterior accessory saphenous vein. This pathway was not refluxing prior to the intervention (in this case, it would have been treated). But for unknown reasons, in some cases a preoperatively non-visible or very thin AASV gets incompetent and feeds the distal GSV with reflux via the communicating vein (see Sect. 6.15.2).

It is important to inform the patients about this fact in case of choosing endoluminal junction treatment prior to intervention. The AASV may need to be closed with either ultrasound-guided sclerotherapy or an endoluminal ablation.

4.12 Documentation of the Findings

The findings of the examination have to be documented as images and as a description of the venous pathways.

The images have to include:

- Compression ultrasound of the deep veins at least at the common femoral vein and popliteal vein site, as well as a flow curve inside these veins prior to therapy. This is important to make sure no pathology was present before the intervention. If a prior pathology is present, its documentation demonstrates that this wasn't provoked by the intervention.
- Diameters of the pathological veins: GSV at the junction and at proximal thigh (10–15 cm distally from the groin) measured in cross-section, SSV below the knee crease.
- A flow curve inside the pathological vein segments in PW mode to demonstrate the fact that there was a reflux prior to intervention.

The description might be with a drawing or as a text (see Sect. 11.2.3 and Fig. 11.4). It is always helpful after the intervention to determine exactly which situation was found before the treatment. This is not only important to analyse possible tactical errors in case of failure or for a scientific investigation in larger series, but it will also help to defend yourself in a legal situation.

Literature

1. Trendelenburg F. Ueber die Unterbindung der Vena saphena magna bei Unterschenkelvaricen. Bruns Beitr Klein Chir. 1891;7(1):195–210.
2. Cavezzi A, Labropoulos N, Partsch H, Ricci S, Caggiati A, Myers K, Nicolaides A, Smith PC. Duplex ultrasound investigation of the veins in chronic venous disease of the lower limbs—UIP consensus document. Part II. Anatomy. Eur J Vasc Endovasc Surg. 2006;31:288–99.
3. Coleridge-Smith P, Labropoulos N, Partsch H, Myers K, Nicolaides A, Cavezzi A. Duplex ultrasound investigation of the veins in chronic venous disease of the lower limbs—UIP consensus document. Part I. Basic principles. Eur J Vasc Endovasc Surg. 2006;31(1):83–92.
4. De Maeseneer M, Pichot O, Cavezzi A, Earnshaw J, van Rij A, Lurie F, Smith PC. Duplex ultrasound investigation of the veins of the lower limbs after treatment for varicose veins e UIP consensus document. EJVS. 2011;42(1):89–102.
5. Mendoza E, Lattimer CR, Morrison N. Duplex ultrasound of superficial leg veins. New York: Springer; 2014.
6. Lattimer C, Azzam M, Papaconstandinou JA, Villasin M, Ash S, Kalodiki E. Neuromuscular electrical stimulation reduces sludge in the popliteal vein.

J Vasc Surg Venous Lymphat Disord. 2017. pii: S2213–333X(17)30448–1. https://doi:10.1016/j.jvsv.2017.09.008. [Epub ahead of print].
7. LattimerCR,FranceschiC,KalodikiE.Optimizingcalfmuscle pump function. Phlebology. 2017:268355517709410. https://doi.org/10.1177/0268355517709410. [Epub ahead of print]. PMID: 28530489.
8. Weskott HP, Mendoza E, Lattimer CR. The ultrasound scanner. In: Mendoza E, Lattimer CR, Morrison N, editors. Duplex ultrasound of superficial leg veins. New York: Springer; 2014.
9. Labropoulos N, Tiongson J, Pryor L, Tassiopoulos AK, Kang SS, Mansour A, Baker WH. Definition of venous reflux in lower-extremity veins. J Vasc Surg. 2003;38:793–8.
10. Habenicht M, Rabe E, Amsler F, Mendoza E. Toe elevation manoeuvre to assess venous reflux in comparison to manual calf compression and release. Vasa. 2016;45(4):299–304.
11. Jeanneret C, Labs KH, Aschwanden M, Bollinger A, et al. Physiological reflux and venous diameter change in the proximal lower limb veins during a standardised Valsalva manoeuvre. Eur J Vasc Endovasc Surg. 1999;17:398–403.
12. Lattimer CR, Azzam M, Kalodiki E, Geroulakos G. Quantifying saphenous recirculation in patients with primary lower extremity venous reflux. J Vasc Surg Venous Lymphat Disord. 2016;4(2):179–86. https://doi.org/10.1016/j.jvsv.2015.09.006. Epub 2015 Nov 24. PMID: 26993865.
13. Franceschi C. Mésures et interprétation des flux veineux lors des manœvres de stimulation. Compressions manuelles et manœvre de Paraná Indice dynamique de reflux IDR et indice de Psatakis. J Mal Vasc. 1997;22(2):1–5.
14. Mendoza E. Diameter reduction of the great saphenous vein and the common femoral vein after CHIVA long-term results. Phlebologie. 2013;42:65–9.
15. Mendoza E. Popliteal reflux in incompetent small saphenous veins. Phlebologie. 2013;42:37–41.
16. Lattimer CR, Mendoza E. Superficial venous reflux duration and cessation with two concurrent duplex probes. J Vasc Surg Venous Lymphat Disord. 2015;3(2):154–60.
17. Lattimer CR, Azzam M, Kalodiki E, Geroulakos G. Venous filling time using air-plethysmography correlates highly with great saphenous vein reflux time using duplex. Phlebology. 2014;29(2):90–7. https://doi.org/10.1258/phleb.2012.012042. Epub 2013 May 6. PMID: 23035010.
18. Mendoza E. The sapheno-femoral junction in ultrasound. Phlebologie. 2014;43:42–5.
19. Zollmann P, Zollmann C, Zollmann P, Veltman J, Kerzig D, Doerler M, Stücker M. Determining the origin of superficial venous reflux in the groin with duplex ultrasound and implications for varicose vein surgery. J Vasc Surg Venous Lymphat Disord. 2017;5(1):82–6.
20. Stücker M, Moritz R, Altmeyer P, Reich-Schupke S. New concept: different types of insufficiency of the saphenofemoral junction identified by duplex as a chance for a more differentiated therapy of the great saphenous vein. Phlebology. 2013;28:268–74.
21. Mendoza E, Stücker M. Duplex-ultrasound assessment of the saphenofemoral junction (Review). Phlebological Review. 2015;23(3):1–8.
22. Mendoza E. Handbuch CHIVA, Arrien GmbH; 2002.
23. Mendoza E, Amsler F. CHIVA with endoluminal procedures: LASER versus VNUS—treatment of the saphenofemoral junction. Phlebologie. 2017;46:5–12.
24. Dwerryhouse S, Davies B, Harradine K, Earnshaw JJ. Stripping the long saphenous vein reduces the rate of reoperation for recurrent varicose vein: five-year results of a randomized trial. J Vasc Surg. 1999;29(4):589–92.

Second-Level Imaging 5

Sergio Gianesini, Paolo Zamboni,
and Erika Mendoza

5.1 Introduction

Technological advancements are bringing awareness of previously underdiagnosed and undertreated pathological conditions such as iliac vein obstruction influencing lower limb venous drainage. A great interest is arising in modern phlebology in the identification of obstructive and compressive causes of venous drainage impairment.

On the other side, an increasing knowledge and awareness has been developed on the pelvic congestion syndrome and on its impact on lower limb chronic venous disease. Vein specialists must be aware of the possible pathological conditions inside and outside the same lower limb site. Moreover, they must be aware of the diagnostic potentials offered today.

S. Gianesini, M.D., Ph.D. (✉)
Vascular Diseases Center, University of Ferrara, Ferrara, Italy

USUHS University, Bethesda, MD, USA

P. Zamboni, M.D.
School of Vascular Surgery and Vascular Diseases Center, University of Ferrara, Ferrara, Italy

Unit of Translational Surgery, AOU Ferrara, Ferrara, Italy
e-mail: zmp@unife.it

E. Mendoza, M.D., Ph.D.
Venenpraxis, Wunstorf, Germany
e-mail: erika.mendoza@t-online.de

5.2 Pathological Scenario: Iliac and Pelvic Venous Drainage Impairment

Chronic venous disease and venous thrombosis have been reported more frequently on the left lower limb rather than on the right one: a fact that already Virchow attributed to the possible compression of the left iliac vein by the crossing iliac artery [1, 2]. At the same time, cadaver dissections reported a surprisingly high percentage of iliac intraluminal lesions that affect iliac venous drainage, in up to 30% of unselected cases [3, 4]. These intraluminal lesions have been described as webs, ridges, velums, bridges, quilted wall adhesions, and even total occlusion [5].

The genesis of these lesions remains a matter of debate, combining the possible traumatic effect of the nearby artery pulsation with a possible ontogenesis. Magnetic resonance imaging points out the possible overlapping presence of intrinsic and extrinsic causes of iliac drainage impairment in up to 66% of patients [6].

Since terms like "iliac compression syndrome," Cockett syndrome, and May-Thurner syndrome are often used wrongly as synonyms, it is suggested to use the term non-thrombotic iliac vein lesions (NIVL) to indicate this kind of iliac vein drainage impairment [7]. As the imaging detection of an obstacle to iliac vein drainage is not sufficient for a non-thrombotic iliac vein lesion (NIVL) diagnosis, clinical findings are

P. Zamboni et al. (eds.), *Saphenous Vein-Sparing Strategies in Chronic Venous Disease*,
https://doi.org/10.1007/978-3-319-70638-2_5

fundamental. Typical presentation includes recurrent deep venous thrombosis, lower limb swelling and pain, ulceration, venous claudication, and chronic venous disease.

Less frequently this condition can lead to phlegmasia cerulea dolens, superficial venous thrombosis, and bilateral- or right-sided symptoms [8–10].

Non-thrombotic iliac vein lesion (NIVL) can present an acute or chronic onset. The first one is easier to detect since it is easily associated with sudden leg edema and redness. The chronic condition is more difficult to be detected and requires a full investigation of patient history, physical examination, and diagnostic imaging. In the diagnostic process, it must be remembered that also trauma, surgery, recent catheterization radiation, and malignancies can be involved in iliac venous drainage impairment.

On the other side, pelvic congestion syndrome (PCS), rightfully already described by Hobbs in 1990, thanks to the diagnostic technological advancements, is now always more linked to its impact on lower limb venous drainage [11].

Such condition must be known both by vein and obstetrics and gynecology specialists dealing with patients presenting pelvic pain and varicose veins fed by pelvic refluxing points. Pelvic heaviness exacerbated by the standing position and particularly present at the end of the day and by the premenstrual period, dysmenorrhea, dyspareunia, postcoital pain, and dysuria are all medical history data suggesting the diagnosis.

In some cases, also hematuria and left low back pain are observed, so suggesting a possible extrinsic compression of the left renal vein between the aorta and the superior mesenteric artery (so-called nutcracker phenomenon). Also, hemorrhoids, vulvar, and gluteal varicosities are clear signs of potential impairment of the pelvic venous system.

Typically, these patients are multiparous women with a history of venous and gynecological disorders.

As suggested by Gaweesh [12, 13], pelvic obstruction could be the reason for varicose veins in patients without a history of deep venous thrombosis, thereby offering stenting of the iliac veins as a solution. If this obstruction hypothesis was true, it would introduce a new industry of treatment for simple varicose veins. Recent investigations with air plethysmography have questioned the obstruction hypothesis by demonstrating improved gravitational venous drainage in patients with varicose veins. The venous drainage index (VDI) in mL/s was faster, presumably because the outflow pathways were larger as a result of the reflux [14]. Further investigations on a tilt table have defined a cutoff point in the venous drainage index (VDI) to differentiate between proximal obstruction on one hand and normal subjects or patients with varicose veins without pelvic obstruction on the other [15]. This simple investigation could be performed as a first step, noninvasive screening test. After demonstrating a prolonged VDI, the site and nature of the obstruction can be investigated further using the more invasive imaging techniques like abdominal or transvaginal ultrasound, contrast venography, CT, MRI, or intravenous ultrasound.

5.3 Second-Level Imaging

In pelvic congestion syndrome, a detailed sonographic analysis must include the assessment of the escape points from the pelvic region (see Chap. 8), together with an evaluation by abdominal scanning. In this last case, the patient must be fasting and have had a residue-free diet. The scanning must include the ovarian veins, which are considered pathological when the reflux last more than 2 s and the diameter is larger than 8 mm in standing position [16].

Endocavitary (transvaginal or transrectal) examination by a 5–7.5 MHz probe is the primary way to visualize pelvic varicosities [17]. Phlebography has been considered the reference imaging technique for pelvic congestion syndrome assessment, to be performed after a preliminary ultrasound assessment [18]. Nowadays, after the improvement of techniques and knowledge around the application of duplex, this method seems to have become the gold standard [19].

Looking at the pelvic congestion syndrome investigation, as well as at non-thrombotic iliac vein lesions (NIVL), computed tomography and magnetic resonance imaging are to be considered in order to rule out the suspect of potentially involved extra- or intraluminal masses exerting compression. They should be performed in specialized centers with experience in venous imaging.

5.4 Third-Level Imaging

The introduction of intravascular ultrasound (IVUS) technique has supported previous finding in demonstrating that the diagnostic sensitivity of venography for non-thrombotic iliac vein lesion (NIVL) is only on the order of about 50% [20]. Considering the absence of radiation and its sensitivity above 90%, intravascular ultrasound (IVUS) is now considered a diagnostic standard in this type of lesions.

The progressive diffusion of intravascular ultrasound (IVUS) has also revealed a broader spectrum of non-thrombotic iliac vein lesion, including multiple distal arterial crossover points. In some cases, the combined use of venography and IVUS is helpful to get oriented in the complex scenario of "para"-physiological iliac lesions, where a certain degree of compression or stenosis is not to be considered pathological.

This is particularly true considering that the same patient can present a degree of compression varying over a short period of time [21]. Even if there is no established diagnostic imaging criterion, studies show that a persistent narrowing of the iliac vein should be demonstrated, associated with permanent spurs, independently of the patient position to state the diagnosis of non-thrombotic iliac vein lesion.

A reduction of more than 50% of the vein caliber is considered a valid indicator of stenosis [22]. A secondary indicator is the activation of collateral circles, intraluminal spurs, and changes greater than 2 mmHg across the stenotic lesion in supine position [23]. The diagnostics involved in this assessment include ultrasonography, plethysmography, computed tomography, magnetic resonance venography, ascending contrast venography, and IVUS.

5.5 Second-Level Consultation

Modern phlebology represents a fascinating and wide medical science, involving skills and expertise far above the simple assessment of lower limb venous drainage. Vein specialists must be aware of the several pathophysiological aspects of venous disease, developing diagnostic and technical skills that overcome the traditional lower limb venous scanning. If this is not possible in their own office, networks with specialized radiologists or phlebologists have to grow with mutual exchange of information.

At the same time, it's fundamental to develop growing interactions among the different specialties involved with venous treatment. Surgeons, obstetricians and gynecologists, radiologists, and dermatologists must promote a constant interaction in order to manage at best conditions iliac vein drainage impairment and pelvic congestion syndrome, which have been underdiagnose and undertreated for too long.

Literature

1. McMurrich JP. The occurrence of congenital adhesions in the common iliac veins and their relation to thrombosis of the femoral and iliac veins. Am J Med Sci. 1908;135:342–6.
2. Virchow R. Uber die Erweiterung kleinerer Gefasse. Arch Path Anat. 1851;3:4279.
3. Cockett FB, Thomas ML. The iliac compression syndrome. Br J Surg. 1965;52:816–21.
4. Ehrich WE, Krumbhaar EB. A frequent obstructive anomaly of the mouth of the left common ilia vein. Am Heart J. 1943;26:737–50.
5. May R, Thurner J. The cause of the predominantly sinistral occurrence of thrombosis of the pelvic veins. Angiology. 1957;8:419–27.
6. Kibbe MR, Ujiki M, Goodwin AL, et al. Iliac vein compression in an asymptomatic patient population. J Vasc Surg. 2004;39:937–43.
7. Raju S. Iliac vein outflow obstruction in 'primary' chronic venous disease. Phlebolymphology. 2008;15(1):12–6.
8. Hurst DR, Forauer AR, Bloom JR, Green eld LJ, Wake eld TW, Williams DM. Diagnosis and endovascular

treatment of iliocaval compression syndrome. J Vasc Surg. 2001;34:106–13. https://doi.org/10.1067/mva.2001.114213. PMID: 11436082.
9. Knipp BS, Ferguson E, Williams DM, Dasika NJ, Cwikiel W, Henke PK, Wakefield TW. Factors associated with outcome after interventional treatment of symptomatic iliac vein compression syndrome. J Vasc Surg. 2007;46:743–9. https://doi.org/10.1016/j.jvs.2007.05.048. PMID: 17903652.
10. Shebel ND, Whalen CC. Diagnosis and management of iliac vein compression syndrome. J Vasc Nurs. 2005;23:10–17; quiz 18–19. https://doi.org/10.1016/j.jvn.2004.12.001. PMID: 15741959.
11. Hobbs JT. The pelvic congestion syndrome. Br J Hosp Med. 1990;43:200–6.
12. Gaweesh AS, Kayed MH, Gaweesh TY, et al. Underlying deep venous abnormalities in patients with unilateral chronic venous disease. Phlebology. 2013;28:426–31.
13. Gaweesh AS. Impeded venous drainage: novel view of chronic venous disease pathophysiology. Med Hypotheses. 2009;73:548–52.
14. Lattimer CR, Kalodiki E, Mendoza E. Gravitational venous drainage is significantly faster in patients with varicose veins. Phlebology. 2016;31(8):546–53.
15. Lattimer CR, Mendoza E. Reappraisal of the utility of the tilt-table in the investigation of venous disease. Eur J Vasc Endovasc Surg. 2016;52:854–61.
16. Park SJ, Lim JW, Ko YT, et al. Diagnosis of pelvic congestion syndrome using transabdominal and transvaginal sonography. Am J Roentgenol. 2004;182:683–8.
17. Haag T, Manhès H. Veines et algies pelviennes chroniques. J Mal Vasc. 1999;24:267–74.
18. Balian E, Lasry JL, Coppé G, et al. Pelviperineal venous insufficiency and varicose veins of the lower limbs. Phlebolymphology. 2008;15(1):17–26.
19. Whiteley MS, Dos Santos SJ, Harrison CC, Holdstock JM, Lopez AJ. Transvaginal duplex ultrasonography appears to be the gold standard investigation for the haemodynamic evaluation of pelvic venous reflux in the ovarian and internal iliac veins in women. Phlebology. 2015;30(10):706–13.
20. Neglen P, Raju S. Intravascular ultrasound scan evaluation of the obstructed vein. J Vasc Surg. 2002;35:694–700.
21. Brinegar KN, Sheth RA, Khademhosseini A, Bautista J, Oklu R. Iliac vein compression syndrome: clinical, imaging and pathologic findings. World J Radiol. 2015;7(11):375–81.
22. Liu Z, Gao N, Shen L, Yang J, Zhu Y, Li Z, Si Y. Endovascular treatment for symptomatic iliac vein compression syndrome: a prospective consecutive series of 48 patients. Ann Vasc Surg. 2014;28:695–704. https://doi.org/10.1016/j.avsg.2013.05.019. PMID: 24559785.
23. O'Sullivan GJ, Semba CP, Bittner CA, Kee ST, Razavi MK, Sze DY, Dake MD. Endovascular management of iliac vein compression (May-Thurner) syndrome. J Vasc Interv Radiol. 2000;11:823–36. https://doi.org/10.1016/S1051-0443(07)61796-5. PMID: 10928517.

Part II

CHIVA

6 Saphenous Sparing Strategy in the CHIVA Context

Erika Mendoza

Abbreviations

AASV	Anterior accessory saphenous vein
GSV	Great saphenous vein
PASV	Posterior accessory saphenous vein
RET	Reflux elimination test
SFJ	Sapheno-femoral junction
SPJ	Sapheno-popliteal junction
SSV	Small saphenous vein

6.1 Evidence-Based Rationale of the Strategy

Varicose veins are still of unknown reason. Though there has been progress in understanding through applied physics and anatomy since the Doppler and later the duplex ultrasound allowed to analyse recirculations, though histology and tissue mediator changes offer possible explanations, the last reason for the dilatation and flow reversion in superficial leg veins is still to be found.

The destruction of reflux pathways was a good solution over many years, when no other instrument was available to stop the consequences of venous reflux, like skin changes, pain and ulceration.

E. Mendoza, M.D., Ph.D
Venenpraxis, Wunstorf, Germany
e-mail: erika.mendoza@t-online.de

Already early investigations about the effect of compression on the venous wall histology which nearly recovered to normal after 7 days of compression hosiery [1] contradicted the dogma that saphenous wall degeneration in varicose disease is irreversible. All the CHIVA research published later (see Chaps. 1 and 10) and a Cochrane review [2] state that recidives are less frequent if saphenous veins are spared during surgery. Thus, and analogous to all the other surgical fields, the organ preservation should at least be given a chance.

6.2 Instructions for Readers

Persons confronted with CHIVA for the first time often argue that it is too much of information to learn the shunt types and then to learn how to treat them. Trying to prevent this confusion, the authors have explained the shunts in Chap. 3 (see Sects. 3.7–3.9). Based on these shunts, Franceschi developed the treatment strategies for haemodynamic flow correction [3–5]. They are based on four principles (see Sect. 6.3.4) and then applied to the shunt types. The schematic flow images throughout the chapter are based on those explained in Chap. 2 (see Fig. 2.5) and also used throughout Chap. 3.

This chapter starts with the international definitions used in the CHIVA context to avoid semantic confusion, which are the bases for

P. Zamboni et al. (eds.), *Saphenous Vein-Sparing Strategies in Chronic Venous Disease*,
https://doi.org/10.1007/978-3-319-70638-2_6

CHIVA (Sect. 6.3). Then, the different approaches to the most frequent shunt types are first analysed "in general" (Sect. 6.4).

Adapting to the usual treatment thinking, which is anatomy-oriented, the different management options of the pathological compartment jumps are described separately first:

- N1 → N2 = deep vein to saphenous vein at the junction (see Sects. 6.5 and 6.7)
- P → N2 or N3 = pelvic reflux into saphenous vein or tributary (see Sect. 6.6)
- Refluxing N2 (Sect. 6.8)
- N1 → N2 = deep vein to the saphenous vein via a perforating vein (see Sect. 6.9)
- N1 → N3 = deep vein into a tributary via a perforating vein (see Sect. 6.9)
- N2 → N3 = saphenous vein into a tributary (see Sect. 6.10)

Please note that re-entry pathways are considered when designing the strategy for the patient but are never treated!

Finally, the acquired knowledge is applied to the treatment decisions in every shunt type in Sect. 6.11 with clinical examples.

The chapter finishes with tips of how to get started, explanation to handle difficult situations like the treatment after superficial vein thrombosis and large varicose veins and outcome evaluation.

6.3 Bases of the CHIVA Strategy and International Terminology

At the World CHIVA Congress in 1998 in Paraná (Argentina), a consensus was reached within the European CHIVA Association to develop a multilingual terminology for anatomical and physiological nomenclature in the context of CHIVA. There had previously been difficulties in comprehension, because of the differing meanings of a given word in different languages. The definitions given below are a basic assumption for international understanding of the CHIVA method.

The recirculation types were further elaborated at the World CHIVA Congress in May 2002 in Berlin/Teupitz; the results of this consensus conference are summarised in Sects. 3.7 and 3.8.

6.3.1 Venous Competence or Incompetence

Venous incompetence is the inability of a vein to provide unidirectional flow towards the heart, appropriate to the heart's functioning, haemodynamic reserves and thermoregulation and independent of the bodily attitude.

Competent venous flow is:

- Unidirectional
- Towards the heart
- Independent of the position of the body

It is adapted to:

- Heart's function
- Thermoregulation
- Haemodynamic reserves

6.3.2 Anatomical Concepts

The muscle fascia covers the muscles. The saphenous fascia covers the saphenous veins and together with the muscle fascia forms the saphenous compartment. The saphenous veins lie directly on the muscle fascia and are covered by the saphenous fascia, so that they course through a fascial tunnel (see Sect. 2.2.3). For this reason, they are also known as "interfascial" veins.

Venous networks: For the purposes of the CHIVA method, veins are divided into four groups according to their position relative to these fasciae, originally with the abbreviation R for "réseau" from French and in English with the abbreviation N for "network".

Classification N1–N4

N1 Network: All the veins which course in the deep compartment delimited by the muscle fascia, like deep veins and perforating veins

N2 Network: All the veins which lie directly on the muscle fascia and below the membranous layer or saphenous fascia, like interfascial veins (saphenous veins, Giacomini vein, proximal segment of the accessory anterior saphenous vein)

N3 Network: All the veins which course between the fasciae and the skin: arch veins, tributaries and all the tiny reticular veins, capillaries and spider veins

N4 Network: These are specific N3 veins that serve to connect N2 veins

- Longitudinal N4: Connections between the same N2 vein (like those connecting two points on the great saphenous vein)
- Transversal N4: Connections between different N2 veins (like those connecting the great saphenous vein with the small saphenous vein)

The vein of Giacomini is sometimes completely interfascial (N2) but functionally connects two different N2 veins (GSV, SSV), so functionally it is a transversal N4 vein.

6.3.3 Haemodynamic Concepts

The blood flow in a vein is defined by:

1. Direction of flow (see Sect. 3.2)
2. Source of its contents (see Sect. 3.4)
3. Volume
4. Pressure

The first two aspects are most important for the purposes of learning about the CHIVA strategy.

6.3.3.1 Direction of Flow

Anterograde or antegrade flow moves in a physiological direction and follows the rule: "big" N to "small" N, superficial to deep:

- N3 – N2 – N1 tributary drains to saphenous vein to deep vein via junction or perforating vein
- N3 – N1 tributary drains to deep vein via perforating vein
- N2 – N1 saphenous vein drains to deep vein via junction or perforating vein

Retrograde flow moves in a pathological or "reverse" direction.

> Note: retrograde is not the same as towards the foot. For example, in the upper veins of the confluence of superficial inguinal veins, flow towards the foot is not pathological.

6.3.3.2 The Source of Its Contents

The usual source of the content of a vein is from superficial veins to deep veins in case of antegrade flow (see Sect. 6.3.3.1).

The reflux source is the point at which blood starts flowing against the compartment rule, it enters one vessel from another in retrograde flow, jumping from a small N into a bigger N.

- N1 → N2 from deep vein into saphenous vein via the junction or a perforating vein
- N2 → N3/N4 from a saphenous vein into a tributary
- N1 → N3 from the deep vein via a perforating vein into a tributary

6.3.3.3 Drainage from the Varicose Vein: Re-entry Points

The re-entry point is the point where the blood in pathological flow re-enters a competent vessel, through which it is drained from the leg to the heart, where the blood changes anatomic compartments again in the physiological way from a big N to a small N (see Sect. 3.5).

- N2 – N1 from a refluxing saphenous vein via a perforating vein to the deep vein
- N3 – N2 from a refluxing tributary into a saphenous vein
- N3/N4 – N1 from a refluxing tributary via a perforating vein into the deep vein

The re-entry point is very often a perforating vein.

The draining vessel, for example, the perforating vein, which is primarily healthy, is thus permanently overloaded by the additional blood volume of the recirculation.

A distended re-entry perforating vein is not primarily diseased but is simply, like the deep veins, overloaded by the reflux volume.

6.3.3.4 Shunts

A shunt is a short circuit or diversion from one vascular region to another, consisting of a reflux source and a re-entry point (see Sects. 3.7–3.9).

A shunt may be open or closed, depending on whether or not the reflux returns to its original starting point.

Closed shunt: The blood returns to its starting point, overloading the venous system. The patient presents recirculation through a closed circuit (see Sects. 3.7.1 and 3.8).

Open shunt: The vein system has a reflux source and a re-entry point, but the blood does not complete a circuit. It can be just diverted (open deviated shunt; see Sect. 3.7.2) or bypassing an obstruction (open bypassing shunt or open vicarious shunt; see Sect. 3.7.3)

Classifying Recirculations (Closed Shunts) into Shunt Types (see Sect. 3.8)

Shunts are classified into six different types, called shunt types, according to their origin, course, implied networks and re-entry pathways, especially with reference to their treatment. The shunt type is defined according to the principal recirculation pathway; subsidiary circuits may be connected to the principal recirculation.

6.3.3.5 CHIVA Strategy

The CHIVA strategy consists of four parts (for further explanations, see Sect. 6.3.4):

- Dividing the hydrostatic pressure column
- Interrupting the recirculations
- Maintaining re-entry points
- Eliminating non-draining N3 networks

1. **Dividing the hydrostatic pressure column**

   Interrupting the reflux source is dividing the pressure column between the next superior deep vein valve and the re-entry point of the recirculation. Note: In case no iliacal valve exists and the sapheno-femoral junction is incompetent, the pressure column in the incompetent N2 (GSV) and depending N3 (varicose tributary) starts at the right heart atrium. Divisions are possible at each pathological compartment jump (N1 – N2, N2 – N3) and at branching points of refluxing tributaries, as well as below a draining perforating vein in the course of a refluxing N2 or N3 segment.
2. **Interrupting the recirculations**

   The main object of the CHIVA strategy is to avoid recirculation circuits by means of ligations and interruptions, so as to remove the patho-haemodynamic cause of varicose veins: the pathological jumps of anatomic compartments.
3. **Maintaining re-entry points**

   Re-entry points allow the blood to drain from the veins of the superficial networks (N2 and N3) into the deep system (N1) and therefore must not be ligated.
4. **Eliminating non-draining N3 networks**

   Large tributaries usually have muscle cells in the wall, allowing a good recovery of diameters after volume overload was interrupted. On the contrary, smaller tributaries or those with slow flow in preoperative conditions (poorly drained) usually do not. The recommendation is therefore to spare saphenous veins (N2), optionally also large tributaries (N3), combined with exhairesis or sclerotherapy of reticular varices. Exhairesis of all tributaries whilst maintaining the saphenous trunk veins and sclerotherapy of varicose reticular and spider veins are both compatible with CHIVA.

6.3.3.6 Different Types of Intervention

CHIVA 1: Interruption of the proximal reflux source of the principal and optionally also the subsidiary recirculations.

CHIVA 2: Interruption of the N2 – N3 jump without interruption of the N1 – N2 jump as a first step in case of shunt type 3 (RET positive; see Sect. 3.8.9). Check up after some months, and if necessary interruption of the primary reflux point, if it has not become competent.

CHIVA 1 + 2: "Conservative, non-haemodynamic procedure"

Simultaneous ligation of the primary and distal reflux sources with shunt type 3 instead of CHIVA 2 and later on second step. The result is an undrained system with numerous superficial vein thrombosis and recurrences in tributaries. Applied in some countries due to reimbursement necessities. The proximal saphenous trunk is left in the leg, but no longer participates in leg drainage. This is therefore described as an undrained system or a non-haemodynamic procedure.

Devalvulation: Resection of the valve in a competent saphenous vein to avoid a non-drained situation in case of CHIVA 1 + 2: The saphenous vein (N2) can then drain into the next perforating vein, avoiding the superficial vein thrombosis and permitting a drained situation for the saphenous vein.

Crossotomy: Interruption of the N1 – N2 jump at the sapheno-femoral junction (SFJ) at the level of the fossa ovalis without interruption of the tributaries of the groin. They are left draining into the great saphenous vein (GSV) avoiding a thrombosis of the latter.

6.3.4 CHIVA Strategy

Claude Franceschi explained four bases of the CHIVA strategy in his first publication in 1988. Since then, they have remained unaltered:

1. Interrupt recirculation circuits by closing the escape point
2. Divide the pressure column
3. Maintain re-entry routes
4. Eliminate non-draining tributaries

The result is:

- Only flow from superficial to deep (N3 – N2 – N1)
- No flow in circles (closed shunts)
- No volume overload in superficial leg veins

Sometimes, to achieve this result, blood will flow towards the food for a short segment in an N3 or N2 vein. The direction of flow plays not a big role, as long as the amount of blood is adapted to the vein diameter, the re-entry for the blood is adapted to the volume and thus a drained situation is created. After the interruption of the SFJ (see Fig. 6.1) and during diastole, blood in the proximal GSV will flow with a flat curve towards the foot (which means the "wrong" direction) until it finds the next perforating vein (see also Sect. 4.11.1 and Fig. 4.40). Blood from tributaries (N3) will drain through the GSV (N2) into the deep vein via a perforating vein (see Fig. 6.1b). There will be no pathologic compartment jumps and no volume overload, as the GSV was designed to drain the blood of the tributaries and the deep veins to drain the blood of the leg.

This fact could be demonstrated by investigations measuring diameters of the common femoral vein beneath the level of the confluence of the GSV (SFJ) 6 months and 5 years after applying CHIVA for GSV reflux. The common femoral vein is dilated in case of chronic venous insufficiency as compared to healthy individuals and reduces its calibre after surgery [6–8]. If the retrograde drainage of the tributaries through the GSV into the deep veins would overload the femoral vein, the diameter would not reduce to normal after CHIVA. At short term (6 months, [7]), the calibre reduction to normal values [9] could be demonstrated; this was still true in midterm evaluation (10 years, [8]), even though 20% of the investigated patients showed a slight recurrence.

6.3.4.1 Interruption of Recirculation Circuits

As with all other surgical options for the treatment of varicose veins, the basic object of the CHIVA strategy is to interrupt the recirculation circuit.

The simplest way to do this is to interrupt the first reflux source. This prevents the blood from flowing from a low N to a higher one. In other words, the blood can no longer flow out of the deep veins into the superficial system nor from the saphenous vein into the tributaries (see Fig. 6.1). In this way, not only the recirculation is interrupted, but volume overloading in the superficial vein system is also eliminated.

As a result of the reflux point interruption, the blood can only flow from a "big N" into a "little N" (see Fig. 6.1b). A certain volume of blood flows down towards the foot in the superficial system below the interruption; however, a downward flow is not necessarily a reflux. Reflux consists of blood flowing antegrade during muscular systole (in the affected vein or another), which flows backwards in the diseased vein during muscular diastole, generally towards the foot. This usually involves mainly the passage of blood from a low N (like a deep vein, N1) into a higher one, for example, to a saphenous vein (N2). Thus, blood flows back into the superficial system after it has already entered the deep system; this is undesirable since its physiological objective should be the most direct route to the heart (see Sect. 3.2.1).

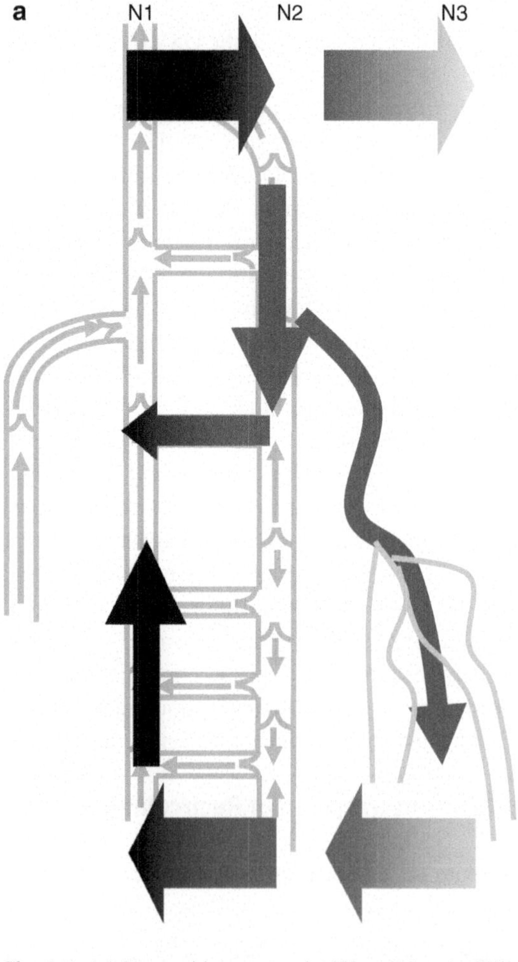

Fig. 6.1 (**a**) Shunt with escape point N1 → N2 at the SFJ, reflux into the GSV (red arrow), second escape point N2 – N3 at knee level into a refluxing tributary (red arrow), re-entry perforating vein on GSV (N2 – N1) and re-entry perforating vein on the tributary (N3 – N1) (blue arrows). (**b**) The base of the CHIVA strategy: Interruption of pathological compartment jumps: – N1 → N2 and N2 → N3. Flow after treatment of a varicose vein with CHIVA: The blood flows towards the foot for a short segment but never from N1 to N2 or N2 to N3. The total blood volume in the leg is reduced to normal. With permission by [10]

Reflux is the basic signal indicating recirculation: blood in circular flow, which never leaves the leg. If the primary reflux source is interrupted however, as by interruption of the SFJ, this will allow the blood from the tributaries of the confluence of superficial inguinal veins to flow towards the foot through the GSV as far as to the next perforating vein. In this case there is flow towards the foot but no recirculation exiting the deep vein and therefore no reflux. The blood from the capillary networks which joins the epigastric and pudendal veins (N3 veins) flows through a saphenous vein (N2) into the deep vein system (N1), without any occurrence of circular flow. The blood simply flows through a slightly longer segment of N2 (see Fig. 6.1).

This footward-directed flow after an interruption of the SFJ is often misinterpreted when investigating patients after CHIVA. The same happened to Dwerryhouse [11] when they aimed to compare stripping with crossectomy without stripping (which is not CHIVA!!). They found a footward-directed flow and described this as a reflux, so all the patients were catalogued as "failure". If the upwards exit is closed and the saphenous vein is still patent, the blood has to leave it at a point downwards. And this necessarily induces a footward flow.

The Italian language has an ideal word for this non-refluxing retrograde flow after interruption of the SFJ: "deflusso", which could be translated into English as "downflow" or "deflux".

The return of varicose veins to their normal calibre is the logical result of this relief from overloading [7, 8]. This reduction in calibre functions best in the saphenous trunks. Perhaps one reason for this is the additional anchorage of the saphenous veins by the saphenous fascia, as well as the fact that the walls of the saphenous veins contain more muscle cells than epifascial tributaries (see Sect. 2.6).

Keeping the saphenous veins is useful not only for later use of the vein as bypass material but also, more importantly, in order to preserve drainage routes for the superficial vein system of the leg and preventing recidives without escape point [12].

6.3.4.2 Division of the Hydrostatic Pressure Column

In the standing subject, varicose veins carry the blood into the deep vein system by the easiest route, as dictated by gravity. Even if the recirculation is stopped, blood from the tributaries will prefer this easier way just down through the superficial vessels. For this reason, it is important, whenever possible, to interrupt refluxing segments below confluences with tributaries or perforating veins, so that the blood is forced to find a route to the deep vein system through perforating veins, instead of remaining in the superficial vein system and flowing down to the foot. Division of the pressure column is particularly important for a good cosmetic result in the calf region.

6.3.4.3 Keeping Re-entry Points Untouched

Re-entry perforating veins must be maintained untouched in order to provide drainage from the superficial vein system. They must be preserved as part of the CHIVA strategy.

The diameter of the drainage pathway, for example, the re-entry perforating vein or the draining tributary, must be sufficient to drain the flow from the refluxing proximal vein, without creating a bottleneck for the backflow. This is one of the most important concepts in CHIVA treatment. In the first days after intervention, the treated vein is still distended and fills with blood from antegrade tributaries when standing. If the blood from this vein cannot drain well through perforating veins after the intervention, superficial thrombosis is very likely to develop.

The Calibre of the Draining Vein Must Match That of the Drained Vein

A velocity profile during duplex examination in PW mode can help in decision-making. If the tributary planned to be interrupted is closed by digital compression, the proximal segment of the vein from which this tributary is filled with reflux must still show a good reflux curve. If the reflux ceases (almost) completely under digital compression of the tributary, the digitally closed vessel is the principal drainage pathway and must not be interrupted in order to prevent a superficial vein thrombosis in the saphenous vein (see Fig. 6.2).

6.3.4.4 Eliminating Non-draining Venous Networks

The non-draining tributary network consists of veins which are distended by reflux with a poor drainage (see Sect. 3.2.3). The blood flows slowly in these veins, and they do not recover to normal calibre properly after volume overloading is relieved. They are mostly veins from the region of the accessory anterior saphenous vein (AASV) or reticular varices. It is sometimes necessary to carry out a mini-phlebectomy to optimise the cosmetic outcome or to apply sclerotherapy later on, if they still persist at time of follow-up. Large, winding saphenous tributaries do not fall into this group. They generally reduce their calibre well after volume overload is relieved. If the patient wants to see immediate results, the tributaries can also be phlebectomised, whilst the saphenous trunks are maintained.

Thus, the mini-phlebectomy or sclerotherapy of tributaries is not contradictory with CHIVA as often supposed. CHIVA aims to preserve the ***saphenous*** draining pathways.

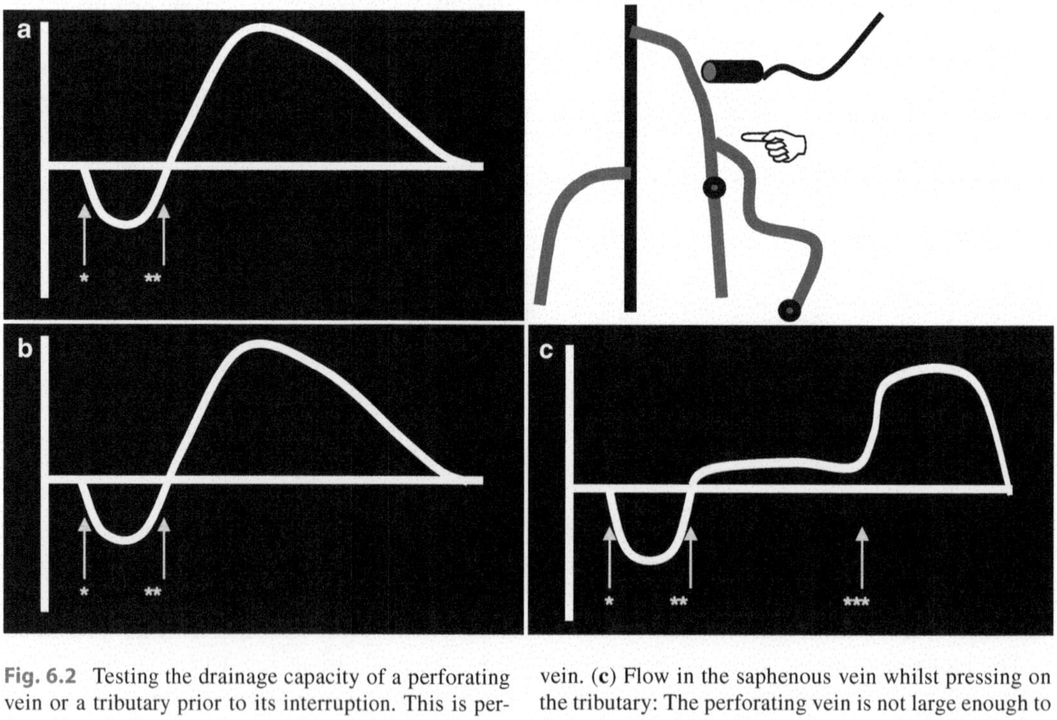

Fig. 6.2 Testing the drainage capacity of a perforating vein or a tributary prior to its interruption. This is performed occluding the tributary with a finger. (**a**) Flow in the saphenous vein without manipulation (left) and setting of veins, finger and probe (right) (as Fig. 3.31). (**b**) Flow in the saphenous vein whilst pressing on the tributary, no alteration in the curve: The perforating vein on the GSV is able to drain the blood from the saphenous vein. (**c**) Flow in the saphenous vein whilst pressing on the tributary: The perforating vein is not large enough to drain the blood from the saphenous vein. This tributary should not be touched simultaneously to the junction in order to avoid a thrombosis in the GSV. *Forefoot elevation, **forefoot goes down again and relaxes, ***finger releases the pressure on the tributary. With permission by [10]

6.4 CHIVA Strategy Depends on the Saphenous Perforating Veins

The most important distinction between two recirculation systems prior to decide which CHIVA strategy to apply is to find out whether there is or not a draining perforating vein link between the refluxing saphenous vein and the deep vein. This will differentiate the most frequent shunt types (see Fig. 6.3): shunt type 1 (with perforating vein drainage) from shunt 3 (without perforating vein drainage). The difference can easily be found with the reflux elimination test (RET; see Sect. 3.8.9 and Fig. 3.31): digitally pressing on the refluxing tributary and testing if the GSV is still refluxing—in case of draining perforating vein on the GSV, the reflux will be persistent also under digital compression of the tributary (RET negative), and in case of no perforating vein, the reflux will stop (RET positive). The same criterion differentiates shunt 4 (with perforating vein, RET negative) from shunt 5 (without perforating vein drainage, RET positive).

After the first description of CHIVA, it soon became obvious that the situation defined as shunt type 3 made some problems: The CHIVA concept proposes to interrupt the veins at their pathological compartment jumps. This would mean to close the SFJ and the origin of the tributary (see Fig. 6.3). This works perfectly in case of shunt type 1 (see Fig. 6.3 left). But when closing the junction and the origin of the tributary, the

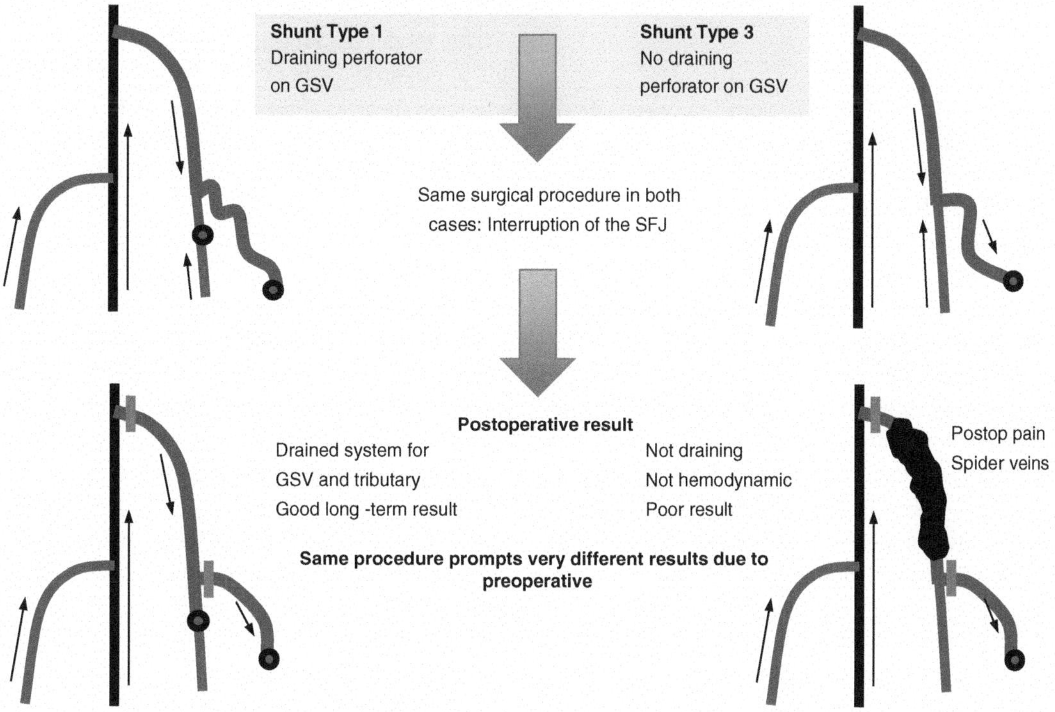

Fig. 6.3 Comparison between results when applying the same treatment to shunt types 1 and 3 (after Cappelli, presented in Boston 2013). With permission by [10]

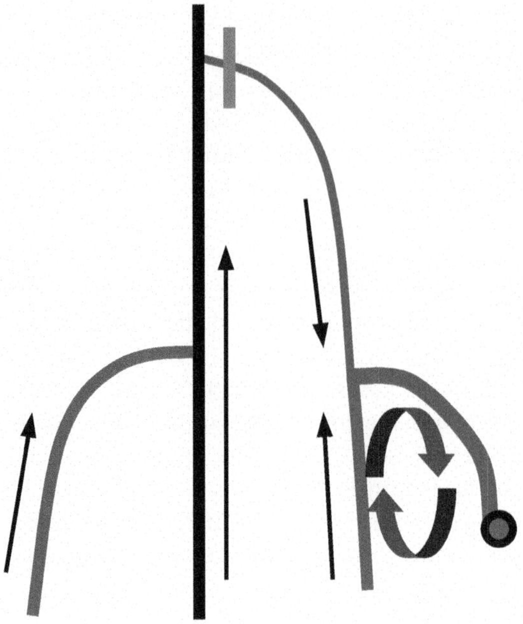

Fig. 6.4 Interruption of the SFJ: The GSV will reduce its diameter and have retrograde, non-overloading flow. As a result, we find a recirculation from the distal saphenous vein into the tributary. N1 | N2 → N3 – N1. With permission by [10]

segment of saphenous vein between both interruptions would remain "non-drained" in case of shunt type 3 (see Fig. 6.3 right) (see also Sect. 6.11.3 shunt type 3).

If only performing crossotomy to the situation on the right part of Fig. 6.3 aiming to avoid the possible GSV thrombosis, a recirculation in the tributary would remain (see Fig. 6.4). Of course, the reflux volume would be reduced significantly, changing the shunt type 3 into a shunt type 2. In case of C4–C6 situation, when an improvement of clinics is the major focus, this will help. But in case the cosmetic result is a priority of the patient, this way will not be not satisfactory, as the tributary would remain visible.

6.4.1 CHIVA in Two Steps or "CHIVA 2"

To solve this problem, CHIVA in two steps was developed and called "CHIVA 2" in the CHIVA meeting in Passenans, 1994. In the first step, only the N2 → N3 compartment jump is treated with interruption of the tributary or tributaries that drain the reflux from the saphenous vein (Fig. 6.5) (see Sect. 6.11.3 Shunt 3). As a result, we will find a flow conversion in the great saphenous vein to antegrade in the days after the intervention (see Sect. 6.4.1.1). This situation can remain stable after some weeks, or a recurrence of reflux through the junction appears either draining through a perforating vein (see Sect. 6.4.1.2) or draining through a new tributary (see Sect. 6.4.1.3). As this remodelling takes some time, the control ultrasound should be performed about 3 months after the intervention or even later on. In case of permanent antegrade flow, patients at the control used to be also clinically free of complaints. On ultrasound, a diameter reduction of GSV can be assessed and antegrade flow. On the contrary, in case of GSV reflux, patients feel some discomfort at the disconnection point (CHIVA 2 point), and in ultrasound, the GSV is still enlarged and refluxing.

This model of "working in two steps" is difficult in countries, where vein surgery is hospital based and the availability of surgical theatre slots is difficult. That is why other options have been developed, like devalvulation or CHIVA 1 + 2 (see Sect. 6.12).

Of course, all expressed ideas concerning "CHIVA 2" apply also to the SSV, but there is no published data to tell about a percentage of cases.

As after the first step of CHIVA 2 there could be a saphenous vein thrombosis in the proximal segment of the GSV ascending into the femoral vein, special attention has to be paid to thrombosis risk factors and to heparin prophylaxis for 10–14 days after intervention. This is especially true in case of diameters of GSV at proximal thigh larger than 8.5 mm (see Pintos, Sect. 10.1.4).

6.4.1.1 Flow Conversion in the Saphenous Vein

Forty-two percent of patients with a shunt type 3 have an antegrade flow after tributary disconnection in shunt type 3 after 1 year; this is stable in

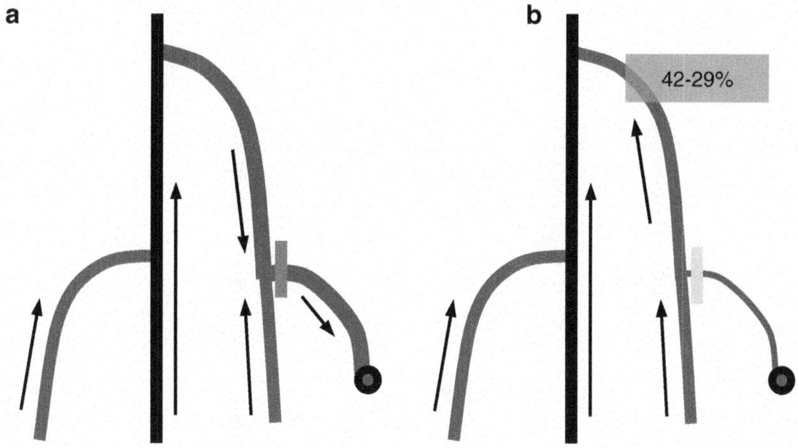

Fig. 6.5 (**a**) First step of CHIVA 2: interruption of the tributary with flush ligation at the jump N2 – N3 (dark green) N1→ N2 ┼ N3 – N1 (**b**) Flow conversion in GSV in 42% (1 year) and 29% (3 years) after first step of CHIVA 2. The tributary drains its physiologic blood load through the perforating vein, no recirculation, no varicose vein. The light green line at the N2 – N3 jump interruption represents the fact that this interruption is "old" N1→ N2 ┼ N3 – N1 results in no reflux—no second step is necessary. With permission by [10]

29% of patients after 3 years [13]. This means that the GSV will be flowing physiologically with antegrade drainage (see Fig. 6.5) in midterm in about a third of all cases treated with CHIVA 2 first. There are some factors favouring this evolution:

- Small diameter of affected GSV
- Short refluxing segment of GSV (refluxing tributary at the proximal thigh)

Obviously, this result is the optimum desirable and really meets the saphenous sparing condition with an evolution to normality after the intervention.

6.4.1.2 Persistent Reflux Draining Through a Perforating Vein

In case of reflux recurrence in the GSV after tributary interruption, the reflux will find a new re-entry pathway. This might be a perforating vein existing on the saphenous vein which enlarges to drain the reflux volume. That means that a shunt type 3 has been converted into a shunt type 1 and can be treated as such with a crossotomy (see Fig. 6.6).

6.4.1.3 Persistent Reflux Draining Through a New Tributary

The other option after the first step of CHIVA 2 with recurrent reflux in the GSV is a new refluxing tributary draining the refluxing blood from the saphenous vein, which most often fills the first existent dilated tributary at some point. The patient returns reporting that nearly nothing happened apart from a slight reduction in the tributary or a disappearance of a part of the tributary and often reduction of symptoms. The reflux amount in the GSV in the months after the first step is most often less than before the intervention (see Fig. 6.7a). Again, a first step of CHIVA 2 can be performed interrupting the new refluxing tributary, expecting antegrade flow in the GSV (see Fig. 6.7b). In the authors' personal experience, more than half of the patients had no flow reversal in the GSV after the second intervention of a tributary.

Another option is to perform a crossotomy and to leave a reflux into the tributary, if the patient is not too bothered by the fact that a tributary will be seen (see Fig. 6.7c).

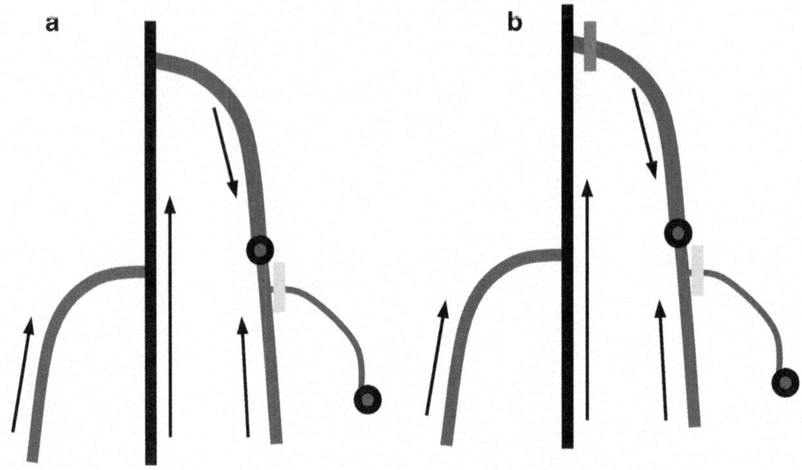

Fig. 6.6 (**a**) After the first step of CHIVA 2 (light green line), the tributary has reduced calibre, draining through a perforating vein. The GSV is still refluxing, draining through a new widened perforating vein on the GSV—which might be proximal to the tributary interruption point (as depicted) or distally. N1→ N2 ⫲ N3 – N1 results in N1→ N2 – N1 (**b**) In this situation, the interruption of the SFJ (dark green line) completes the treatment and is called the second step of CHIVA 2. Blood from the proximal segment of the GSV will then drain through the perforating vein. N1 ⫲ N2 – N1. With permission by [10]

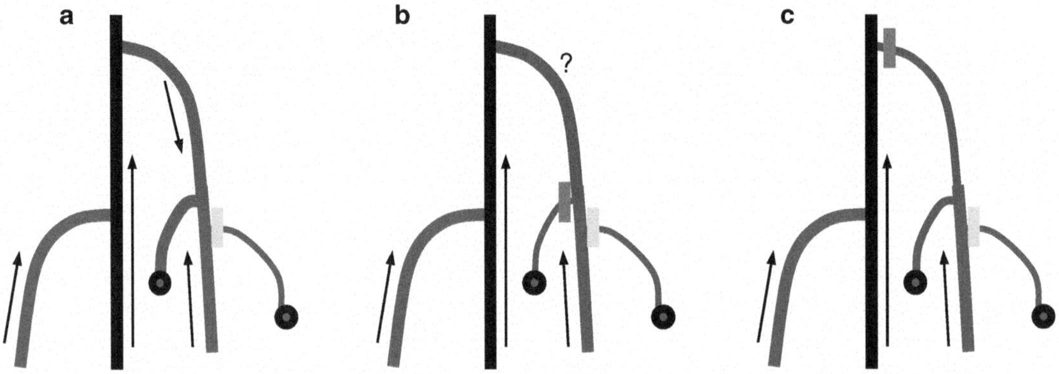

Fig. 6.7 (**a**) After the first step of CHIVA 2 (light green line), the tributary has reduced calibre, draining through a new refluxing, which might be proximal to the tributary interruption point (as depicted) or distally and that might join the pre-existent tributary (not shown). N1→ N2 ⫲ N3 – N1 results in N1→ N2→ N3 – N1 (**b**) One option is the interruption of the new refluxing tributary with the problem of the uncertain flow reversal in the GSV. (**c**) The third option is the interruption of the SFJ, resulting in poor cosmetic results (see Fig. 6.4). With permission by [10]

6.4.2 Devalvulation of GSV

To avoid the treatment in more than one step in case of shunt type 3 and fearing proximal thrombosis in the GSV after applying first step of CHIVA 2, the "devalvulation" was proposed by Claude Franceschi in the CHIVA Meeting (1994 Passenans, France) and has been further developed. The aim is to create a draining situation for the GSV destroying the valve(s) in the GSV further down to the draining tributary until the level of the next GSV perforating vein (see Sect. 7.9). Depending on the preoperative finding, there are three situations to use a devalvulator, called Type

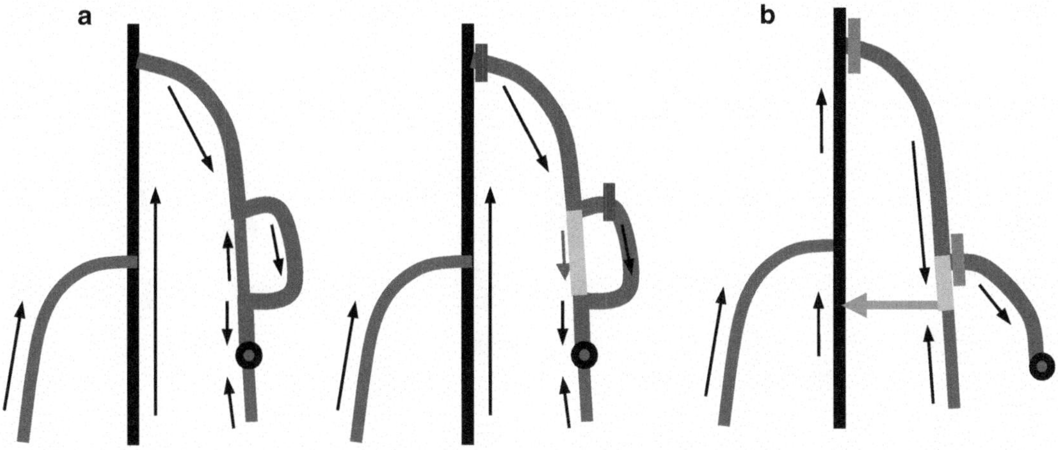

Fig. 6.8 Devalvulation in shunt 3. (**a**) Devalvulation Type A left: preoperative situation with two refluxing segments on the GSV and one interposed competent segment, as well as a perforating vein draining the distal segment located on the GSV. Right: crossotomy and tributary disconnection (green lines) and devalvulation (orange) of the competent segment between the two refluxing GSV segments. The upper GSV is now drained through the distal re-entry perforating vein. N1 ┼ N2 ┼ N3 – N2 – N1 (**b**) Devalvulation Type Bp and B: management of shunt type 3 (as in Fig. 6.3 upper right) with crossotomy, tributary disconnection and devalvulation (orange line) of the GSV between the tributary disconnection point and the next perforating vein (blue arrow). If there is a large perforating vein preoperatively, this type of devalvulation is called Bp, and if not, it is called B. N1 ┼ N2 ┼ N3 – N1. N1

With permission by [10]

A, Type Bp and Type B (see Fig. 6.8), based on the presence or not of a draining perforating vein.

- Type A is the case of a multisegmental reflux in GSV. The devalvulation will be applied on the competent GSV segment between the two refluxing segments (see Fig. 6.8a).
- Type Bp applies to a shunt type 3. Distal to the refluxing tributary, on the antegrade segment of the GSV, a perforating vein is visible (most often the proximal paratibial or Boyd) (see Fig. 6.8b).
- Type B: Same situation as Bp (shunt type 3), but no visible distal perforating vein on the GSV. In this case, we assume the presence of the perforating vein at the typical locations (see Fig. 6.8b).

According to the results of the group in the Vall d'Hebron University Hospital (Barcelona) presented 2011 in Napoli by JM Escribano, the devalvulation worked in all three groups without statistical significant differences. They developed draining re-entry perforating veins achieving a drained system after one step.

The devalvulation has some advantages: It allows to treat a shunt type 3 in one session, being sure to achieve a drained situation.

6.5 Management of the Sapheno-femoral Junction

The great saphenous vein (GSV) is very often affected in varicose disease. The reflux source can be located at the groin with different variations, depending on the conditions of the terminal and preterminal valve, as well as of the competence of the groin tributaries at the sapheno-femoral junction (SFJ) [19, 20] (see Fig. 6.9a and Sect. 4.4).

Treatment decisions depend not only on the described conditions but also on the draining

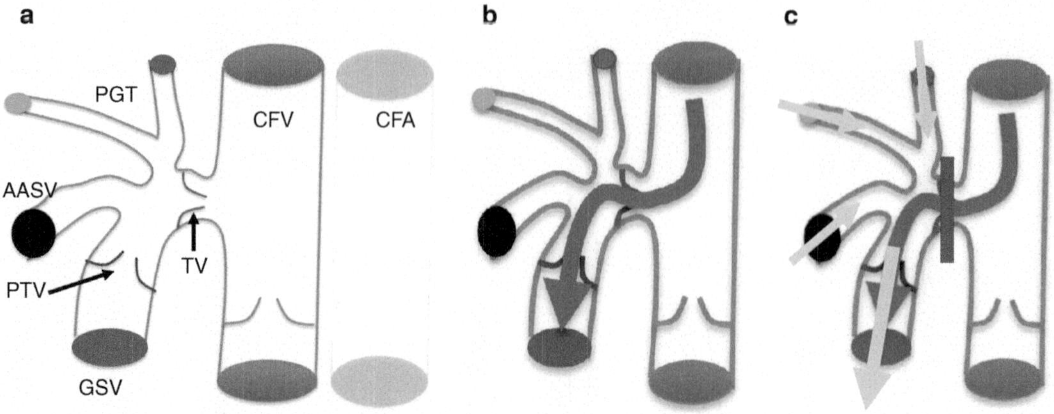

Fig. 6.9 (**a**) Schematic representation of the sapheno-femoral junction: CFA, common femoral artery; CFV, common femoral vein; PGT, proximal groin tributaries; AASV, anterior accessory saphenous vein; GSV, great saphenous vein; TV, terminal valve; PTV, preterminal valve. This schematic representation is the basis of the next figures. It has to be remarked that there are lots of anatomic variations in the sapheno-femoral junction and not always all the tributaries are present and or there is more than one of each. (**b**) Incompetent terminal and preterminal valve at the SFJ (for legends, see figure **a**). The reflux emerges from the femoral vein (blue) and trespasses the terminal valve and the preterminal valve. The GSV (green) is filled with reflux. The accessory anterior saphenous vein (violet) and the other tributaries of the groin (pudendal, epigastric and circumflex veins—yellow and orange) are competent. (**c**) The crossotomy is represented by a red line: interruption of the GSV at the very level of the ostium. The reflux path is interrupted; the draining path from the tributaries into the patent GSV is possible (yellow arrows) and washes the distal GSV avoiding thrombosis. With permission by [15]

pathways of the reflux (see Sect. 6.4). In case no draining perforating vein is found on the saphenous vein, possibly the tributary will be treated first and the SFJ later on only in case it is still refluxing (see "CHIVA in two steps", Sect. 6.4).

6.5.1 Incompetent Terminal and Preterminal Valve

This section deals with the treatment of a reflux in the GSV caused by incompetent terminal and preterminal valves (see Fig. 6.9b).

Claude Franceschi introduced the concept of "crossotomy" in 1988 [5], which means to interrupt the saphenous vein from the deep vein at the level of the ostium, leaving the groin tributaries untouched (see Fig. 6.9c). The groin tributaries drain retrogradely through the saphenous vein and further down into the deep vein via a perforating vein. They wash out the GSV avoiding a thrombosis (see Sect. 7.2). This interruption was described as double ligation with interruption between both—later on modified adding clips, with and without interruption but always leaving the drainage of the junction tributaries into the distal GSV.

In some countries, this technique is not reimbursed by the public health-care system (like in Germany); thus the crossectomy with ligation of all the groin tributaries excepting the posterior accessory saphenous vein is often performed, surprisingly with little superficial thrombosis as a consequence, but destroying the drainage pathway of the pudendal, epigastric, accessory anterior and circumflex veins. This is not CHIVA at its pure form.

Further developments, like endoluminal heat or glue application, are studied in the context of CHIVA [14]. Long-time results are still missing. For further information, see Sect. 7.13.

The SFJ will be treated in the CHIVA concept in case of:

- Incompetent terminal and preterminal valve.
- In addition: draining perforating vein further down on the saphenous vein (RET negative).
- If no draining perforating vein is found on the GSV (RET positive), consider first to treat the tributary or apply devalvulation (see Sect. 6.4).

6.5.2 Incompetent Anterior Accessory Vein

In case of an incompetent terminal valve and competent preterminal valve, the reflux from the deep vein fills a short segment of the GSV and then escapes into the anterior accessory saphenous vein. The AASV is one of the most important tributaries of the GSV. Its pathology is often cosmetically bothering. There are lots of possible combinations of reflux with the GSV and thus lots of treatment options at groin level. Usually the AASV feeds a long visible tributary net, which often does not disappear completely after reflux abolition. So, a simultaneous sclerotherapy or phlebectomy should be proposed to the patient; alternatively the sclerotherapy could be applied after some months, as the AASV will have reduced its calibre (see Sect. 7.12).

The anterior accessory saphenous vein (AASV) has a proximal interfascial segment (N2). Along its course, it pierces the fascia to become extrafascial (N3) in most cases. Sometimes it stays interfascial. It has an inter- or epifascial communicating vessel to the GSV. This connecting vessel has to be considered when applying CHIVA.

A classification into a shunt type 1 or 3 is difficult, because the vein is interfascial in its origin (N2) and only in its course it turns epifascial (N3) sometimes without any branching.

6.5.2.1 Incompetent Terminal and Competent Preterminal Valve

Reflux from the common femoral vein (N1) with incompetent terminal valve into the GSV (N2), escaping into the AASV. Competent preterminal valve with no reflux down the GSV. The AASV is always subfascial in the first segment, becoming extrafascial at a certain point of its course; thus it might be considered an N3 with a first segment as N2, using N2/N3 to signal this (Fig. 6.10a).

The treatment is a flush ligation of the AASV at the confluence with the GSV, also called lateral crossotomy. The SFJ itself must not be ligated, since in that case the distal, antegrade GSV would have no drainage, causing a non-drained situation for the GSV and possibly thrombosis in a healthy vessel.

6.5.2.2 Incompetence of a Subfascial AASV with Refluxing Tributary Leaving the Fascia

Incompetent terminal valve with reflux from the femoral vein (N1) into the GSV (N2). Competent preterminal valve with reflux escaping through refluxing AASV. In this case, the AASV has a complete subfascial course; thus it is an N2 vessel. Further down the reflux drains into an extrafascial tributary (N3); the AASV is competent in the footward segment (see Fig. 6.11a).

In this case the AASV may be considered as an N2 with reflux into a tributary. The interruption of the tributary “en niveau” is often enough to cause a flow reversal in the AASV (see Fig. 6.11b). Otherwise the vein has to be treated as described in Sect. 6.5.2.2: lateral crossotomy.

6.5.2.3 Incompetence of the AASV with Simultaneous Incompetence of the GSV and Draining Perforating Vein on GSV

Reflux from the common femoral vein (N1) with incompetent terminal and preterminal valve, into the GSV (N2) above or above and below the

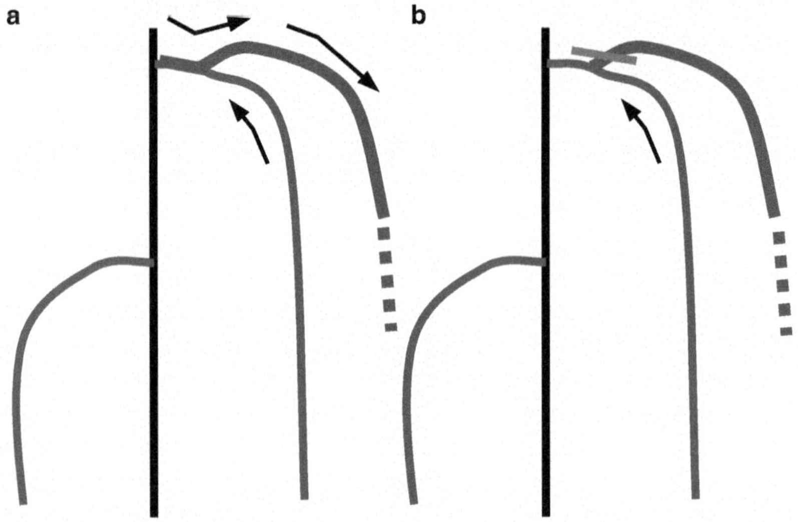

Fig. 6.10 (**a**) Incompetence of the terminal valve, competence of the preterminal valve with reflux escaping through AASV. N1 → N2 (GSV) → N2/3 (AASV) – ... (**b**) Treatment option: flush ligation of the AASV at the GSV, sometimes called "lateral crossotomy". N1 ← N2 ∤ N2/3 – ... With permission by [10]

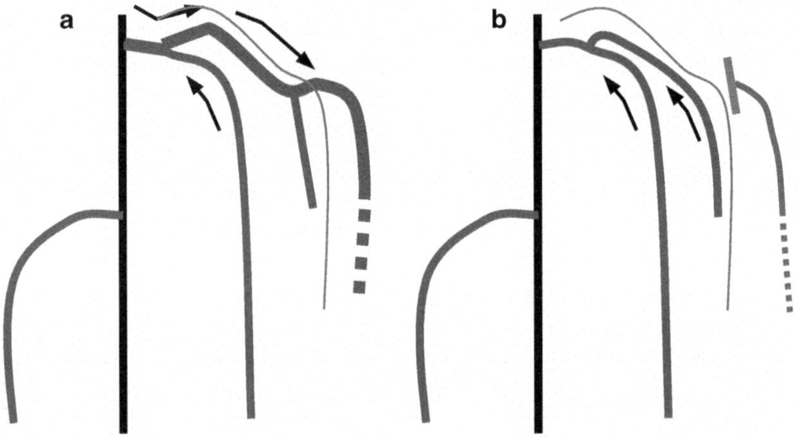

Fig. 6.11 (**a**) Incompetence in the proximal section of the AASV. The reflux leaves the AASV and exits from the fascia (brown line) through a tributary. N1 → N2 (GSV) → N2 (AASV) → N3 (**b**) Situation after interruption at the tributary with flush ligation at the level of the AASV. The interfascial lateral accessory saphenous vein and the SFJ have become competent again. N1 ← N2 (GSV) ← N2 (AASV) ∤ N3 With permission by [10]

knee. Drainage through perforating vein from the GSV (shunt type 1). In addition, reflux into the AASV (N2/N3) as refluxing tributary (see Fig. 6.12a).

The treatment consists in the interruption of the SFJ (crossotomy) with simultaneous interruption of the AASV (see Fig. 6.12b).

6.5.2.4 Incompetence of the AASV with Simultaneous Incompetence of the GSV and No Draining Perforating Vein on the GSV

Reflux from the common femoral vein (N1) with incompetent terminal and preterminal

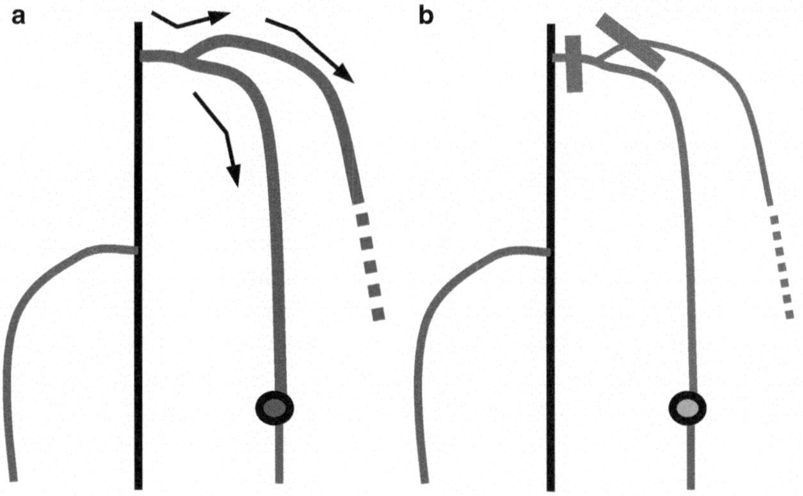

Fig. 6.12 (**a**) Reflux in GSV and AASV with incompetent terminal and preterminal valve, draining perforating vein on the GSV. N1 → N2 – N1 ↘ N2/3 – N1 (**b**) After crossotomy with additional interruption of the AASV calibre reduction in GSV and AASV. N1 ⊣ N2 – N1 ↘ N2/3 – N1. With permission by [10]

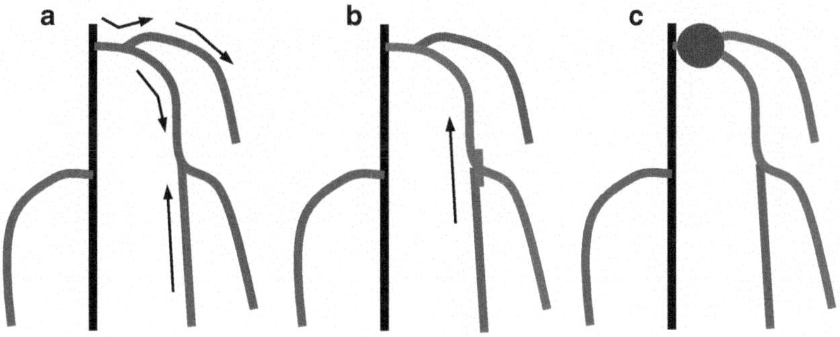

Fig. 6.13 (**a**) Shunt type 3 with two tributaries: one at distal thigh and one is the AASV. N1 → N2 → N3 – N1 ↘ N2/3 – N1 (**b**) Treatment in case of little reflux: interruption of the tributary with flow reversal in the GSV in about 50% of cases. Later the AASV could be treated with sclerotherapy in case of little reflux or with interruption at the confluence with the GSV. N1 → N2 ⊣ N3 – N1 ↘ N2/3 – N1 (**c**) Treatment in case of dilated veins: crossotomy including the interruption of the AASV and perhaps later sclerotherapy of the tributary. N1 ⊣ N2 → N3 – N1 ↘ N2/3 – N1. With permission by [10]

valve, into the GSV (N2) above or above and below the knee. Drainage through a tributary from the GSV (shunt type 3). In addition, reflux in the AASV (N2/N3) as refluxing tributary (see Fig. 6.13a).

Usually in case of shunt type 3, the treatment is flush ligation of both tributaries, followed by crossotomy after some months in over 50% of cases (see Sect. 6.4.1). As the AASV has to be ligated in the groin itself, in case of a further need of a crossotomy after some months, a re-intervention in the groin would be necessary and has to be performed in scarred tissue. That is why this approach is no good option.

There are two alternatives:

- In case of little reflux in GSV and AASV, with small diameters (Fig. 6.13b), perform first flush ligation of the distal refluxing tributary (at the thigh or calf), but not touching the AASV. Follow-up: In case of competent GSV, then perform a phlebectomy or sclerotherapy of AASV. In case of still refluxing GSV (terminal and preterminal valve), perform a crossotomy and interruption of the AASV in a second step.
- Dilated GSV and AASV with large amount of reflux (Fig. 6.13c): treatment of the SFJ as first step with crossotomy and interruption of AASV. Depending on the calibre reduction of the tributary, it may be treated after some months with sclerotherapy or phlebectomy or flush ligation.

6.5.2.5 Reflux in the AASV with Drainage into the GSV at Mid-thigh via a Communicating Vein

Reflux from the common femoral vein (N1) through the SFJ into the GSV (N2), escaping into the AASV. The preterminal valve is competent; thus the GSV at proximal thigh is competent but is filled refluxingly via a connecting vein from the AASV at mid-thigh (See Fig. 6.14a).

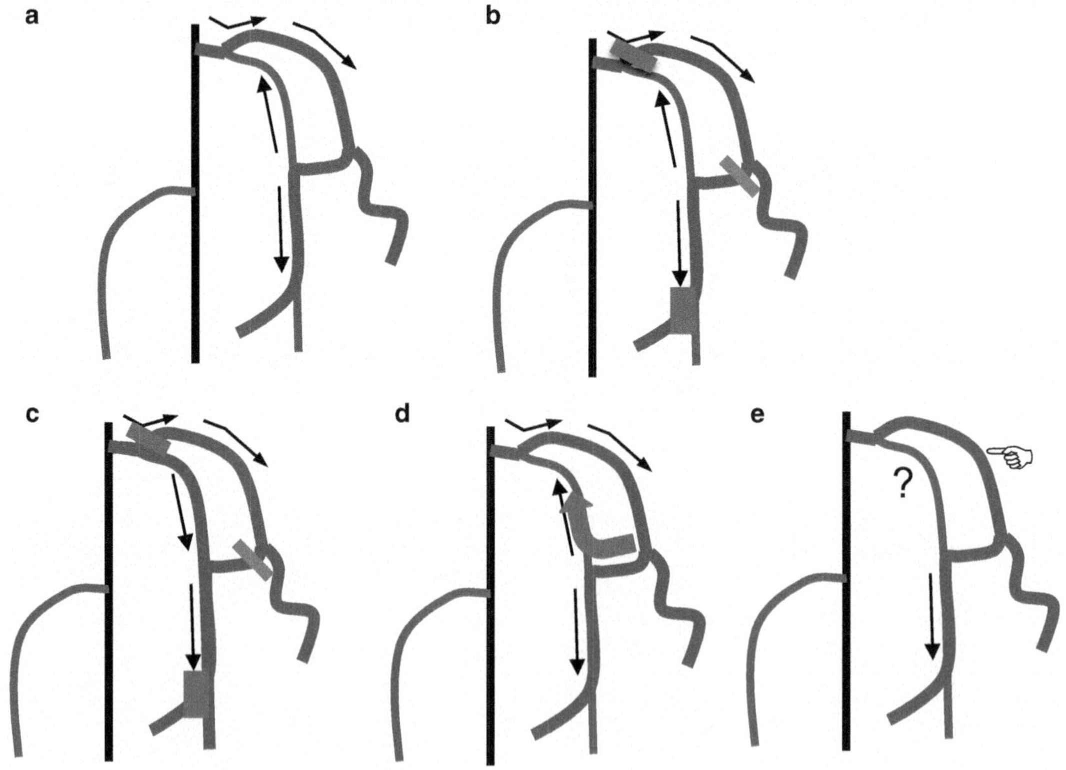

Fig. 6.14 (**a**) Reflux from deep vein into GSV and AASV, competent GSV at proximal thigh. AASV branches, one tributary fills the GSV with reflux. N1 → N2 → N3 – N1 ↘ N2 → N3 – … (**b**) Treatment of the situation in a: interruption of the AASV at its junction with the GSV, interruption of the branch feeding the GSV and of the distal GSV tributary. N1 ⊬ N2 → N3 – N1 ↘(crossed) N2 ⊬ N3 – … (**c**) Failure of the strategy with development of an apparently new reflux in the proximal GSV. (**d**) In the preoperative investigation, usually we find a diastolic flow from refluxing AASV into GSV, assuming the GSV at the proximal thigh is competent. (**e**) Manoeuver to discover the flow direction in the GSV at proximal thigh digitally closing the AASV during exploration. With permission by [10]

The treatment consists in a flush ligation of the AASV at the GSV in the groin and an interruption of the tributary feeding the GSV to diminish the flow into the GSV and flush ligation of the tributary distal at the GSV (Fig. 6.14b).

Very seldom the proximal GSV becomes incompetent after this strategy (Fig. 6.14c). Possibly it was already dilated but when measured with duplex, a reflux did not occur, because the amount of blood refluxing via AASV was more important, provoking an antegrade diastolic flow in the GSV (Fig. 6.14d). To unmask this latent reflux in the GSV prior to the first treatment step, the AASV has to be occluded (e.g. with a finger) during the ultrasound exploration, and then the GSV at proximal thigh has to be explored during a provocation manoeuver. Only if still there is no reflux in muscular diastole, the GSV at this level has to be assumed as competent (Fig. 6.14e).

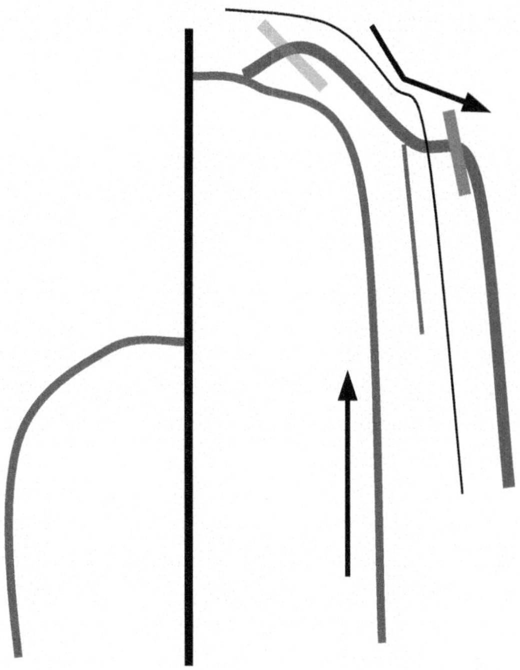

Fig. 6.15 Surgical procedure for isolated incompetence of the AASV. The brown tiny line represents the fascia. Either interruption of the AASV at the level of the GSV (surgically or with endoluminal devices) or after emerging the fascia in case of the existence of a competent distal AASV segment. Alternatively, the AASV without reflux from the deep veins can be treated with foam sclerotherapy. With permission by [10]

6.5.2.6 Isolated Incompetence of the AASV

Sometimes we find an isolated reflux in the AASV with competent terminal and preterminal valves. The reflux source might be the competent GSV or a reflux from pelvine tributaries into AASV (see Fig. 6.15).

Classically and following CHIVA principles, an interruption of the AASV in the groin should be performed (half-coloured green interruption point in Fig. 6.15). As the amount of reflux is little (not emerging from the deep vein), the author generally treats these patients with foam sclerotherapy, if a treatment is really necessary (e.g. for cosmetic reasons). Alternatively, the interruption at fascial level with or without phlebectomy of the subcutaneous part of the vein may be performed (full-coloured green interruption point in Fig. 6.15). In theory, the AASV could be closed with endoluminal techniques.

6.6 Management of Pelvic Reflux

Pelvic reflux has its origin in an incompetent pelvine network, filling tributaries at the groin, the ventral, inner or posterior part of the thigh and this finding a retrograde pathway to fill leg veins. The classification and treatment of the pelvic leak points are extensively discussed in Chap. 8.

The refluxing pathways originated by a pelvic reflux are:

- Pelvic reflux feeds the GSV via a tributary of the sapheno-femoral junction.
- Pelvic reflux feeds the GSV via a tributary at the thigh or the calf.
- Pelvic reflux feeds the SSV via a long tributary at the calf or the Giacomini vein.
- Pelvic reflux fills only tributaries, not involving a saphenous vein in the pathology.

The first situation is discussed in Sects. 6.6.1 and 6.6.2 and the last three in Sect. 6.6.3.

6.6.1 Competent Terminal and Incompetent Preterminal Valve

This condition is only known since the introduction of ultrasound to the diagnostics of superficial vein insufficiency. When applying saphenous vein ablative procedures, the source of the reflux is indifferent. It is always the same procedure: crossectomy and stripping. This is the reason why even after the introduction of ultrasound, the distinction of the source of reflux at the SFJ was not important for lots of phlebologists or vascular surgeons [16–18].

And this is the reason why often colleagues do not understand what is meant, when CHIVA appliers talk about competent terminal valve and incompetent preterminal valve or para-ostial reflux, referring to the fact that the reflux does not trespass the ostium, like the case described in Sect. 6.3.1, but comes from the tributaries in the groin (see Fig. 6.16).

This is why it is strongly recommended to gather further information in Sect. 4.4 and in additional books or articles, in case of not being familiar with the exploration of the groin tributaries. The terminal valve is competent; neither with dynamic provocation manoeuvres nor with Valsalva or compression release of the calf, a reflux from the femoral vein into the GSV can be generated. The reflux source is found in the supra-inguinal region, summarised as pelvic reflux (see Fig. 6.16a and Sects. 6.6, 6.11.4.2, and 6.11.4.4 and Chap. 8).

In these patients, no pathologic compartment jump is found at the level of the groin cease. But a pathologic amount of blood is drained into the GSV. The pelvic compartment ("P") feeds a tributary. This is the pathologic compartment jump. And this tributary meets the saphenous vein at the groin level (P → N3 – N2).

The drainage of groin tributaries into the saphenous vein is a physiologic condition. The amount of blood makes the difference (see Sect. 4.5). The origin of the reflux has to be found and possibly treated, depending on the drainage pathways (see shunt types 4 and 5 and Sects. 3.8.5, 3.8.7, 6.11.4, and Chap. 8).

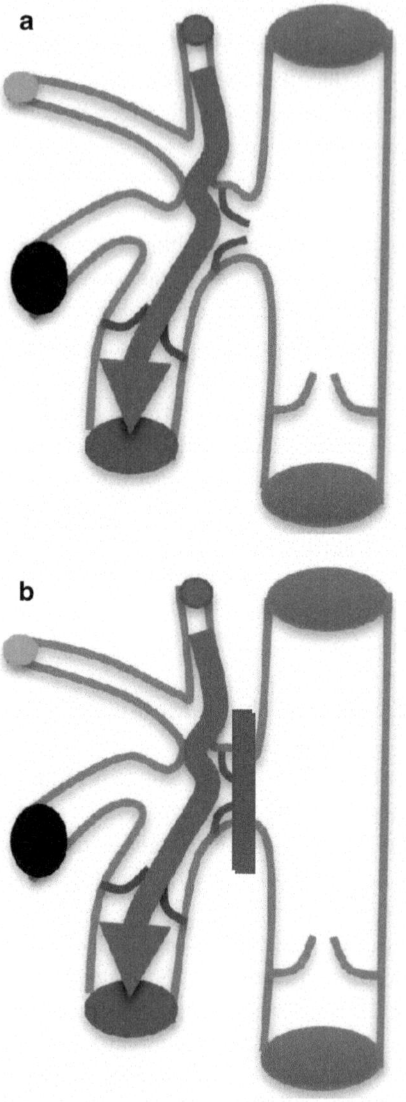

Fig. 6.16 (**a**) Para-ostial reflux that means competent terminal valve and incompetent preterminal valve. The reflux does not flow from the deep vein into the GSV. The origin is another network, in this case pelvic reflux. (**b**) Result after applying a crossotomy, an interruption of the GSV at the level of the ostium and leaving the reflux filling the GSV: The reflux situation is exactly the same as prior to the intervention (Compare Figs. 4.10–4.12 and 4.43). With permission by [15]

How to treat this condition? Thinking as usual in classical phlebology, as the GSV is refluxing starting at the SFJ, the "crosse" has to be treated. But when applying a crossotomy to a para-ostial reflux and leaving the GSV in situ (we are doing saphenous vein sparing surgery!), this interruption would not change anything in the haemodynamic situation (see Fig. 6.16b, red line and Fig. 4.43).

> In this condition and in the CHIVA context, a crossotomy is not an option.

The optimum would be to establish a drained situation, where either the reflux would be abolished at its origin (at the level of the pelvic network, see Chap. 8) or the reflux from the pelvic network would be drained into the deep veins in a proper way creating a stable drained circuit without a compartment jump in the leg that would cause a volume increase in any venous network of the leg.

Depending on the drainage situation of the GSV, different possibilities would be at choice:

If there is a draining perforating vein on the GSV (shunt type 4; see Fig. 6.17a) and a refluxing tributary at the leg, the tributary at the leg can be treated (see Fig. 6.17b), leaving the pelvic reflux drained through the GSV and the perforating vein. The GSV would suffer a discreet overload with pelvic blood, but often this situation remains stable throughout many years. If the amount of pelvic reflux is too high, the pelvic leak point should be treated (see Fig. 6.17c and Chap. 8).

Experimentally some colleagues have interrupted the GSV distally to the junction that means at the level of the preterminal valve. In classic venous surgery, this always has been thought to be malpractice leading to recidives. These procedures are only anecdotes, as the colleagues never published their results. Having a close look at the endoluminal thermal ablation therapies, the closure distally to the preterminal valve leaves exactly the same situation: the groin tributaries drain into the deep veins via the SFJ. Possibly in the future this could be an option as alternative to the surgical interruption of pelvic leak points, which is not a familiar routine method for every vascular surgeon (see Fig. 6.17d) [14].

If there is no draining perforating vein on the GSV (shunt type 5; see Fig. 6.18a), the interruption of the distal tributary will lead to a competent GSV in 97% of cases, stable throughout the time (see Fig. 6.18b) [13].

This is one of the optimum situations to apply CHIVA: A GSV with reflux and feeding refluxing tributaries is reverted to a competent vein, stable throughout time. The benefit for the patient is obvious: preservation of the complete untouched N2 system and no scar in the groin (neither surgical nor endothermal). And it is the optimal "starter" setting for hesitating colleagues: The flow reversion in a refluxing GSV is a strong "convincer".

To discriminate between the presence or not of a draining perforating vein along the refluxing GSV, the RET (reflux elimination test) is performed (see Sect. 3.8.9 and Fig. 3.31).

6.6.2 Incompetent Terminal and Preterminal Valve with Additional Reflux in Groin Tributaries

Sometimes, in addition to a reflux from the femoral vein into the GSV via an incompetent terminal and preterminal valve, an additional pelvic reflux joining in through a groin tributary is found. For this situation, as seen in Sect. 6.5.1, CHIVA proposes the crossotomy. The problem is that this would leave a reflux from the groin tributary into the GSV (as depicted in Fig. 6.16b).

There are some options:

- The pathologic tributary is interrupted in the context of the crossotomy. This would leave a non-drained situation for the pelvic reflux (groin tributary), which could lead to recidives fed by the pelvic leak point.
- The crossotomy is performed in addition to an interruption of the pelvic leak point (see Chap. 8).

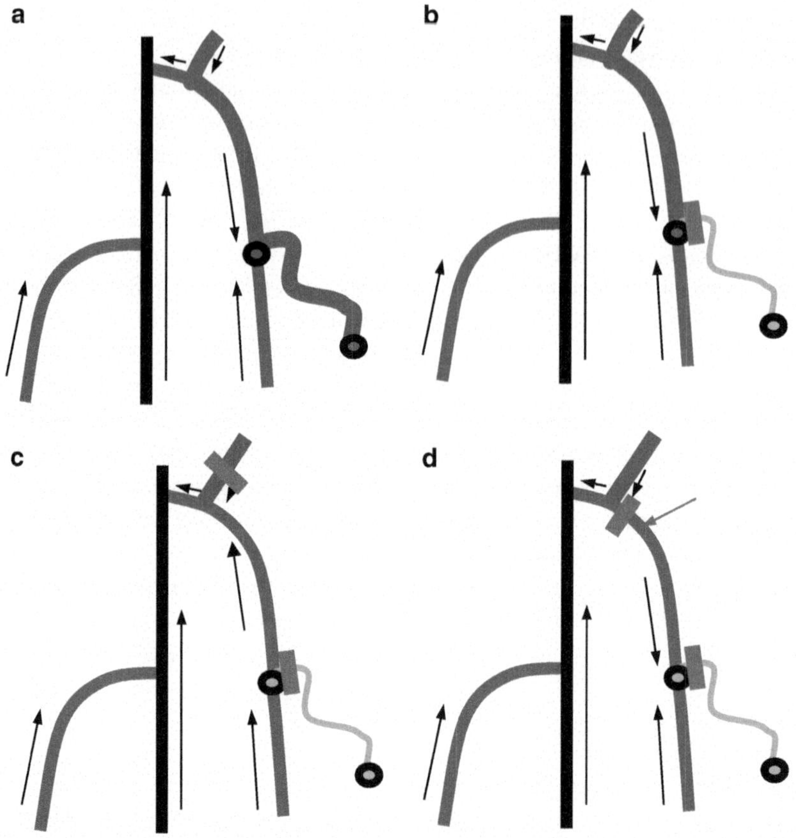

Fig. 6.17 (**a**) Shunt type 4 with pelvic reflux, filling the GSV retrogradely, draining through a perforating vein on the GSV and in a tributary. The terminal valve is competent and the preterminal valve incompetent. P → N2 – N1 ↘ N3 – N1 (**b**) One option is the interruption of the tributary. The tributary will reduce its calibre; otherwise it could undergo phlebectomy or sclerotherapy. The pelvic reflux will still fill the GSV and drain through the perforating vein. P → N2 – N1 ✕↘ N3 – N1 (**c**) If the volume overload in the GSV is too high, the pelvic leak point could be interrupted. As a result, the GSV would become competent. P ┼ N2 – N1 ✕↘ N3 – N1 (**d**) Another option would be the closure of the proximal GSV distal to the preterminal valve with endoluminal thermal ablation of a short segment (e.g. 7 cm) in addition to the tributary interruption. This leaves the junction as drainage for the pelvic reflux, avoiding a reflux into the GSV. This option has the disadvantage that it disrupts the GSV instead of leaving it with antegrade flow as shown in c, and it leaves it with a retrograde flow filled by draining tributaries. P → N2 ┼ N2 – N1 ✕↘ N3 – N1. With permission by [10]

- In case of a perforating vein draining the GSV, the pelvic leak point is left without treatment when performing a crossotomy, expecting a good drainage retrogradely through the GSV and the perforating vein, achieving a drained situation for the pelvic leakage.

6.6.3 Pelvic System Feeding Tributaries

A pelvic reflux feeds a tributary. The tributary is enlarged and can be seen through the skin at the inner thigh, ventral thigh or dorsal aspect of the

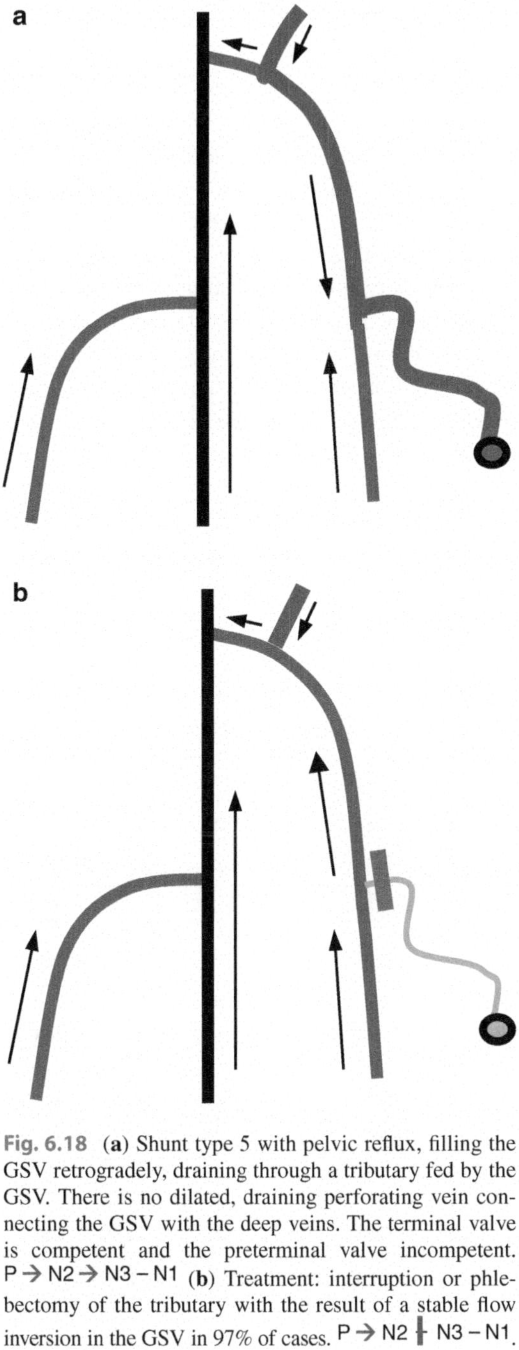

Fig. 6.18 (a) Shunt type 5 with pelvic reflux, filling the GSV retrogradely, draining through a tributary fed by the GSV. There is no dilated, draining perforating vein connecting the GSV with the deep veins. The terminal valve is competent and the preterminal valve incompetent. P→ N2→ N3 – N1 (b) Treatment: interruption or phlebectomy of the tributary with the result of a stable flow inversion in the GSV in 97% of cases. P→ N2 ǂ N3 – N1. With permission by [10]

thigh. These tributaries can either meet an accessory or saphenous vein or be drained into a perforating vein.

Depending on the reflux amount, a surgical interruption of the pelvic leakage point is advised (see Chap. 8), or in case of lesser diameters, a sclerotherapy should be considered. Sometimes the sclerotherapy of the tributary will reverse the reflux in the affected saphenous or accessory veins.

6.7 Management of Incompetent Sapheno-Popliteal Junction

The considerations about reflux sources, treatment depending on the distal drainage explained for the GSV, also apply to the small saphenous vein (SSV). Still there are some differences. In the SSV, we do not find a terminal and preterminal valve, neither a complex tributary system. The pelvic reflux can feed the SSV via the Giacomini vein or a superficial tributary; this is however a very seldom condition that should be treated in the same way as explained for the GSV. In this chapter, only the special features of the SSV regarding to its anatomical and functional criteria will be exposed.

6.7.1 Anatomic Features of SSV

The small saphenous vein (SSV) shows only one tributary, the Giacomini vein or thigh extension of the SSV present in 60% of cases. The Giacomini vein begins at the SPJ and courses up the back of the leg to the mid-thigh and then turns medial and ventral to meet the GSV. It carries blood from the back of the thigh to the SPJ and/or the GSV; the direction of flow under physiological conditions has not been clearly established.

The SSV drains into the popliteal vein at different levels, in the knee-fold or above it, seldom below it via a muscle vein (see Sect. 4.6). These anatomic variations of the sapheno-popliteal junction (SPJ) have to be taken into account when deciding the treatment modalities in the CHIVA context.

Figure 6.19 shows the different anatomical elements of the SPJ (see also Sect. 4.6). A particularity of this junction, as compared to the SFJ, is that both the SSV itself and its "junction tributary", the vein of Giacomini, are covered by a very thick fascia. This means that the SSV, the muscle veins and the vein of Giacomini are all directly subject to the same pressure as the popliteal vein.

6.7.2 Treatment of the SPJ Depending on the Giacomini Vein and Muscle Veins

The treatment of the SPJ depends on the anatomy. This has to be considered when planning the CHIVA strategy for the following reasons:

- Muscle veins from the gastrocnemius musculature drain directly into the SPJ and can have connections with the last 5–10 cm of the SSV. Thus, they may maintain recirculation after the SPJ has been interrupted as shown in Fig. 6.20a.
- Another source of permanent reflux can be found in the Giacomini vein, which can have connections to the deep venous system at the back of the thigh or even being refluxing fed by the GSV (see Fig. 6.20b).
- The vein of Giacomini may also present an excessively high blood column even without pathological reflux from the muscle veins, preventing a good cosmetic outcome after interruption of the SPJ leaving the Giacomini vein draining into the distal SSV (see Fig. 6.20b).

In the presence of reflux from the popliteal vein into the SSV, with no confluence of the vein of

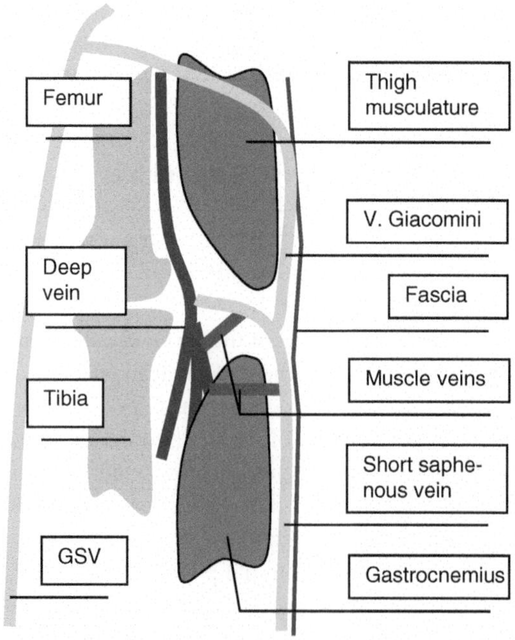

Fig. 6.19 Anatomic components of the junction of the small saphenous vein with the popliteal vein. Bones are represented in grey and muscles in orange. The deep venous system (N1) is in dark blue, muscle veins in turquoise and interfascial veins (N2) in light blue. The superficial fascia is very strong in the dorsal part of the leg, covering the N2—veins and the muscles, as well as the fossa poplitea like a tent. It is represented in green. The muscle-fascia wraps the muscles and is represented as black line covering the orange muscle (compare Fig. 4.25). With permission by [10]

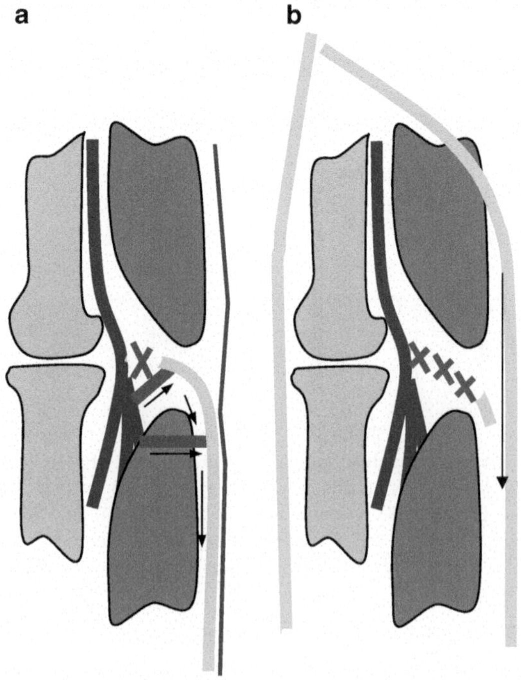

Fig. 6.20 Persistent reflux in post-operative examination after interruption of the junction of the SSV directly at the level of the popliteal vein. (**a**) Reflux persists through the muscle veins which wasn't identified prior to the intervention. (**b**) Persistent reflux through a long segment of the vein of Giacomini after interruption of the SPJ without treatment of the Giacomini vein. With permission by [10]

Giacomini or the muscle veins into the SSV, a classic flush ligation of the SSV at the confluence with the popliteal vein is recommended (no figure).

However, if the vein of Giacomini or muscle veins also flow into the SSV, examination a few weeks after interruption at the deep vein might show that the SSV is still filled refluxingly out of one of these sources (Fig. 6.20). That is the reason why in these cases it is best to interrupt the SSV distal to the vein of Giacomini as a first option, considering the SPJ as a perforating vein that is "terminalised" (see Sect. 6.9.2) with this strategy (see Fig. 6.21a) or distal to the muscle veins (see Fig. 6.21b red cross). Alternatively, the centimetres of SSV with confluence of muscle veins may be completely extracted, performing flush ligation at the popliteal vein and interrupting the muscle veins at the point they join in the SSV (see Fig. 6.21c, red lines and Fig. 6.22 for further details).

In case the SSV drains directly into a muscle vein and not into the SPJ, which is very often, the

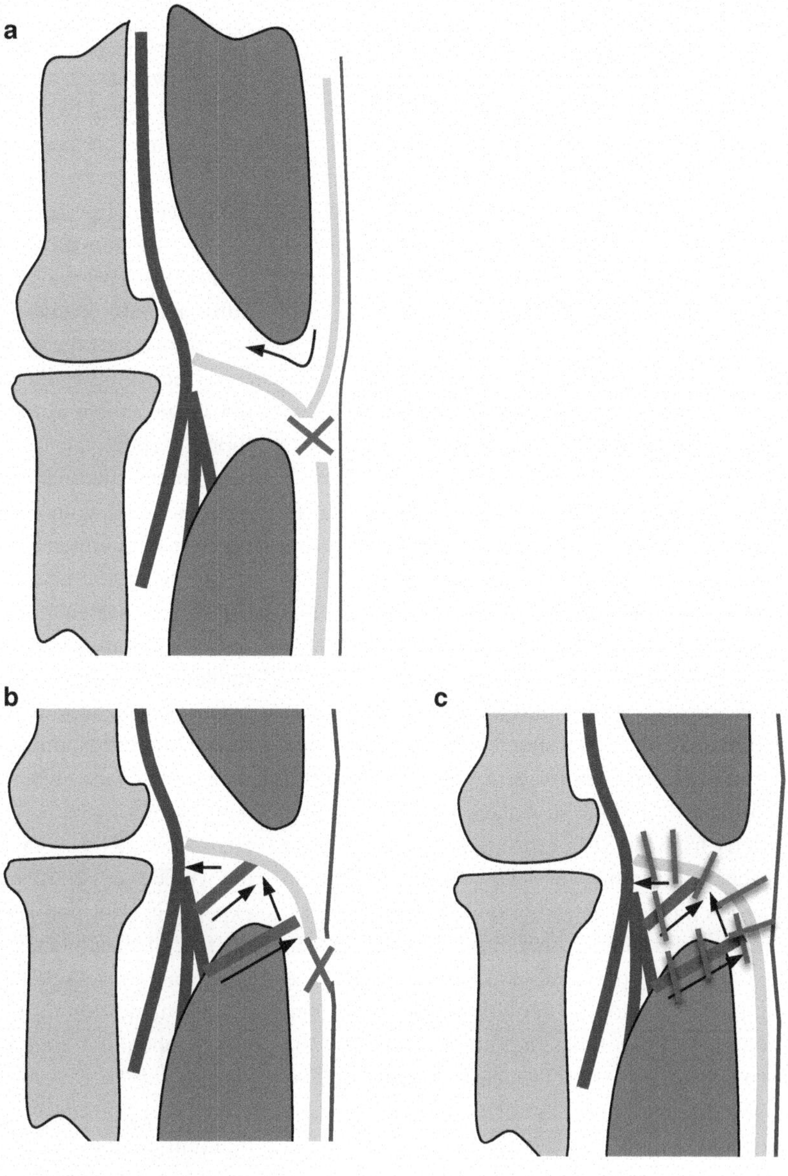

Fig. 6.21 Flow situation after interruption of the SSV not at the junction with the popliteal vein but (**a**) after interruption of the SSV below the vein of Giacomini confluence, allowing the blood of the Giacomini vein to drain into the deep vein through the junction, (**b**) after interruption of the SSV below the last muscle vein (red x) or (**c**) exhairesis of the junction (red lines). With permission by [10]

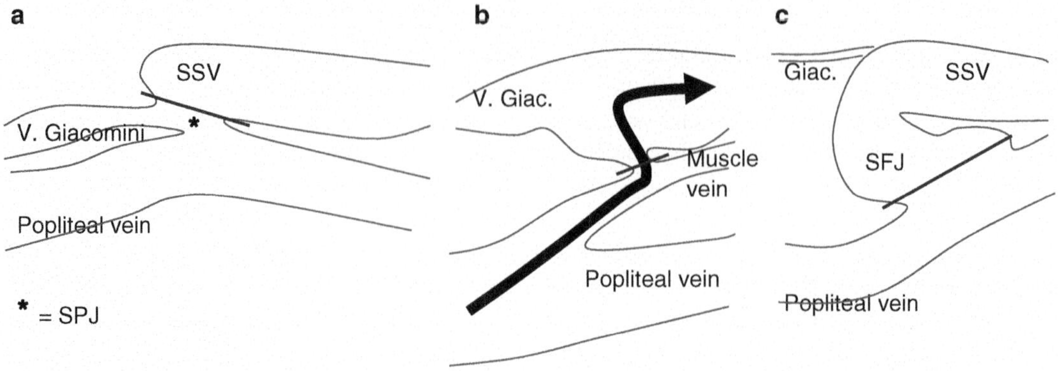

Fig. 6.22 (**a**) The vein of Giacomini drains directly into the popliteal vein. Interruption of the SSV is further distal, green line to allow drainage of the Giacomini vein. (**b**) (Corresponds to Fig. 4.27b) Reflux from the popliteal vein via a muscle vein into the SSV (red arrow). Treatment: interruption of the SSV at its confluence with the muscle vein (green line). (**c**) (Corresponds to Fig. 4.26a): Reflux from the popliteal vein into the very dilated SSV. Interruption of the SSV with flush ligation directly at the popliteal vein (green line). The thin vein of Giacomini will not bring a clinical relevant reflux into the SSV, so it may be left as perfusion of the SSV to avoid thrombosis. With permission by [10]

interruption level should be between the SSV and the muscle vein, not at the level of the popliteal vein, as then a deep vein (muscle vein) would be interrupted (See Fig. 6.22b).

6.7.3 Recurrences at the Sapheno-popliteal Junction

Unfortunately, recurrence after ligation distal to the junction may sometimes occur through a tributary in the popliteal fossa region (see Fig. 6.23): After interruption of the SSV below the confluence of the vein of Giacomini or the muscle veins, refluxing tributaries may appear in the popliteal fossa despite initial flow reversal, especially in case of mixed shunts with systolic reflux in the short saphenous vein. The blood flows from the SPJ into the subcutaneous vessels either directly from the SPJ or through the distal section of the Giacomini vein. The strategy may be sclerotherapy or interruption of the tributary. Before performing a flush ligation of the SSV at the level of the popliteal vein, it has to be sorted out that the Giacomini vein is not part of an open bypassing shunt replacing the function of the deep vein (see Fig. 6.45) in case of strong reflux.

In rare cases, in the absence of any connection between the SSV and the deep venous system in the fossa poplitea, the Giacomini vein takes over as the only vessel carrying drainage from the SSV. If the SSV is refluxing in these patients, the reflux usually originates from the GSV or a perforating vein at the back of the thigh. In the first case, the reflux in the GSV has to be treated. In the latter, the perforating vein should be interrupted (see Sect. 6.9.1).

Another specific problem of the SSV is very seldom found in the post-operative development years after the interruption of the SSV either next to the deep vein or distal to the confluence with the Giacomini vein. The SSV occasionally suffers a recanalisation or new anastomosis in the saphenous compartment, despite resection of some centimetres and use of non-absorbable suture. In ultrasound, a vessel like the SSV is seen at a place, where the first post-operative control demonstrated a correct interruption. Histology of the vein shows no muscle cells in the wall demonstrating a neovessel (author's own experience, not published). It almost seems as if the fascial sheath leads as guidance for the reconstruction of a vessel. To avoid this, it may be necessary in addition to sew the two fasciae (muscle and saphenous) together to close this virtual space.

All these difficulties must be considered when planning a strategy for the SPJ. The problem of

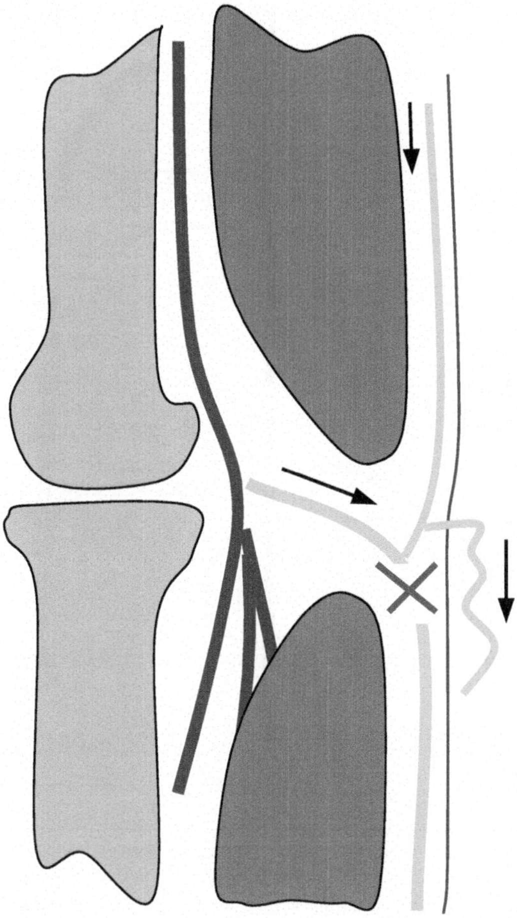

Fig. 6.23 Possible recurrence from the proximal V. Giacomini after distal interruption of the SSV. With permission by [10]

surgical treatment of the SSV using the CHIVA method is not finally solved however, as this condition is rarer than a reflux in the GSV and no randomised studies have been performed or published.

6.7.4 Alternatives to Surgery of the SPJ

Sometimes the surgical approach to the SPJ is not easy. The proximal centimetres of the SSV could then be closed with endoluminal applications (heat or glue) as an alternative. Another option to have in mind is to leave the SPJ untouched and to treat only the tributaries from the SSV. The SSV is covered by a strong fascia and reacts particularly well with calibre reduction after interruption of tributaries (see Sect. 6.4.1). Thus, even if muscle veins or thin perforating veins are present, the interruption of tributaries as only procedure should be considered. At the post-operative examination, the SSV might show antegrade flow or reduced reflux, draining into a perforating vein. This situation could be stable over years. If recurrent tributaries appear or clinics are still present, the SPJ must be treated in a second step.

If both saphenous veins are refluxing in the same patient, a connection often develops between them through a connecting tributary (transversal N4), either the Giacomini vein or a distal tributary. For management, see Sect. 6.11.6.

6.8 Management of Incompetent Saphenous Veins (N2)

The saphenous veins themselves are spared one of the most important targets of CHIVA. Thus, they are touched as little as possible. Depending on the situation, the proximal escape point filling the saphenous vein is interrupted (see Sect. 6.8.1), the escape point is interrupted (see Sect. 6.8.2) or the saphenous vein itself is interrupted (see Sect. 6.8.3).

6.8.1 Management of Incompetent Saphenous Veins Without any Interruption

In case of reflux along the saphenous vein without a draining perforating vein (RET positive), all the reflux of the saphenous vein will be drained into tributaries. An interruption of these refluxing tributaries N2 → N3 will be followed by antegrade flow (see Sect. 6.4.1.1) or volume reduction with the need of further steps (see Sects. 6.4.1.2–6.4.1.3 and 6.4.2).

Another situation, rarely found, is when the escape point is a perforating vein and not a junction (scc Fig. 6.28c). In this case, the flow in the saphenous vein can be corrected without touching the saphenous vein itself.

6.8.2 Interruption of the Escape Point

The interruption of the sapheno-femoral or sapheno-popliteal junction is the most frequent treatment in case of refluxing saphenous vein and has been explained in Sects. 6.5 and 6.7.

A refluxing perforating vein feeding the saphenous vein is also to be interrupted—this would be an interruption of the escape point, but without touching the saphenous vein, and has been explained in Sect. 6.8.1.

6.8.3 Interruption of the Saphenous Vein Along Its Course

An interruption of the saphenous vein itself apart from its junction is seldom performed. The vein regenerates very successfully once the reflux is eliminated. This regeneration is surely supported by the saphenous fascia, as well as the large number of muscle cells in the vein wall. The cosmetic outcome is also better if the tributary is ligated at its confluence with the saphenous vein, instead of ligating the saphenous vein and leaving the tributaries to drain the reflux via a perforating vein.

The interruption of the saphenous trunk plays a role treating refluxes above and below the knee, especially in case of skin changes (see Sect. 6.3.4.2). The interruption can only be performed if there is a draining perforating vein along the refluxing GSV. Fractioning of the pressure column in the GSV will lessen the venous hypertension at the skin areas of the ankle leading to better regeneration after intervention.

Usually the interruption is best set below a knee perforating vein, where a large draining direct perforating vein is mostly found (Boyd or proximal paratibial perforating vein) (see Fig. 6.24). Note that in this case it is not the perforating vein that is interrupted but the GSV distal to the perforating vein. If the Boyd perforating vein would be interrupted instead, we would leave the long pressure column un-fractioned and take drainage possibilities away from the system, both counteracting the CHIVA strategy.

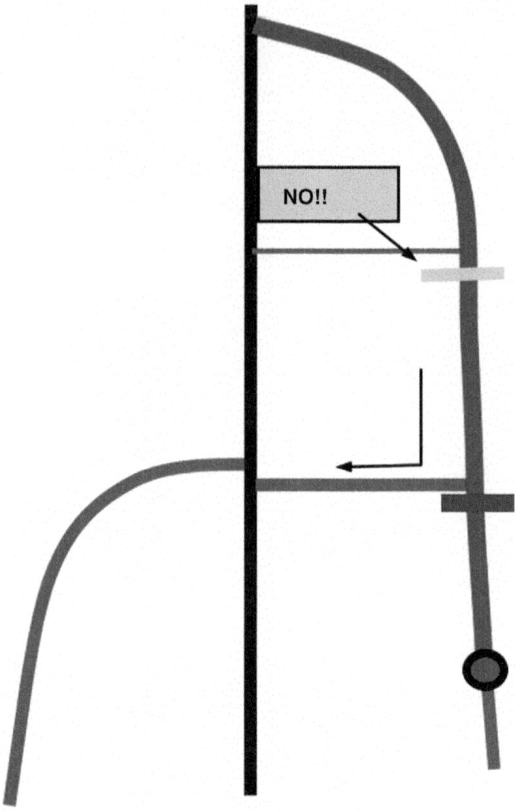

Fig. 6.24 Refluxive GSV with three perforating veins (blue lines along the refluxing segment of the GSV: thin line for thin perforating vein, thick line for large perforating vein and black circle as distal, draining or terminalising perforating vein). The first perforating vein, at the thigh, is too thin to drain the volume from the GSV. If the GSV was interrupted below this perforating vein (the position of the theoretical interruption is marked with an orange line), an undrained situation would be created in the proximal segment. The perforating vein below the knee has a large calibre (thick blue line). The GSV can be interrupted below it (green line) but only because distally to this point we find still a refluxing GSV and a third re-entry perforating vein (black circle), allowing the drainage of the GSV segment distal to the green ligation. With permission by [10]

This procedure is called "terminalising" a perforating vein: The vein was attached to a refluxing segment and now has become the end of the reflux in this segment: it finishes the reflux conducting the blood from the proximal segment to the deep vein and thus "terminalises" the reflux.

6.9 Perforating Veins

The third pillar of the CHIVA strategy is maintaining re-entry points: These re-entry points are usually distended perforating veins, which carry the reflux back to the deep veins and so complete the circuit in the varicose veins. As explained in Sects. 3.5 and 4.7, it is rare to find a perforating vein as a reflux source. Mostly they are draining pathways along the refluxing vein segment or they are at the end of the refluxing vein.

As a rule, a perforating vein should not be interrupted if:

- It has a flow towards the deep vein in diastole: it is a draining perforating vein.
- It has a flow towards the superficial vein in systole: it is the beginning of an open bypassing shunt and is part of the drainage of the leg.

6.9.1 Perforating Veins as a Reflux Source

A perforating vein can be considered a reflux source, if it has a flow towards the superficial vein in diastole. Only these will be interrupted in CHIVA. The flow can be:

- N1 → N2 from the deep vein into a saphenous vein
- N1 → N3 from the deep vein into a tributary

The classical case of a refluxing perforating vein as reflux source for the saphenous vein (N1 → N2) is an incompetent perforating vein at the medial thigh feeding the GSV with refluxing (see Fig. 6.28c as an example). As a treatment, the interruption of the perforating vein is mostly recommended, though sometimes it is not necessary, if the diameter is not too large.

Another more frequent situation is an incompetent perforating vein at the back or lateral aspect of the thigh filling a tributary (N1 → N3). In this case, the treatment of the perforating vein can be surgical with phlebectomy of the tributary or both could be treated with sclerotherapy, depending on the diameter.

6.9.2 Perforating Veins Along the Refluxing Segment

Perforating veins along a refluxing segment usually serve as drainage paths. Blood flow is from superficial to deep. So, they play the role of a re-entry for the shunt (N3 – N1 or N2 – N1). If there are several perforating veins, one of them is the last one in the row, and the others are "intermediate", because there is reflux in the drained way above and below the perforating vein. In these "intermediate" perforating veins, it is possible to apply an interruption of the superficial vein (N2 or N3) **below** the perforating vein (see Fig. 6.24). This procedure is called "terminalisation". The perforating vein then is the end of the refluxing segment, draining the refluxing blood to the deep venous system thus interrupting the pressure column. Terminalisation refers to the fact that this perforating vein is converted from a perforating vein along the refluxing segment into the end of the refluxing segment.

For a perforating vein to be used as part of the CHIVA strategy, its calibre must always be sufficient to drain the refluxing blood, which flows from the superficial vein to the perforating vein (see Fig. 6.24).

Rule of Thumb: The diameter of the perforating vein must be at least half that of the vein to be drained.

Examples:

1. Refluxive GSV, diameter 9 mm. Perforating vein of the adductor canal (formerly Dodd), diameter 2 mm: It cannot be considered as part of the strategy; therefore the GSV must not be

interrupted below this perforating vein (see Fig. 6.24 orange line).

2. Refluxive GSV, diameter 9 mm. Perforating vein below the knee, diameter 6 mm: The GSV can be interrupted distal to the perforating vein (see Fig. 6.24 green interruption).

If the lumen of the drainage route (here the perforating vein) does not bear the correct relation to the lumen of the vessel to be drained (here the proximal GSV), thrombosis may occur in the GSV as the consequence of an undrained situation.

The further distal the perforating vein is in the leg, the less likely it is to be a reflux source. If there is any doubt, decisions over the treatment of perforating veins should always be deferred to the post-operative examination. The patient often understands that the treatment is performed in two steps: First interruption of the primary reflux source and later, perhaps, a further interruption of a tributary or saphenous vein distal to a perforating vein, or an interruption of the perforating vein itself, if it has become refluxing.

This is sometimes the case when a refluxing SFJ and a large perforating vein in the adductor canal are found (see Fig. 6.25). In the first investigation, reflux from SFJ fills the GSV, the pressure columns of GSV and deep vein are competitive, and as in the femoral vein the valves are competent, we observe an inward flow through the perforating vein. After interruption of the SFJ, the pressure column in the superficial vein is reduced, and the flow through the perforating vein reverts and becomes clearly refluxing. In that case an interruption of the perforating vein in a second intervention is necessary.

Another aspect to take into consideration if we find several perforating veins along a tributary or a saphenous vein is the distance between them. If they are at a long distance with a large pressure column, the interruption below the "intermediate" perforating vein is a good option (see Fig. 6.26a). If they are close together and the

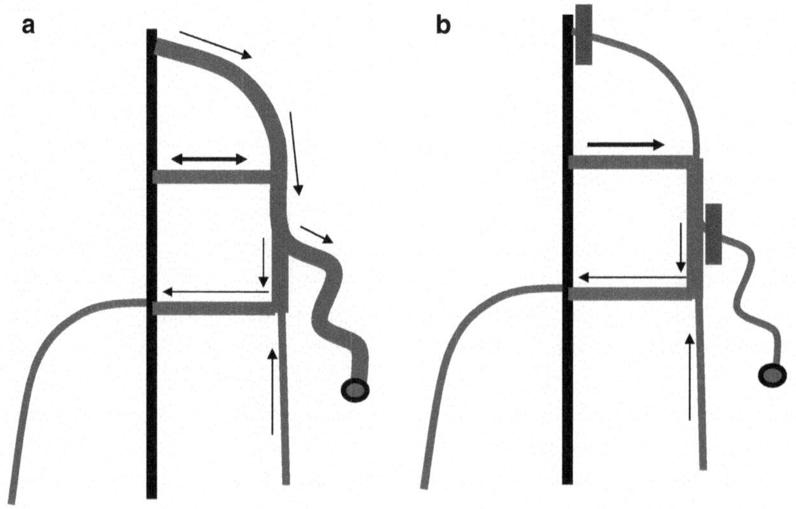

Fig. 6.25 (**a**) Reflux N1 → N2 at the SFJ with in and outflow over a proximal thigh perforating vein. Drainage from the GSV into the deep vein through a below knee perforating vein (N2 – N1) as well as through a tributary. (**b**) Treatment with crossotomy and tributary disconnection (green lines). The interruption of the thigh perforating vein deserves a large scar and so it is possible to wait and see the behaviour after some months. In this case, the flow has become obviously outward, filling the GSV and draining through the below knee perforating vein; thus the proximal now refluxing perforating vein can be disconnected in a second step (not shown). With permission by [10]

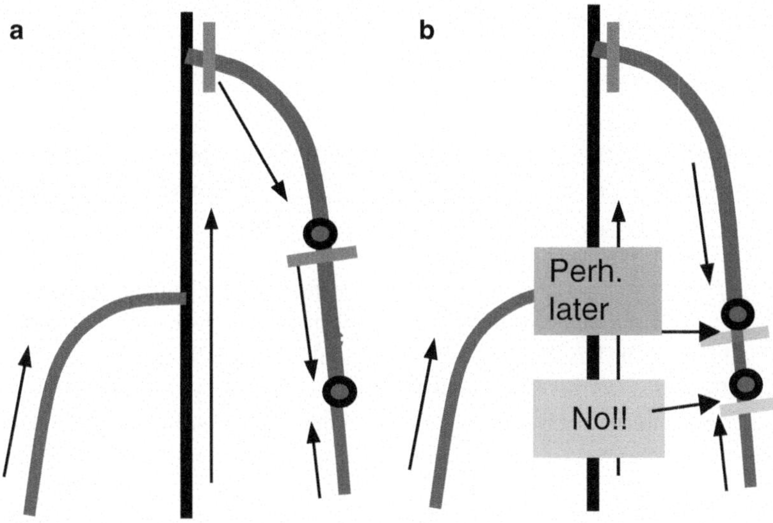

Fig. 6.26 (**a**) Recirculation N1 → N2 – N1 with two well-separated draining perforating veins. The treatment is the interruption at the SFJ (green line), and it can be added by an interruption below the proximal perforating vein (green line). (**b**) Recirculation N1 → N2 – N1 with two draining perforating veins that are close together: interruption at the SFJ only (green line). Just in case the skin should be severely damaged and does not recover properly after the SFJ interruption, the interruption below the proximal perforating vein will improve the situation (light green line). Cave: Never interrupt below the lowest draining perforating vein (orange line); otherwise the distal antegrade draining GSV will lose its drainage, which also is through this perforating vein. These explanations apply also to perforating veins along refluxing tributaries. With permission by [10]

distance between the "intermediate" perforating vein and the last draining perforating vein is very short, the interruption is not worth the scar, because we are just leaving a very short segment—this would only make sense, if we are dealing with an ulceration or severe skin changes—and then only in a second step situation, after skin has partially recovered in consequence of the interruption of the primary reflux source (see Fig. 6.26b). These explanations are true for N2 and N3 vessels drained by perforating veins.

6.9.3 Perforating Veins at the End of the Refluxing Segment

Most of the time at the end of a shunt, we find a perforating vein, draining either a refluxing saphenous vein or a tributary. This one should never be interrupted. It is the drainage of the reflux, and most often it is also the drainage of the distal vessel, which is not affected by the recirculation, especially in case of a GSV reflux (see Fig. 6.26b).

6.10 Management of Tributaries

Tributaries are all the superficial veins running in the subcutaneous tissue. When they become incompetent, they get enlarged and meandering. Physiologically they play the role of the superficial venous reservoir which seems to trigger a progression of varicose disease in case of dilated veins. Tributaries are the mediators of the pathological volume overload and provoke skin changes and proliferate to cope with the pressure (see Sects. 2.2.2 and 2.5). And they are responsible for the cosmetic complaints. In case of little disease, the treatment of tributaries can restore the flow in the saphenous veins (shunt type 5, Sect. 6.4.1.1 and ASVAL, Chap. 12).

If only tributaries (N3) are refluxing, without N2 reflux, the disease is little. We find this in the following situations:

- N2 → N3 – N2/N1 (no reflux from the deep vein): The treatment is the interruption or sclerotherapy of the tributary until the junction with the saphenous vein (see Sect. 6.11.2).
- N1 → N3 – N1: The tributary is fed by a perforating vein, which has to be interrupted. Most often this can be done with a foam sclerotherapy, alternatively with a surgical interruption (see Sects. 6.9.1 and 6.11.5).

6.10.1 Management of N2 – N3 Jump in Case of Positive RET

The reflux elimination test "RET" was designed to examine the drainage paths of the refluxing saphenous vein. It is described in Sect. 3.8.9. In case the RET is positive, this means that on the saphenous vein, there is no draining perforating vein. Interrupting the N2 → N3 jump will be the final treatment, if the terminal valve is competent, resulting in 97% of competent GSV after 3 years. In case of incompetent terminal valve, GSV competence will still be achieved in 29% of cases [13]. As described in Sect. 6.4, the further evolution can be challenging, for the surgeon and for the patient's patience.

6.10.2 Management of N2 – N3 Jump in Case of Negative RET

A negative RET tells us that on the saphenous vein filling the tributary, we find other draining paths—this can be a perforating vein or another tributary or both.

In case of a draining perforating vein, we can interrupt the junction and all the present refluxing tributaries, knowing that the saphenous vein will be drained. This is the optimum situation for a long-lasting, stable CHIVA result.

6.10.3 Management of Refluxing Tributaries Along Their Course (N3)

The treatment of tributaries is often the most important step from the point of view of the patient. The fourth column of CHIVA explicitly includes tributary exhairesis in case of poor drainage. The combination of CHIVA 1 or 2 in the saphenous trunk with simultaneous phlebectomy of all the tributaries offers the possibility of proceeding to achieve quick cosmetic results whilst preserving the saphenous vein.

Tributaries may be removed, but this is not inevitable. With tributaries, it is true to a certain extent that the thicker the vein, the more likely it is to regenerate. But if the diameter is clearly greater than 1 cm, or the tributary has already presented thrombosis, there is a greater probability of poor venous retraction or thrombosis developing after the intervention.

A more important criterion for the removal of tributaries is the flow that they carry. If the retrograde flow is fast and of short duration, which means that they are well-drained, they will in all probability regenerate quickly and without thrombosis. If the retrograde flow is long-lasting and the curve relatively flat, the vein is poorly drained and may be removed.

After performing CHIVA with the main focus on the saphenous veins, the tributaries may reduce their calibre making no more treatment necessary because they have disappeared to the rough eye observation or because the patient has no high cosmetic demands. This is especially true for large recirculation volumes with distal skin changes in elderly patients. Sometimes it is obvious that the tributaries meander through long segments and have lots of divisions, or run specially near under the skin, which makes a calibre reduction leading to a macroscopic disappearance improbable. In these cases, interruption has always to be considered at a point where tributaries branch.

The following possibilities of interruption at branching points exist:

- Same calibre of vessels, both courses of equal length: The tributary causing the bigger cosmetic problem is interrupted.
- Same calibre of vessels, courses of different lengths: One branch soon runs into a perforating vein, the other after a longer distance—interruption of the longer branch (see Fig. 6.27, green line). This keeps the pressure column as short as possible.
- Unequal calibre, but the thinner vessel is still able to drain the proximal section if the other tributary is closed by compression in ultrasound (see Fig. 6.2): interruption of the larger vessel.
- Unequal calibre: The thinner vessel is not sufficient to drain the larger—ligation of the smaller vessel, if any.

It may be said that tributaries can always be interrupted below a branch point or perforating vein, so long as the calibre of the branch or perforating vein is sufficient to drain the reflux coming from proximal on its own (see examples on Fig. 6.27). And the decision to treat tributaries can always be postposed to the control visit, as often then less tributaries will be treated than planned in the first session.

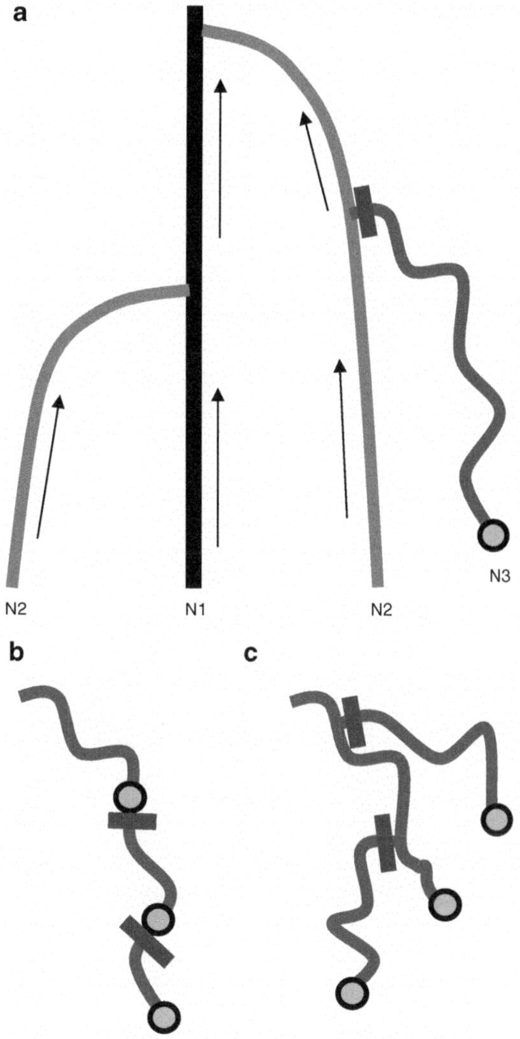

Fig. 6.27 (**a**) Refluxive N3 tributary filled by competent GSV: no branching, no perforating veins apart from the last one (black circle). The interruption will be made at the level of the junction between the tributary and the GSV (green line). No possible interruption along the tributary. (**b**) Same situation than in (**a**), only the tributary is shown. There are three perforating veins along the tributary, and so the tributary can be interrupted below both tributaries on its course, as shown. The last tributary is the re-entry for the last segment. No interruption has to be performed here. Please note that the interruption will be performed on the tributary, not on the perforating vein. (**c**) Branching with different length of segments: interruption of the longer tributary to achieve the best cosmetic result. The interruption has to be performed next to the branching point, without leaving blind sacks to avoid thrombosis. With permission by [10]

6.11 Management According to the Shunt Type

6.11.1 Shunt Type 1

Remember: N1 → N2 – N1 (Fig. 6.3 left and Fig. 6.28)

Recirculation from the deep vein (N1) into the great or small saphenous vein (N2). A distended perforating vein carries the recirculation volume directly out of the affected saphenous vein into the deep vein system (black circle on the vein).

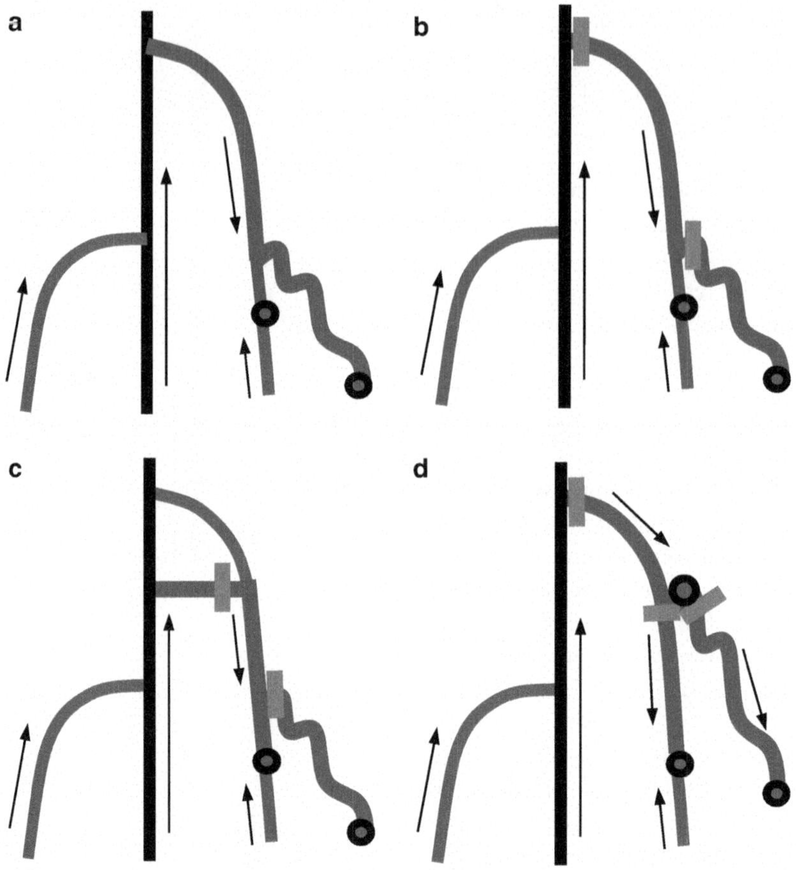

Fig. 6.28 (**a**) Shunt type 1 with tributary or shunt type 1 + 2. (**b**) Interruption of the tributary and the junction in presence of a well-draining perforating vein. (**c**) Competent SFJ, reflux into the GSV through a thigh perforating vein (N1 – N2) with drainage through a perforating vein at the GSV below the knee and through a refluxing tributary. Interruption of the perforating vein and the tributary: Attention the GSV is not interrupted!! (**d**) Refluxive GSV with refluxing tributary. There is a good perforating vein on the tributary just after its confluence with the saphenous trunk. Interrupt at the green lines if a reduction in the pressure column in the distal GSV is to be achieved. With permission by [10]

The principal recirculation runs: Deep–Saphenous–Deep, with no intermediate tributary. One or more tributaries may be involved in the recirculation. Then, this shunt type is also called type 1 + 2 (see Fig. 6.28a).

The strategic decision will depend on where the reflux source is and how many re-entry points there are. The following possibilities exist, **depending on the reflux source**:

- **Highest reflux source is the sapheno-femoral or sapheno-popliteal junction**: Always treat the saphenous junction (see Fig. 6.28b)
- **Highest reflux source is a perforating vein**:
- Interruption of the perforating vein (which is very seldom in CHIVA, as a perforating vein is very seldom the reflux source!) (see Fig. 6.28c)

The following possibilities exist, **depending on the re-entry points**:

- **One perforating vein and no tributaries** Interruption of the highest reflux source only
- **Several perforating veins and no tributary** Interruption of the highest reflux source and the refluxing saphenous vein below the perfo-

rating vein (see Figs. 6.24 and 6.26 and Sect. 6.9.2). The saphenous trunk must never be interrupted below the most distal perforating vein, as this eliminates the drainage from the healthy distal saphenous vein (see Fig. 6.26b orange line). There are no haemodynamic benefits for the GSV in dividing the pressure column by creating short segments.

- **One perforating vein and one or several tributaries**
  If the perforating vein presents with a large calibre, the highest reflux source and all the incompetent tributaries are interrupted close to the saphenous vein. If the calibre of the perforating vein is not very large but is draining the saphenous vein, the situation may be treated as a shunt type 3: in other words, applying CHIVA 2. First only the tributaries will be interrupted with flush ligation at the saphenous vein. At the post-operative examination, the junction will still be refluxing and the saphenous vein calibre lessened. The perforating vein will have adapted its calibre to cope with the remaining reflux from the junction. The second step of CHIVA 2 will then be the interruption of the junction.
  Alternatively, the SFJ can be interrupted, leaving one tributary untreated so that it serves to drain the saphenous vein in addition to the perforating vein. If it is found in the post-operative examination that the calibre of the saphenous vein has diminished, then the last incompetent tributary can be treated. In this situation (thin calibre perforating vein), a second operation is very often needed also in shunt type 1, regardless of what treatment is used, if a superficial thrombosis shall be avoided.
- **Several perforating veins and several tributaries**
  This may be assumed as a situation with good drainage of the saphenous vein as there is more than one perforating vein on the saphenous vein. The junction and all tributaries can be interrupted, and if appropriate, the saphenous vein can be disconnected below a perforating vein to fractionate the pressure column.
- **Perforating vein on a tributary close to the saphenous trunk**
- This condition often occurs at the thigh. Treat the SFJ and other tributaries as usual. In case of dilated perforating vein on the tributary (see Fig. 6.28d): interruption of the saphenous vein below the confluence with the tributary (which then drains the blood from the saphenous trunk into the very short segment of the tributary and then into the perforating vein) and interruption of the tributary distal of the perforating vein. Afterwards the proximal saphenous vein is drained through the perforating vein situated on the tributary. Neither the tributary nor the distal saphenous vein is connected any more to the proximal reflux source. In case no fractioning of the pressure column of the GSV is wished, the tributary is disconnected at the saphenous vein and the perforating vein is interrupted, to avoid feeding of the distal tributary (no image).

6.11.2 Shunt Type 2

Remember: N2 → N3 – N2/1

Recirculation from a (healthy) saphenous vein into a refluxing tributary (see Fig. 6.29).

The calibre of these refluxing tributaries is not very large, since the recirculation volume cannot be very great if no deep veins are involved. In shunt type 2, only blood from the superficial vein system can be part of the incompetence, by definition. As a rule, treatment by interruption of the highest reflux source is enough. That means interruption at the level of the confluence between tributary and saphenous vein. In some cases, additional interruptions need to be done at other branching points of the refluxing tributaries to other junctions (see Sect. 6.10.3).

Alternatively, an isolated mini-phlebectomy of the refluxing tributary (N3) can be performed. The saphenous trunk is not harmed, which is a principal object of CHIVA. A third option is the application of sclerotherapy to the tributary without any surgery in an attempt to abolish reflux.

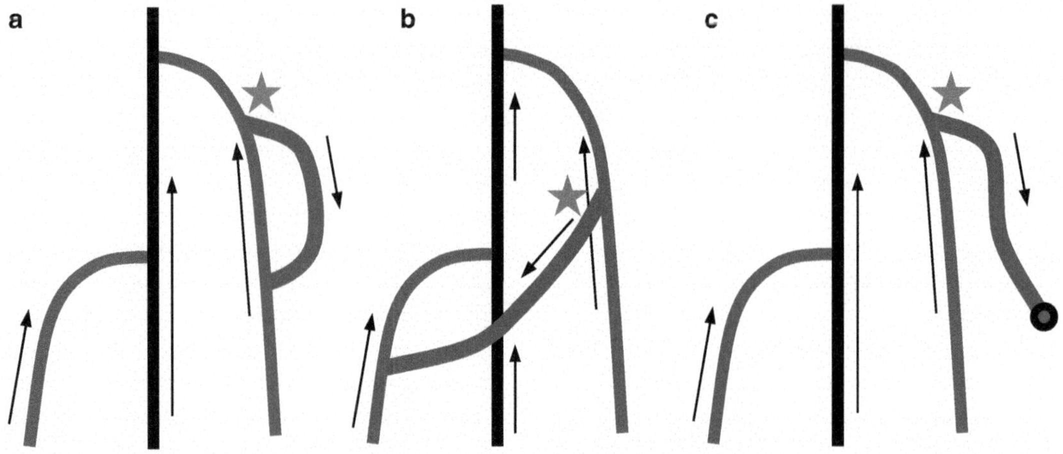

Fig. 6.29 Different forms of shunt type 2. (**a**) Closed shunt type 2 N2 → N3 (=N4L) – N2. Remember: N4 stands for N3 connecting two saphenous veins, in this case the same, thus "L" for longitudinal. (**b**) Open deviated shunt type 2: N2 → N3 (=N4T) – (different) N2. Remember: N4 means N3 connecting two saphenous veins, in this case different ones, thus "T" for transversal. (**c**) Open deviated shunt type 2: N2 → N3 – N1. All three cases would be treated with interruption at the reflux start (green star) (N2 ǂ N3). With permission by [10]

This is the easiest option for sure. But it has the risk of damaging the saphenous trunk by foam propagation if not properly done (see Sect. 7.12).

6.11.3 Shunt Type 3

Remember: N1 → N2 → N3 – (N2) – N1.

Recirculation from the deep veins into one of the saphenous veins and then through one or more tributaries back into the deep vein system. There is no distended perforating vein on the saphenous vein which could act as drainage between the reflux source and the first competent segment of the GSV further down (see Fig. 6.30). This is the commonest form of recirculation together with the shunt type 1.

The highest reflux source is the junction or, very rarely, a perforating vein filling the saphenous vein directly. The treatment is described in detail in Sect. 6.4.1. The fact that it cannot be treated leaving a stable, drained situation in one session without devalvulation (see Sect. 6.4.2) makes this shunt the more complex to understand or deal with.

As with shunt type 1, this strategy depends on the source and re-entry point of the reflux.

6.11.3.1 Shunt Type 3 with the Highest Reflux Source in a Junction

During the preoperative duplex ultrasound, be sure to document the flow profile in PW in the saphenous vein and its diameter. Apply the first surgical step: interruption with flush ligation of all refluxing tributaries where they join the saphenous vein (first step of CHIVA 2).

Follow-up with duplex after at least 6 weeks:

- Proximal saphenous vein is competent: Follow-up in further 6–12 months
- Proximal saphenous vein with diminished reflux (PW record is less than preoperatively or reflux appears only in the Valsalva manoeuvre and not in dynamic provocation manoeuvers) and the patient has no cosmetic complaints: Tell the patient to come back in 6 months or earlier if varices reappear or in the event of distress. In case of progression, see next step.
- If the reflux is unchanged to the preoperative situation (which occurs if a perforating vein opens, or a new tributary or bypass round the ligation forms), the junction must be treated.

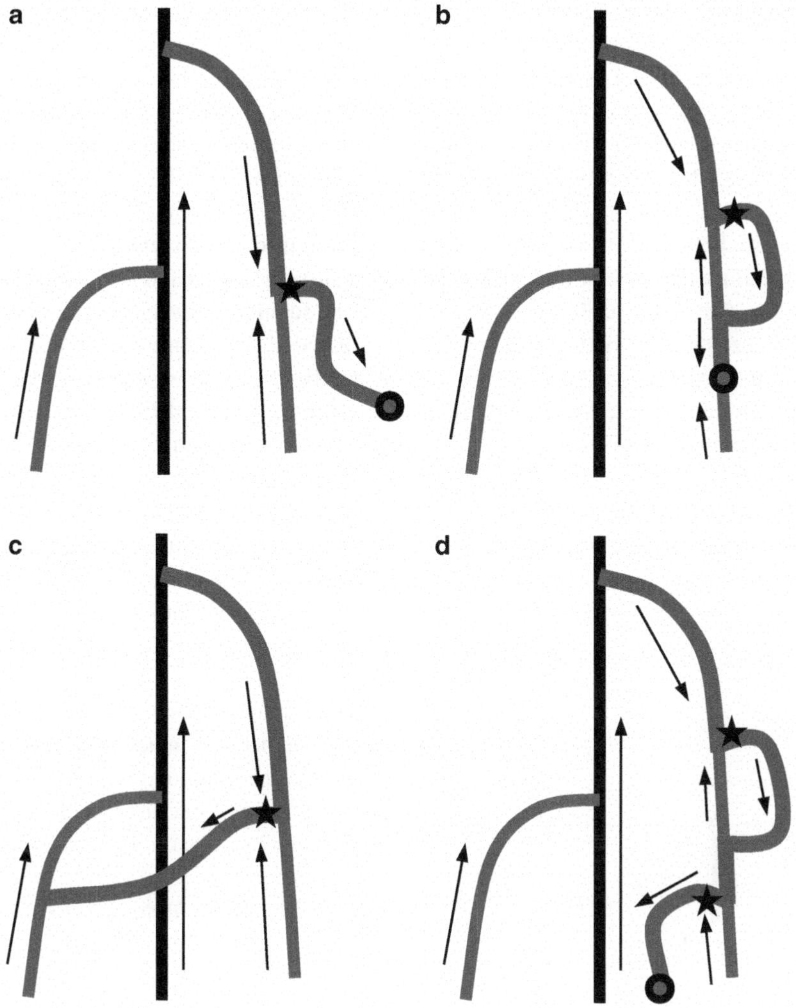

Fig. 6.30 Shunt type 3 with different draining pathways. The black star marks the point, where the first step of CHIVA 2 would be performed, the so-called CHIVA 2 Point. (**a**) Shunt type 3: N1 → N2 → N3 – N1. (**b**) Shunt type 3: N1 → N2 → N3 (=N4 L) – N2 – N1. (**c**) Shunt type 3: N1 → N2 → N3 (=N4 T) – N2 – N1. (**d**) Shunt type 3: N1 → N2 → N3 (=N4 L) – N2 → N3 – N1 (N4 L means N3 connecting the same saphenous vein, longitudinally; N4 T means N3 connecting different saphenous veins, transversally). With permission by [10]

6.11.3.2 Shunt Type 3 with the Highest Reflux Source Is a Perforating Vein

This is a rare condition, mainly through a perforating vein at the thigh. Usual procedure at shunt type 3.

- In case of little reflux and small perforating vein: flush ligation of the CHIVA 2 point only and control of perforating vein at follow-up. Only if there is still a reflux in the perforating vein and a new tributary has developed, perform the interruption of the perforating vein in the second step.
- In case of large reflux amounts and dilated perforating vein, perform flush ligation of the tributary and interruption of the perforating vein in the first session, but never touch the GSV itself.

6.11.3.3 Management in Case of Aplastic Segments of GSV

Sometimes the GSV itself has aplastic segments with a superficial accessory longitudinal vein acting as a bypass (see Sect. 4.5.1). In case of reflux and in the absence of a functional interfascial saphenous trunk, this accessory vein may be seen as a "functional saphenous vein" (Fig. 6.31), and a CHIVA 2 procedure may be applied. However, the regeneration rate after CHIVA 2 in the author's experience is not so good. Depending on the diameter of the proximal saphenous vein, an interruption at the junction in the first session may be the better option for dilated veins.

6.11.3.4 Management Depending on the Drainage Pathways

The "CHIVA 2 point" is always interrupted at the saphenous vein; only subsequent drainage variants are discussed here:

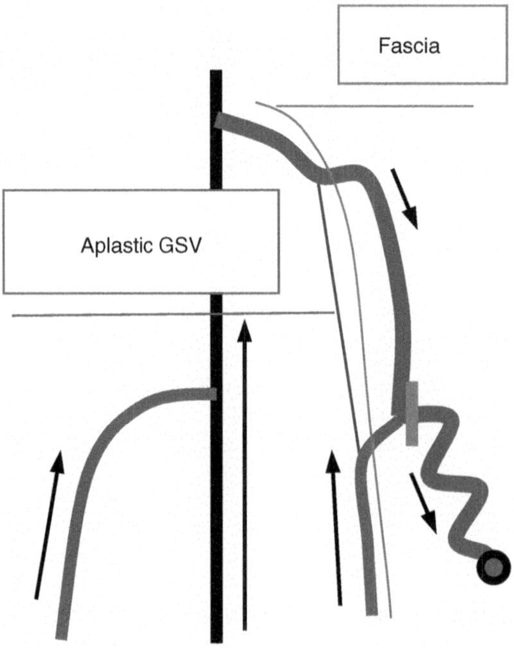

Fig. 6.31 Shunt type 3 with an aplastic segment of the GSV and bypass via a superficial rectilineous accessory vein, draining the reflux into a tributary. The distal GSV is competent, no drainage through a perforating vein from the GSV itself. Interruption at the origin of the tributary leaving the rectilineous bypass of the GSV is a treatment option. With permission by [10]

- **Drainage through a** tributary with re-entry into a perforating vein: Interruption at the CHIVA 2 point is sufficient (Fig. 6.32a).
- **Drainage through several tributaries (not shown)**: Every tributary must be interrupted at its junction with the saphenous vein.
- **Drainage through a tributary which drains back into the distal GSV**: The distal GSV is refluxing and drains into a perforating vein. The segment between both refluxing segments of GSV is competent. Interruption at the CHIVA 2 point is sufficient. After this interruption, the distal GSV should no longer be filled in retrograde flow, allowing it to regenerate (Fig. 6.32b).
- **Drainage as before, with a new draining tributary for the distal segment of GSV**: Both refluxing junctions with flow from the saphenous vein into the refluxing tributary are treated as CHIVA 2 points (see Fig. 6.32c).

The small saphenous vein (SSV) in the authors' experience reacts particularly well to the CHIVA 2 procedure (which is a different experience as compared to other groups). Unfortunately, no CHIVA 2 results on SSV are published so far.

6.11.3.5 Shunt Type 3 in Combination with Shunt Type 1

Sometimes a combination of shunt types 1 and 3 can be found in the same recirculation: in the upper part, we find a shunt type 1 with a perforating vein on the saphenous vein; but, below the perforating vein, the blood drainage corresponds to shunt type 3 (see Fig. 6.33). The saphenous vein is still refluxing distally to the perforating vein and drains then through a tributary. If a ligation of the GSV below the perforating vein is performed, as shunt type 1 procedure expects, the tributary is obliged to serve as drainage for the distal, antegrade section of the GSV. This will not produce a good cosmetic outcome. The upper section should therefore be treated as shunt type 1 with interruption of the SFJ. The section below the perforating vein should be treated as shunt type 3, using CHIVA 2: The tributary must be interrupted with a flush ligation at the GSV.

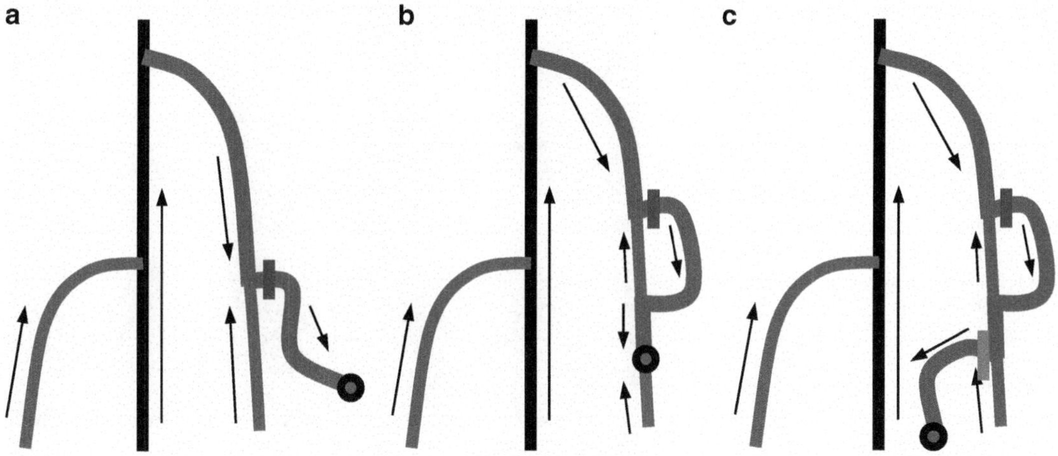

Fig. 6.32 Treatment options for the first step of CHIVA 2 in shunt type 3. (**a**) One draining tributary—interruption of the draining vessel at its junction with the saphenous vein. N1 → N2 ┼ N3 – N1 (**b**) One draining tributary, which itself drains back to the distal GSV and there into a perforating vein. Treatment as **a**). N1 → N2 ┼ N3 – N2 – N1 (**c**) One draining tributary, draining back into the distal GSV and there again into a draining tributary and a perforating vein. N1 → N2 ┼ N3 – N2 ┼ N3 – N1. With permission by [10]

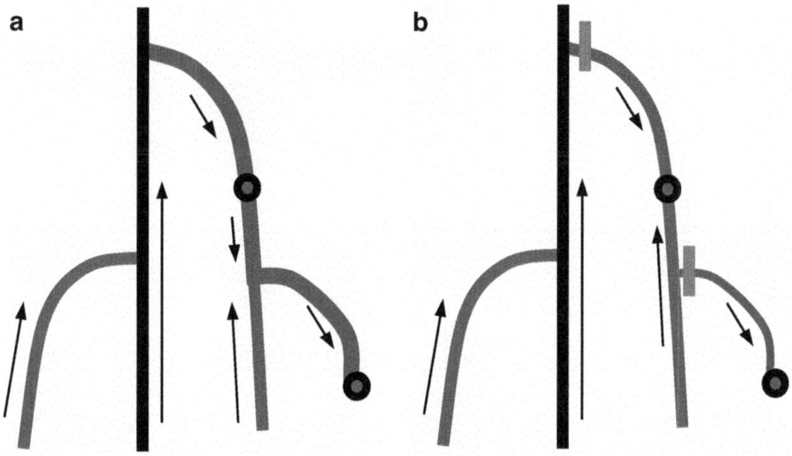

Fig. 6.33 (**a**) Shunt types 1 and 3: The proximal recirculation is a shunt type 1 with refluxing SFJ and draining perforating vein on the GSV (N1 → N2 – N1). The GSV continues to be refluxing downwards, draining through a tributary a perforating vein (N1 → N2 → N3 – N1). N1 → N2 – N1 ↘ N2 → N3 – N1 (**b**) The treatment option is the interruption of the junction and of the tributary; the flow in the distal GSV will get reverted and drain into the perforating vein. N1 ┼ N2 – N1 ↘ N2 ┼ N3 – N1. With permission by [10]

6.11.3.6 Examples of Shunt Type 3 Cases

As shunt type 3 and CHIVA 2 are the most revolutionary innovations to replace stripping, some examples are explained in the figure legends (Figs. 6.34, 6.35, 6.36, and 6.37).

A problem when starting with CHIVA 2 is that many doctors do not like to tell patients that they may have to return in some months for a junction operation, in other words, that they still may have the most serious part of the operation ahead of

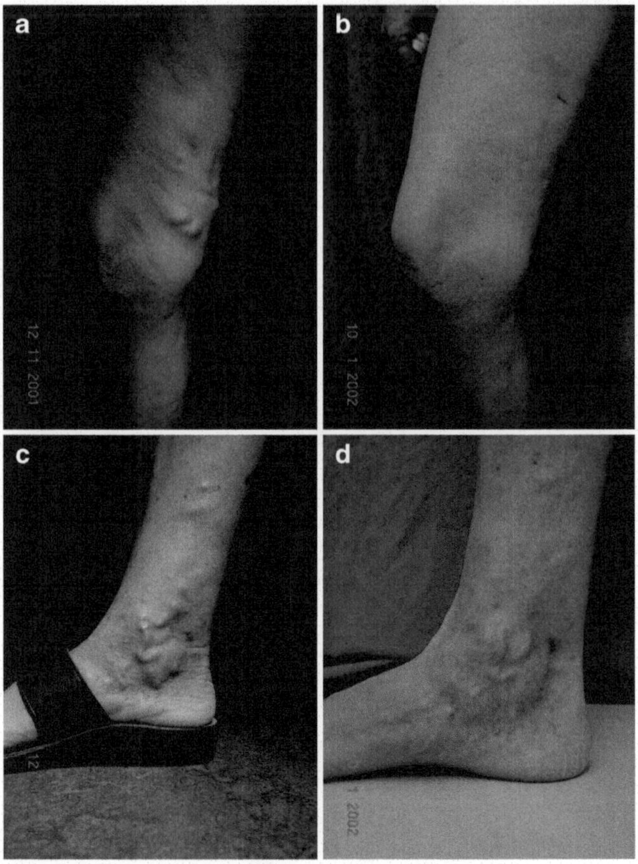

Fig. 6.34 (**a**) Top left (12.11.2001) preoperative photograph: shunt type 3 with flow pattern as in Fig. 6.32a. (**b**) Bottom left: Preoperative image of the foot. (**c**) Top right post-operative control (10.01.2002): After exposure of the GSV at the thigh with disconnection of the tributary as the only treatment. SFJ is competent in post-operative examination; tributary has reduced its calibre and is no longer visible. (**d**) Bottom right: Post-operative image of the foot. This post-operative situation was still stable at the follow-up 15 years later. With permission by [10]

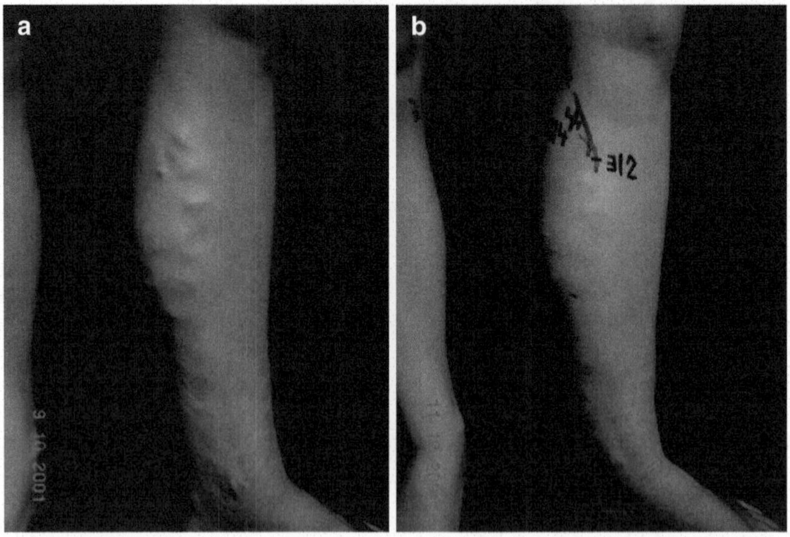

Fig. 6.35 (**a**) 02.10.2001: Preoperative photograph—shunt type 3 with flow pattern as in Fig. 6.32a. (**b**) 11.12.2001: Follow-up 9 weeks after exposure of the GSV in the calf (scar visible under the green line, above the mark 3/2) and ligation of a tributary further distal. Cosmetic result: less veins but still visible. Duplex result: The SFJ was (less) incompetent in the post-operative examination, with new reflux through tributary above the previous CHIVA 2 point. The patient wanted a second attempt with interruption of the new CHIVA 2 point and not an interruption of the junction, so we proceeded as drawn: Exposure of the newly formed CHIVA 2 point and interruption of another tributary. (Not shown: Finally, the SFJ had to be interrupted, because always new tributaries were formed). With permission by [10]

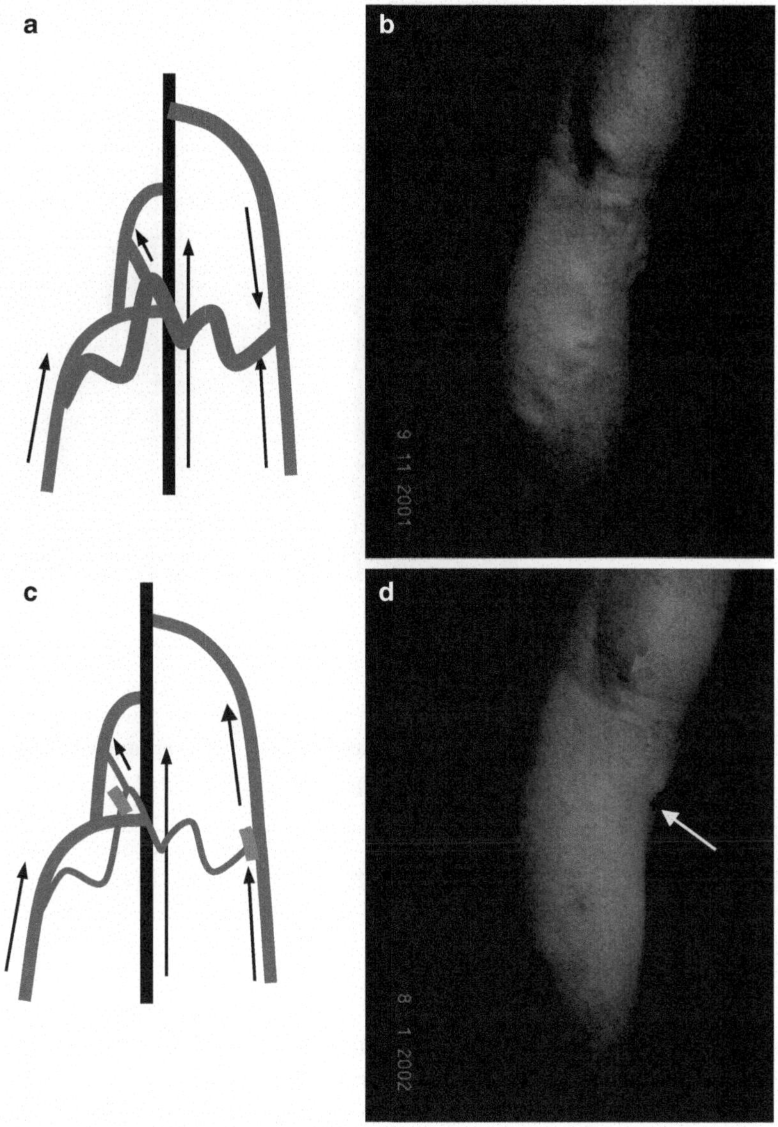

Fig. 6.36 (**a**) Shunt type 3 of the GSV with drainage of the tributary through a competent small saphenous vein and a connection to the competent thigh extension of the SSV. (**b**) 09.11.2001: Preoperative photograph. (**c**) Flow scheme after interruption of the tributary at the junction with the GSV and after branching and draining into the thigh extension of the SSV. Competent SFJ, calibre reduction in the tributary. (**d**) 08.01.2002 Photograph at control after flush ligation of the tributary (yellow arrow) and further interruption of the tributary above the knee crease (blue arrow) as the only measures. Cosmetic disappearance of the tributary without phlebectomy. With permission by [10]

them and that in the meantime there may be no cosmetic improvement.

In Germany, where the doctor is payed per procedure, the dissociated technique (CHIVA 2 with two steps) was not a problem at all. If the patient is properly informed that he is going to have a very little surgery, touching only a tributary, which might resolve the problem with his saphenous vein in approximately 30% of cases, normally the patient will accept the idea. It is most often not a problem of the patient but of the surgeon, who is used to "resolve" things in one session.

A consensus of 21 CHIVA-applying doctors in Germany found out that, in case of shunt type 3 with reflux in GSV ending above-knee, all of them performed the first step of CHIVA 2, because it is highly probable to have a stable anterograde flow situation, and this is just the most important achievement of the technique to allow a refluxing GSV to revert to antegrade flow again [19].

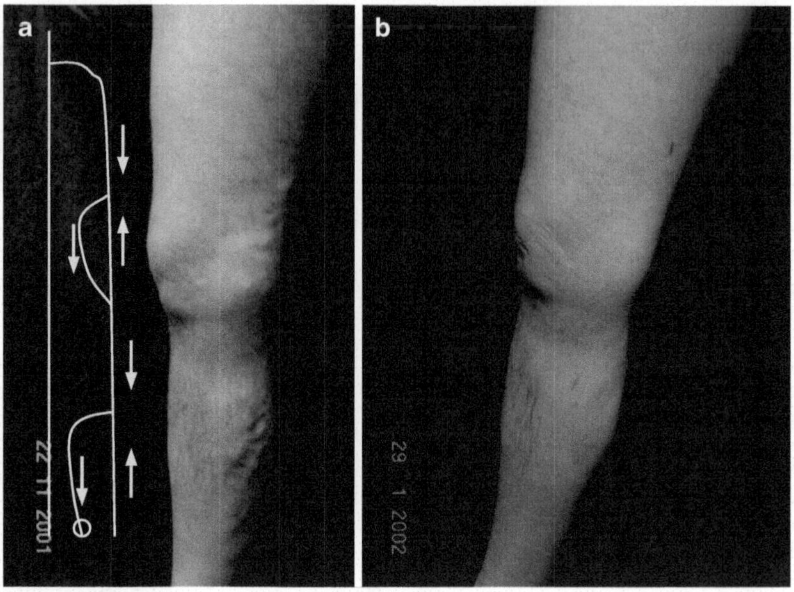

Fig. 6.37 (**a**) 22.11.2001 Preoperative photograph: shunt type 3 with flow pattern as in Fig. 6.32c, which is also shown on the left border of the picture. (**b**) 29.01.2002: Follow-up after exposure of the GSV in the thigh and lower leg with disconnection of the tributaries as the only measures. The SFJ is competent in post-operative examination. With permission by [10]

6.11.4 Shunt Types 4 and 5

As the strategy in case of shunts 4 and 5 have some common points, they will be described together.

Shunt type 4:
Remember: Pelvine shunt type 4: P → N3 – N2 – N1
Perforating vein shunt type 4: N1 → N3 – N2 – N1

Recirculation in the saphenous vein with origin not directly from the deep venous system, but through a tributary, which may conduct reflux from pelvine vessels (Pelvine shunt type 4) or from perforating veins (perforating vein shunt type 4). Drainage directly from the saphenous vein to the deep vein via perforating vein analogous to drainage in shunt type 1 (Fig. 6.38).

Shunt type 5:
Remember: Pelvine shunt type 4: P → N3 – N2 → **N3** – N1
Perforating vein shunt type 4: N1 → N3 – N2 → **N3** – N1

Recirculation in the saphenous vein with origin as shunt type 5. Drainage from the saphenous vein to the deep vein via a tributary. No dilated perforating vein on the saphenous vein, analogous to drainage in shunt type 3.

Variations of these shunt types are described in Chap. 3 (Fig. 6.39).

Following the CHIVA methodology, the correct procedure would be to interrupt the **reflux source**. In case of a perforating vein reflux, this is easy to perform by interruption of the perforating vein (shunts 4 and 5); see Sect. 6.9.1.

In case of pelvic reflux, the reflux source will never be touched within the leg. Even an interruption of the pelvic tributary in the groin with phlebectomy as far as you may go through the groin incision will not reach the proximal reflux point.

Franceschi and Bahnini first described the interruption at the P point (perineal reflux) and the I point (inguinal reflux) which was later elaborated by Delfratre, described in Chap. 8.

If the pelvic reflux source shows as a net of tributaries emerging from the labia or visible at the inner part of the proximal thigh or a long epigastric vein visible on the skin proximal to the inguinal ligament, then it might be enough to treat this net with sclerotherapy to reduce the proximal reflux in the same session as the distal tributary interruption.

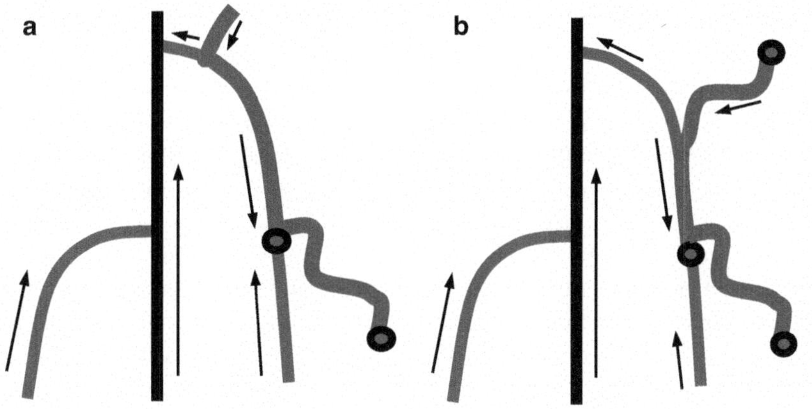

Fig. 6.38 Shunt type 4 is defined by the drainage from the GSV through a perforating vein on the GSV (mandatory). Additionally, there can be a drainage through a tributary. (**a**) Pelvic shunt type 4. (**b**) Perforating vein shunt type 4. With permission by [10]

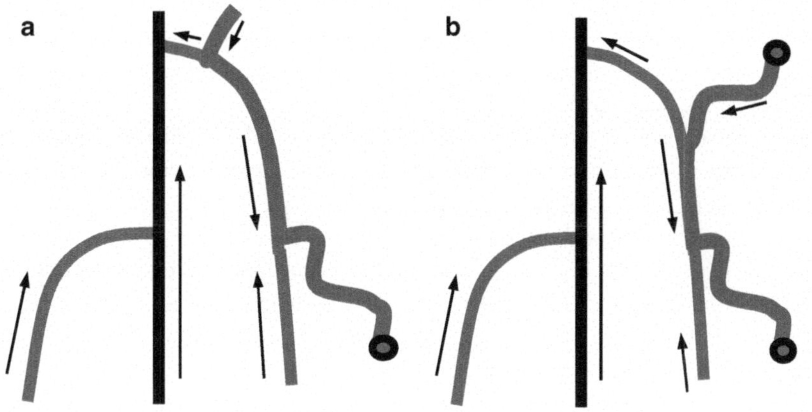

Fig. 6.39 Shunt type 5: It is defined by no draining perforating vein on the GSV. Reflux drains via a tributary. (**a**) Pelvic shunt type 5. (**b**) Perforating vein shunt type 5. With permission by [10]

In case the sclerotherapy is not feasible and no surgeon with experience in interrupting pelvic leakage points is available, this supra-inguinal reflux will be always a source of recidives, independently of the technique applied. In the eyes of the author, the treatment of the GSV distal to the confluence of the refluxing pelvic branches with endoluminal thermal ablation of some centimetres may be one option and is being investigated. It would allow a drainage of the pelvic reflux to the deep veins through the junction, perhaps avoiding the natural evolution to new varicose veins in the groin or via inner, dorsal or ventral aspect of the thigh.

Sometimes not treating the junction in case of little reflux drained via a perforating vein (shunt type 4; see Fig. 6.17b) is an option: The little reflux might take years to develop, whilst the recidives after interruption often develop to bothering tributaries on the proximal thigh after some months. In any case, the patient must be informed that the highest reflux source is pelvic and will not be treated in this case.

Treatment of tributaries: In both cases (shunt types 4 and 5), the tributaries will always be disconnected from the saphenous veins as described for shunt types 1 and 3, respectively.

6.11.4.1 Perforating Vein Shunt Type 4

(a) *No distal tributaries present* (Fig. 6.40a): Interruption of the refluxing perforating vein
(b) *Tributaries present* (Fig. 6.40b): Interruption of the refluxing perforating vein and distal tributaries. The refluxive tributaries can be interrupted in any case and independently of the drainage capacity of the draining saphenous vein perforator, because saphenous vein can also be drained through its untouched and antegrade junction.

6.11.4.2 Pelvic Shunt Type 4

(a) *No distal tributaries present* (see Fig. 6.41a): Prior to any treatment, it has to be considered, if a treatment is necessary. This is a typical case of a "stable" reflux. It exists, but normally it does not harm the patient (no cosmetic complaints because no tributaries are visible, normally no pain as the reflux amount is not too large). If a decision to treat the vein was made, interruption of the pelvic reflux must be performed (sclerotherapy, interruption of leakage point, closure of the GSV distal to the preterminal valve with endoluminal heat).
(b) *Distal tributaries present* (see Fig. 6.41b): In case of *little amount of reflux*, perform interruption of the tributaries to meet cosmetic exigencies. If reflux in saphenous vein is little (e.g. diameter of saphenous vein at proximal thigh less than 4–6 mm), an interruption of the tributary might be enough to achieve a stable situation without touching the proximal source. The result after interruption only of the tributary in Fig. 6.41b will be shown in Fig. 6.41a (prior to treating the pelvine reflux). With little reflux, this situation can keep stable over years. In case of *large amounts of reflux*, an interruption of the pelvic reflux with all its variant forms and their limitations as described above will be necessary, as well as the interruption of the tributary.

6.11.4.3 Perforating Vein Shunt Type 5

In this situation, the treatment is very easy: interruption of the refluxing perforating vein and interruption of the refluxing tributary or tributaries with flush ligation (see Fig. 6.42).

6.11.4.4 Pelvic Shunt Type 5

This is the perfect situation to apply CHIVA 2 tactic.

First step: Interruption of the refluxing tributary (Fig. 6.43a). In case of subfascial net of pelvic tributaries emerging from the labia or visible at the medial aspect of the proximal thigh (see above), a sclerotherapy of these tributaries

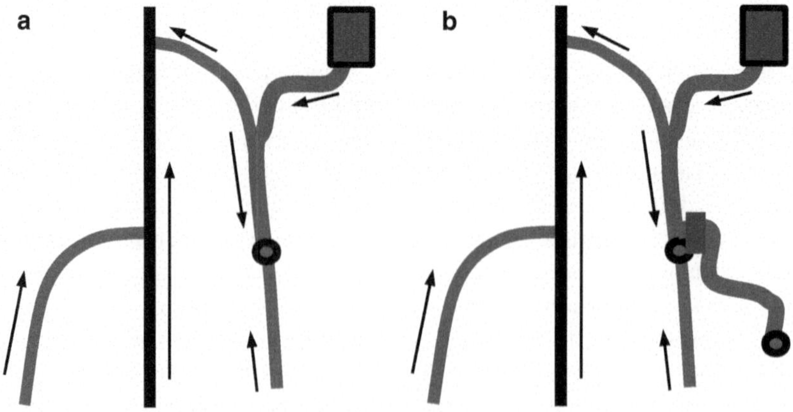

Fig. 6.40 Shunt type 4 perforating vein without tributary (**a**) and with tributary (**b**). The perforating vein has to be treated with subfascial closure (green rectangle), the tributary only if present. With permission by [10]

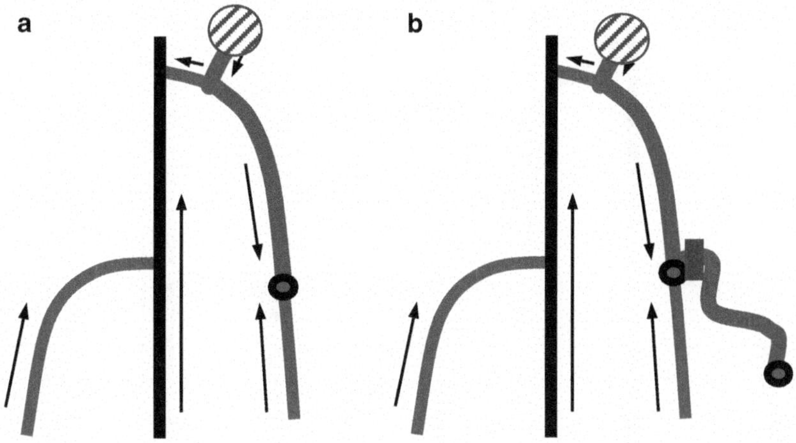

Fig. 6.41 Shunt type 4 with pelvine reflux without additional refluxing tributary (**a**) and with additional refluxive tributary (**b**). (**a**) Consider not to treat anything or deal with the pelvine reflux (see text), represented with a green and white lined circle. (**b**) Consider interrupting only the connection between tributary and GSV (green line) and treat the pelvine reflux (green and white lined circle) only if clinics make this step necessary due to large amounts of reflux. With permission by [10]

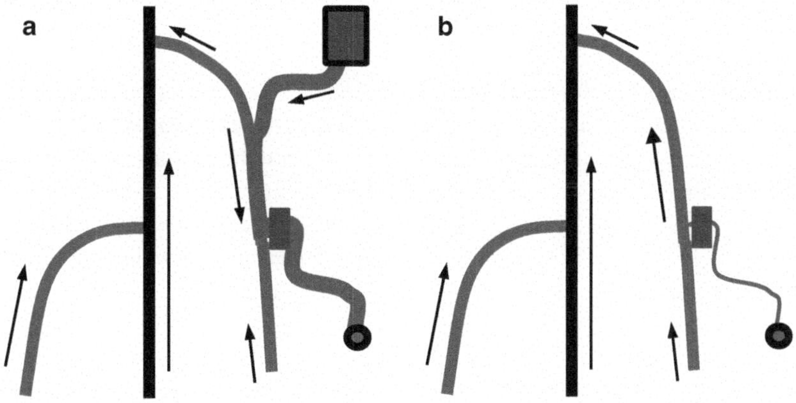

Fig. 6.42 Shunt type 5 perforating vein: (**a**) Interruption of the perforating vein (green rectangle) and the tributary. (**b**) In almost all cases, antegrade flow in GSV. With permission by [10]

may be done in the same session with the tributary disconnection.

Second step: Follow-up after 8 weeks to some months with two possibilities:

- *In 97% of cases, saphenous vein has no reflux* (see Fig. 6.43b):
  Refluxive pelvic tributary drains through the junction to the deep vein. No need of further interruption. Follow-up after 6 and 12 months just to make sure the saphenous vein does not develop a new reflux fed by the pelvic tributary.
- *Saphenous vein has reflux* (3%; see Sects. 6.4.1.2–6.4.1.3). Reflux in saphenous trunk after tributary disconnection is only possible, if a new draining point has opened. There are two options:
  - Drainage through a new refluxing tributary proximal or distal from the interruption point. We find again a pelvic shunt type 5. The tributary could be disconnected again. However, our experience teaches that in almost all the situations, the reflux from the groin will

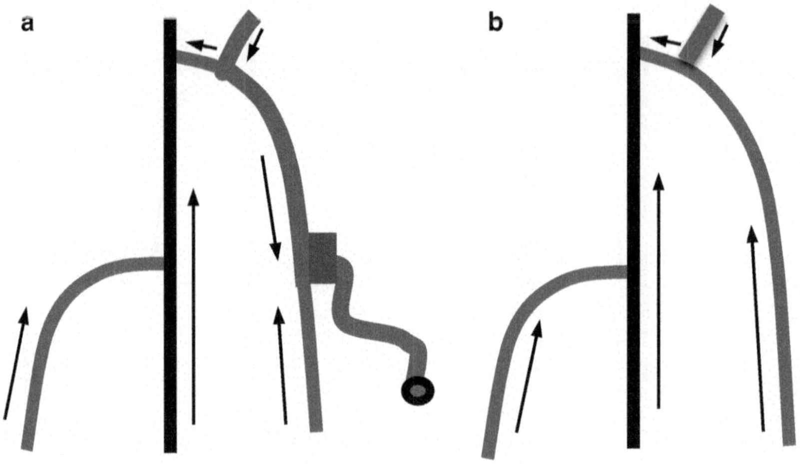

Fig. 6.43 Pelvic shunt type 5: (**a**) First step disconnection of the tributary (green line). (**b**) Result in 97% of cases: Pelvic reflux is drained via the competent terminal valve into the deep vein; GSV is competent. With permission by [10]

reappear, so it is the best to treat the pelvic reflux with one of the options as described above.

- Drainage through a perforating vein on the saphenous vein. In this case we have a pelvic shunt type 4. Further treatment is described there.

6.11.5 Shunt Type 6

Remember: This is a conglomeration of all reflux situations not covered by shunt types 1–5. The saphenous vein is not involved in the recirculation. It is mostly the situation with a reflux emerging from perforating veins or pelvic reflux that feed tributaries without saphenous vein involvement in the reflux.

The treatment depends on the extension of the disease. Often the cosmetic bothering veins are so tiny that a sclerotherapy is sufficient, even to treat the refluxing perforating vein.

Following the CHIVA principles, the reflux source should be interrupted: disconnection of the perforating vein or interruption of the pelvic leak point. The visible tributaries at the leg may be left in situ waiting if they reduce after interruption of the reflux source. If the cosmetics are the principal reason for the patient to ask for a treatment, the tributaries may be treated by sclerotherapy, phlebectomy or interruptions at branching points.

6.11.6 Shunt Involving Both Saphenous Veins

Sometimes patients present with reflux in both saphenous veins of one leg. Mostly these refluxes are interconnected. It is very seldom to find independent refluxes affecting both superficial collectors. In this case, they have to be treated isolately considering each as one recirculation circuit.

Often, especially in persons after sports with trauma on the calf, different muscle perforating veins with reflux feeding superficial N3 vessels independently are found. This is another situation with lots of independent recirculations, but not affecting saphenous veins.

The two scenarios most often found is the connection of great and small saphenous vein either through the Giacomini vein or through a tributary below the knee. In both situations, either vein can serve as drainage for the other.

6.11.6.1 Connection via the Giacomini Vein

Reflux starting at the sapheno-popliteal junction (SPJ) can feed the Giacomini vein and then the great saphenous vein (GSV) as shown in

Fig. 6.44. This is not too rare. The shunt is interesting from different points of view:

- It is the combination of an open and a closed shunt.
- It can be composed by a systolic and a diastolic shunt (see Fig. 3.31, Sect. 3.9.1).
- Concerning the closed shunt, the re-entry is further down in the leg than the escape point, but the path runs much higher in the leg than the reflux source.

With the upcoming of duplex investigation, lot of early recidives after stripping of GSV were identified as caused by Giacomini vein reflux. Thus, also in the ablative setting, this vein needs to be directed with special care.

The shunt classification is difficult, because two saphenous veins are involved: The reflux source is the SSV, draining the reflux in the proximal prolongation under the fascia (or epifascial in a tributary). The pathologic amount of blood ascends to join the GSV at the proximal thigh via the posterior accessory saphenous vein or a tributary, with sub- or epifascial course (N2 or N3, classified as transversal N4, as it connects two saphenous veins). The GSV is competent in the groin and gets incompetent fed from the blood from the SSV recirculation. Usually the refluxing blood drains into a tributary at knee level (above or below it). The most distal perforating vein is at the calf.

In case of diastolic reflux only, we find the following shunts (see Fig. 6.44):

- A shunt type 3 for the SSV (**N1** → **N2** → **N3** – N2 – N1)
- A shunt type 5 for the GSV—considering the SPJ as a perforating vein in this case: N1 → N2 → **N3 (Giacomini vein)** – **N2** → **N3** – **N1**

During the investigation of the reflux in the SPJ, it is important to discriminate between systolic and diastolic reflux—often both are present. This is fundamental for the treatment decision. In case of obstruction of the deep veins in the thigh after thrombosis or muscular dysfunction, the Giacomini vein is a good draining path for the blood of the calf. During systole, the blood will be expelled through the SPJ and the SSV into the Giacomini vein, drained via the GSV and SFJ into the proximal common femoral vein. This is an open bypassing or vicarious shunt, which should not be interrupted to avoid bothering recurrences at the knee level. It can be combined, with a closed diastolic shunt, concerning the

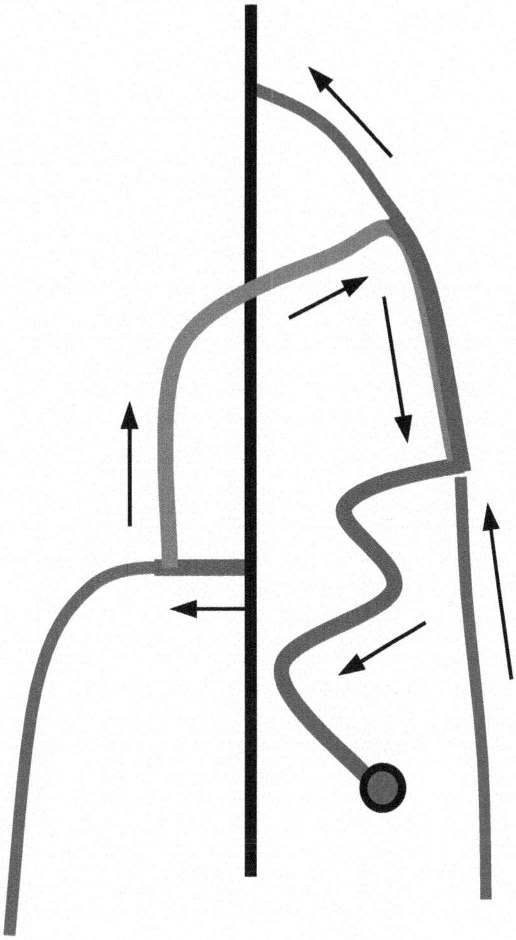

Fig. 6.44 Incompetent SPJ with reflux into the SSV, feeding the Giacomini vein (coloured in orange for differentiation). At the junction with the GSV, some of the blood drains antegrade via the SFJ into the common femoral vein (open deviated shunt if diastolic, open bypassing or vicarious shunt if systolic) and some of the blood fills the distal GSV retrogradely, draining to the deep vein via a tributary (closed shunt). N1 → N2 → TN4 (GV) – N2 – N1 ↘ N2 → N3 – N1. With permission by [10]

GSV—which can easily be treated without interrupting the open shunt (see Fig. 6.45a, b).

As the treatment options are varied, they shall be analysed in detail.

In case that the Giacomini anastomosis runs under a fascia: The treatment is to disconnect the tributary from the GSV with flush ligation (green line in Fig. 6.45a). The whole recirculation then usually regenerates producing antegrade flow in SPJ as well as in the preoperatively refluxing segment of GSV. Sometimes after this tactic, no reflux is seen in the tributary or the GSV, but there is still an open shunt (Fig. 6.45b): reflux from the SSV into Giacomini anastomosis draining into GSV and flowing antegrade to the SFJ. If there is no pain in the fossa poplitea, this condition will not be noticed by the patient nor shall it bother the leg circulation and might be left untouched but observed regularly.

In case the Giacomini anastomosis has extrafascial segments, perform flush ligation of the tributary when emerging the fascia. Figure 6.45c shows the situation in case the tributary emerges directly from the SSV. It might also emerge on the running of the proximal extension of the thigh higher up; in that case the flush ligation has to be performed at this branching from the subfascial to the epifascial vein. Then, the post-operative examination will show an antegrade flow in the SPJ.

If the SPJ is very dilated preoperatively with SSV diameters higher than 10 mms, it should be considered to perform a flush ligation of the SSV at the popliteal level—but only if there is no systolic reflux, which would lead to a high recurrence rate and an impairment of leg drainage.

Of course, attention has to be paid to possible perforating veins in the course of the Giacomini anastomosis on its running on the back of the thigh—these should be treated according to CHIVA principles (see Sect. 6.9).

6.11.6.2 Connection via a Calf Tributary

As presented in Sect. 3.5.4 and Fig. 6.46, the reflux from the GSV can be drained via a con-

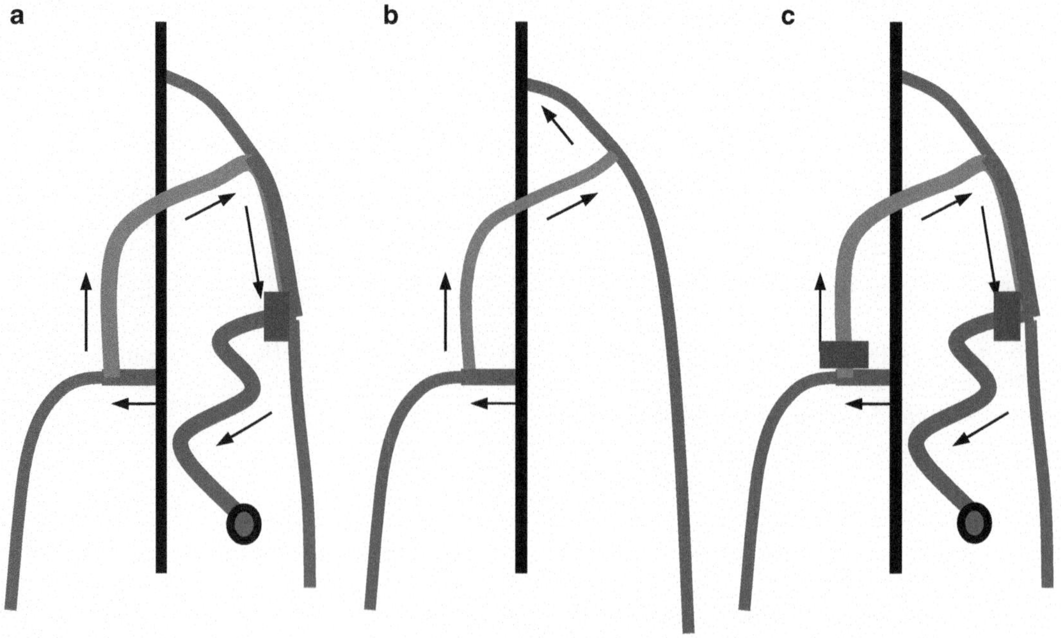

Fig. 6.45 Recirculation via the Giacomini anastomosis coloured in orange for differentiation. (**a**) Treatment option with subfascial Giacomini anastomosis. (**b**) Possible result after strategy described in **a**. (**c**) Treatment option with epifascial Giacomini anastomosis (and after excluding an open bypassing shunt). With permission by [10]

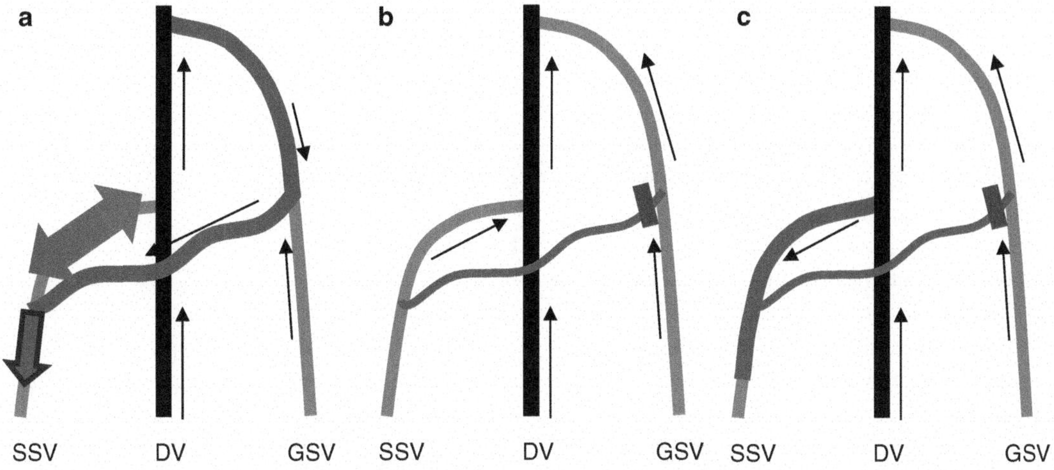

Fig. 6.46 Drainage from a refluxing GSV through a connecting vein between GSV and SSV. (**a**) Preoperative situation: Proximal SSV is enlarged, with antegrade and retrograde flow during diastole. (**b**, **c**) Situation after interruption of the tributary at the level of the GSV, assuming a flow correction in the GSV, which is not relevant to the evolution of SSV. (**b**) The SSV has recovered completely, no reflux. (**c**) The SSV is still refluxing, a second treatment session will be necessary to treat the persisting reflux. With permission by [10]

necting tributary (N3 or transversal N4) with the SSV. Initially the reflux might be drained via the junction, but after some time and with progressive dilatation of the proximal SSV, this will become incompetent, too. Another scenario would be an open systolic bypassing shunt starting at the sapheno-popliteal junction, feeding the SSV and the calf transversal N4 and thus the GSV, which might be competent and draining the flow, until it dilates too much, reverting the flow in diastole and becoming incompetent, too.

Thus, it is very important to double check systolic and diastolic flow when both veins are involved and to try and find out which vein was the first one with reflux, for example, asking the patient, where the first veins were observed on the leg. Another technique is comparing the PW reflux curves in both saphenous veins. The draining ones will show antegrade flow during diastole or a flow to and for.

The vein suspected as secondary filled should not be treated in the first session, as it often recovers completely (see Fig. 6.46).

Another possibility is a primary reflux source in the SPJ, filling the SSV, draining through a tributary into the distal GSV—the proximal aspect of this vein is competent. Usually the treatment of the SSV will solve the reflux situation in the GSV.

6.11.7 Remodelling a Refluxing System

In some cases, there is a very large reflux amount through a junction or a perforating vein with a great number of divisions along the tributaries. In other cases, the tributaries and re-entry perforating veins are large, meandering and difficult to analyse. Obviously, these patients do not have high cosmetic claims, otherwise they would not have allowed the veins to develop to this point. In these cases, the treatment is required for pain or discomfort or skin changes. And in these advanced cases, we always find a shunt type 1 or 3 with reflux from the deep venous system.

Applying the four standard requests for CHIVA—interruption of the reflux source, subdivision of the pressure column, saving the re-entries and eliminating the non-draining tributary system—lots of divisions should be applied. But the larger the vessels, the higher the risk of a superficial vein thrombosis (see Sect. 10.1.4).

It is possible to treat the system in two or more steps: Starting with the interruption of the reflux source (junction or perforating vein), apply low dose heparin for 2 weeks and compression for some weeks or months and wait for calibre reduction in the system [5]. Often patients are so happy to have lost the symptoms just with this step that they do not want to undergo further steps. Or in the post-operative visit after some months, it becomes obvious that some further interruptions make sense—which can then be carried out in a second step.

This strategy is especially useful in patients with skin changes at the calf, allowing a recovery of the skin and incisions with less risk of infection or bad healing.

6.12 Non-haemodynamic Saphenous Vein Sparing Treatment

Sometimes decisions in medicine are subjected to extern necessities, like rules by health-care insurances or other socio-economic reasons. Thus, the treatment of varicose veins in some countries has to be successful after one session; re-interventions or re-investigations are not possible.

As described in Sect. 6.4.1, the treatment of shunt type 3 is not possible in one step—over 70% of the cases will need a second step intervention if starting with first step of CHIVA 2 [13] or a poor cosmetic result if starting with crossotomy.

6.12.1 CHIVA 1 + 2

Performing both steps of CHIVA 2—the tributary interruption and the crossotomy—is called CHIVA 1 + 2.

Applying crossotomy (interruption of the SFJ) and tributary interruption simultaneously, the primary reflux source is interrupted and the tributary will no longer be filled. The cosmetic result will be achieved and the reflux source interrupted (see Fig. 6.3 right and Fig. 6.47).

The problem is that in 38% of cases, the GSV between both interruptions will suffer thrombosis (see Sect. 10.1.4). And as a consequence, spider veins can appear at the thigh due to poor drainage of skin veins, the same as observed after stripping (see Sect. 10.2.2). In some situations, the risk of matting is not the central problem but the quick treatment of an ulceration or severe skin changes, e.g. in adipose persons. In these cases, a CHIVA 1 + 2 procedure might be an option to make sure the target will be reached soon.

To avoid these thrombosis/matting problems, the devalvulation of a segment of the GSV was developed to be applied in the same session with CHIVA 1 + 2 (see Sect. 6.4.2).

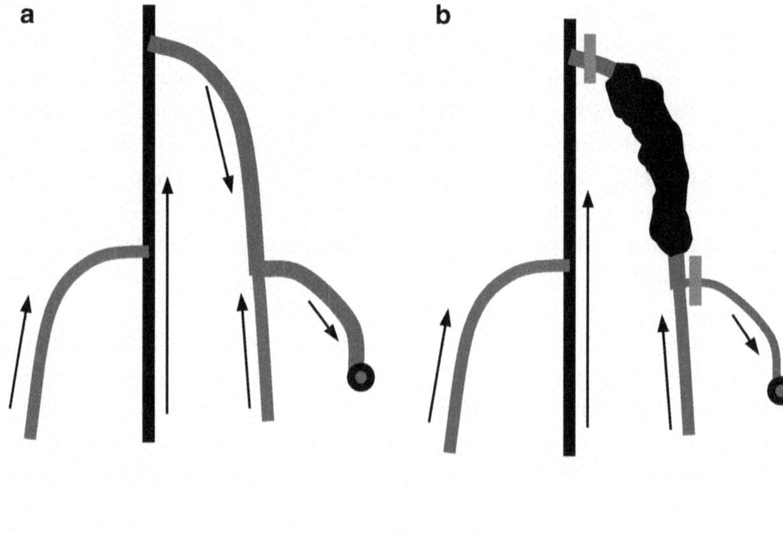

Fig. 6.47 (**a**) Shunt type 3. (**b**) Non-haemodynamic treatment with crossotomy and tributary interruption (CHIVA 1 + 2), leaving the GSV without drainage. This leads to thrombosis or poor drainage of GSV. With permission by [10]

6.12.2 How to Avoid Non-Drained Systems

Non-drained systems lead to spider veins and early recidives through subcutaneous vessels, mostly bothering the patient. The advantage of stable draining vein situation after regular CHIVA is lost might be the one responsible for less recurrence rate as compared to stripping.

In the situation of shunt type 3, the devalvulation was the answer to the unsatisfactory non-drained situation after CHIVA 1 + 2 (explained in Sects. 6.4.2 and 6.12.1).

Thus, especially during the learning curve, seeking for good drainage of all treated segments should be a high goal. As a first step, the analysis of the preoperative situation is very important, also to verify after a failure what could have gone wrong.

If a perforating vein or tributary does not seem to be sufficient to deal with the drainage of a segment, it is best not to do all the possible interruptions in the first step. This is especially important when starting to do CHIVA. Usually surgeons are used to do lots of incisions and tend to plan too much interruptions to achieve a result as good as possible. But just in the learning situation and in doubt if an interruption is necessary, it would be best just to close the most important insufficiency point and leave all the others for a second moment, months later, if they still seem necessary to be treated.

In any case, apply the manoeuver described in Fig. 6.2 before treating a tributary.

6.13 Management in Cases of Preoperative Thrombosis of Superficial Veins

Occlusion due to thrombi makes diagnosis of reflux more difficult, because thrombi close the veins partially or completely. This falsifies the drainage scheme from varicose veins, which is one of the most important bases for decision-making in CHIVA. It is therefore advisable always to try to clear up the thrombosis first by treatment with conservative measures. However, this is not always possible, and the patient must then be treated despite the thrombosis.

In such cases, the recommendation is to limit treatment to interruption of the proximal reflux source. Since the result of this is to further reduce the velocity of blood flow in the occluded region, it is likely that the thrombosis will get worse immediately after the operation. It is therefore recommended to treat these patients with low molecular prophylactic heparin for 10–14 days after the intervention and non-steroidal anti-inflammatory drugs for the first week and then to explore the patient again and to decide whether to give more heparin depending on the calibre reduction of the saphenous vein: good reduction (no more heparin) and no reduction (go on with heparin).

Superficial vein thrombosis after CHIVA will be discussed below (see Sect. 6.14.5). CHIVA treatment in case of deep vein thrombosis is addressed in Chap. 9.

6.14 The Post-operative Examination

The patient should come in for a duplex ultrasound post-operative examination after some months, the earliest to see changes 8 weeks after the operation. Earlier than these changes in the venous system are not established—in some patients it takes even longer.

Apart from examining the vein calibre reduction, the doctor must also find out whether the patient's preoperative distress has changed.

Patients can sometimes feel when new connections open which previously did not exist or were not refluxing. So, it may occur that the clinic, cosmetic and duplex ultrasound findings after a surgery are good, but the patient complains of pains, for example, at the inner thigh after interruption of the SFJ. He can even put his finger on the exact spot. Almost always a (still) thin but refluxing perforating vein can be found, which in a few weeks will again deliver reflux into the GSV. It should be interrupted immediately before it provokes cosmetic complaints. It is not necessary to await development. If the patient wants to postpone the complementary operation to a later date, however, it has to be explained to the patient that new visible varicose veins will appear.

6.14.1 Post-operative Examination of the Junctions After Interruption

The documentation must record (even if only as a note in the file without an image) whether the SFJ or SPJ was closed and how much flow entered the saphenous trunk vein from the superficial inguinal tributaries or the vein of Giacomini. Otherwise it will be impossible later to find the correct cause in the event of recurrence. If the SFJ or SPJ is not closed, it will have to be re-treated. This is very important in CHIVA, as different from the ablating techniques, a residual reflux will very soon express as new visible veins using the non-destroyed pathways. In case of a non-complete crossectomy in the stripping context, it takes years until veins visible in ultrasound after the intervention are clinically relevant.

6.14.2 Post-operative Examination of the SFJ and SPJ After CHIVA 2

After CHIVA 2, the SFJ and SPJ are examined under the same criteria as in the preoperative examination. If the junction is competent, the patient will be called in for regular check-ups. If the junction is incompetent, further procedure will depend on the finding (see also Sect. 6.4.1):

- If there is only minimal reflux, perhaps only under Valsalva, and the patient is otherwise free of distress and satisfied, it is safe to wait a couple of months before carrying out an interruption of the junction. The GSV sometimes requires rather long to further reduce the diameter and may get competent later.
- If there is still a reflux and a new tributary has opened to carry the reflux, the junction must be closed without long delays, because any delay may allow the condition to become aggravated unnecessarily.
- If there is still a reflux and a perforating vein has opened to drain this reflux from the saphenous vein to the deep vein without cosmetic visible branches and no distress for the patient, the situation may be stable for a long time and could be observed until new problems occur, which may then be treated as a shunt type 1. This has to be explained to the patient. If the patient is not able to come in for follow-ups, the immediate interruption of the junction might be the better option.
- If the ligated CHIVA 2 point has reopened or small bypasses have formed, the SFJ must also be treated. A new interruption in the same spot makes little sense as we have noticed in our experience. However, if the CHIVA 2 point was not interrupted properly as flush ligation at the saphenous vein (see Sect. 4.11.2), the correct procedure is to interrupt it again right at the saphenous vein. This extends the treatment considerably for the patient, as he must now wait another 8 weeks to see whether junction needs to be operated.

6.14.3 Post-operative Examination of the Saphenous Veins

If a saphenous trunk vein was refluxing before the operation, the velocity profile and the diameter must be compared with preoperative findings. Some little flow allowing drainage of tributaries to the next perforating vein is normal. In PW mode, the curve will be slow and not long-lasting—about 1 or 1.5 s, this was called "deflusso" in Italian to differentiate it from "reflusso" (reflux; see Sects. 4.11.1 and 6.3.4.1), but a long-lasting reflux of great amounts of blood is no good outcome. If reflux still exists after the operation, the proximal reflux source which was interrupted in the first operation must be examined, and the whole course of the tributaries and perforating veins must be checked for participation in the reflux. If a perforating vein has become refluxing, the saphenous vein must be interrupted below it or the perforating vein itself (see Sect. 6.9). If the vein is filled from a tributary, the reflux source in the tributary must be treated.

6.14.4 Post-operative Examination of the Tributaries

In tributaries, which continue to carry reflux, the same strategic criteria apply as in the first operation. If a tributary is still visible but not carrying large amounts of reflux, it may not be able to reduce its calibre due to wall damage as a consequence of prior thrombosis or wall lesions. Phlebectomy or sclerotherapy can be recommended, because a calibre reduction may then no longer be expected.

In case of residual reflux with partial calibre reduction but with a long segment (high pressure column), an interruption at a branching point can be planned, a phlebectomy or a sclerotherapy.

6.14.5 Post-operative Superficial Vein Thrombosis

Superficial veins may develop a thrombosis after CHIVA that is why in some cases prophylactic doses of heparin are applied post-operatively (see Sect. 10.1.4).

In case of a thrombotic occlusion of the saphenous vein after CHIVA 2, the risk of ascension to the deep vein is given, and it has to be treated to avoid deep vein extension via a junction or patent perforating vein. As found by Pintos (see Sect. 10.1.4), GSV with diameters at proximal thigh over 8.5 mm are more prone to thrombosis. That is why in these patients the SFJ should be treated in the first step in case of shunt type 3 to avoid this possible ascension of thrombi to deep veins. In the author's experience, giving heparin for 10 days as a rule after CHIVA 2 and avoiding CHIVA in two steps in case of large, aneurysmatic veins have made proximal thrombosis anecdotal.

Surprisingly thrombotic occlusion of saphenous veins after CHIVA crossotomy rarely causes pain to the patient, so often it is an incidental finding of the duplex investigation.

Thrombotic occlusions may falsify the outcome of the post-operative examination. Thrombosis in the GSV in the thigh region makes it impossible to measure the post-operative flow of the GSV. Furthermore, if the saphenous trunk is incompetent, a tributary occluded with thrombosis can falsify the evaluation of the proximal segment, since any reflux which might exist in this tributary cannot be measured in the presence of thrombosis.

Therefore, in cases of superficial vein thrombosis, the situation must be evaluated with caution. It is better to call the patient back for examination once the thrombosis has healed. Usually, in asymptomatic patients after crossotomy, no medicaments are necessary: A progression to the deep vein via the junction is no longer possible, in the absence of large perforating veins, a progression via a perforating vein neither. The thrombosis will resolve spontaneously within the longest 12 months.

6.15 Recurrence Management

6.15.1 Recurrence After CHIVA

Complementary interventions after 6–8 weeks, which are necessary in some patients and are consciously planned when deciding the strategy, are not a recurrence treatment but a completion of the CHIVA treatment.

Recurrent veins are situations in which patients who had no varices and no distress when released after CHIVA present new varices in the same places or at other points after some time.

6.15.1.1 Recurrence at the Saphenofemoral Junction

A recurrence after crossotomy can be noted clinically (new visible veins) or by duplex: a reflux re-appears in the GSV which was "draining" in the first exploration after the intervention. Duplex examination can indicate the new reflux source: recanalisation of the interruption of the junction or refluxing pelvine vessels meeting the GSV distal to the groin, perforating veins or other tributaries.

Recanalisation of junction: Redo the interruption and consider what went wrong. Remember: At this site, non-absorbable suture material is mandatory.

Reflux from supra-inguinal vessels: A treatment of these vessels at their origin may be planned at P or I point. Alternatively, multiple vessels seen on the proximal aspect of the thigh (medial or inguinal) may be treated with sclerotherapy to reduce the reflux into the GSV. Another option—in case a pelvine leak point surgery is not available and the vessels are too large to be treated with sclerotherapy—could be the closure of the proximal 5 cm of the GSV with endoluminal heat devices, applying sclerotherapy through the device into the supra-inguinal feeding vessels. This avoids sclerosing damage to the distal GSV.

In 20 years of experience, the author has never seen a "cavernoma" with multiple little vessels in the groin after CHIVA crossotomy as it is observed after crossectomy and stripping, excepting for one case of an obese, diabetic person under corticoids for rheumatic disease that developed an infection of the groin after surgery for C6 varicose veins. In this case, the vessel neoformation possibly was triggered by the infection.

When performing CHIVA with endoluminal heat closure of the proximal segment of the GSV (see Sect. 7.13), the most frequent recurrence is from pelvic vessels or the junction into the anterior accessory saphenous vein (AASV) (see Sect. 4.11.4). The best form to prevent this is treating the AASV during the intervention (e.g. with 0.5 cc of 1% foamed sclerosing agent), if it is visible and dilated. In any case, the patient has to be informed that possibly this vein will be treated in the second appointment, which can easily be done with a little amount of ultrasound-guided sclerotherapy into the AASV when the reflux is first noted to avoid clinical recidives.

6.15.1.2 Recurrent Veins Along the Saphenous Veins

As the GSV is left in situ, any pathologic amount of blood meeting the vein will be transported. In antegrade direction, if the valves have recovered and only first step of CHIVA 2 was performed, but retrograde if the SFJ was closed. Clinical recurrence will not last years until vessels develop. Thus, as soon as tributaries develop, the reflux source should be looked after and treated, given the consent of the patient. Recurrences after first step of CHIVA 2 are explained in Sect. 6.4.1.

Reflux from tributaries at the thigh into the GSV: Treat the tributaries (close origin, miniphlebectomy, sclerotherapy) and the flow into the GSV will reduce back to physiologic.

Reflux from a perforating vein into the GSV: Consider interrupting the perforating vein or the GSV distal to the perforating vein to provoke a change of flow to the deep vein, depending on the position of the perforating vein (the higher, the better it is to close it, the nearer to the foot, the better it is to use the perforating vein to drain the blood from the GSV) (see Fig. 6.26).

Drainage of the reflux into a new cosmetic disturbing tributary: In this case the optimal solution can be given if a perforating vein is found on the GSV—the tributaries can be disconnected from the GSV, leaving the perforating vein untouched as physiologic drainage for the GSV (see Fig. 6.25).

6.15.2 Recurrence Management After Ablative Procedures

After ablation of the saphenous trunk, CHIVA can only be used under certain conditions. The normal N2 drainage routes are no longer available. However symptomatic patients can be helped by volume relief by applying the rules of "interruption of the escape point" and "preserving draining routes" to the recidive.

The following situations may arise in recurrence of varices:

- **Recurrence at the sapheno-femoral or sapheno-popliteal junction with left stump and visible valves**:
  - (Re-)Crossectomy of the junction as the sole treatment. Plenty of dilated and visible tributaries regenerate by themselves as a result, and clinical complaints disappear. At the post-operative examination after 6–8 weeks, residual reflux sources may be found in the rest of the leg; they can be treated under local anaesthetic or with sclerotherapy.
  - Consider sclerotherapy if the stump is short, and the new tributaries have small diameter.
- **Recurrence at the SFJ or SFP with no stump but diffuse little vessels**:
  - Often these diffuse vessels ("cavernoma") are not filled by the deep veins but by pelvine refluxing vessels [20]. Consider treating the pelvic leakage points.
  - Alternatively, ultrasound-guided foam sclerotherapy of the refluxing vessels in the groin with no surgical intervention to reduce the pressure in the leg superficial veins. Wait and see for the rest of the visible vessels, which may disappear afterwards.
- **Recurrence from perforating veins**: This kind of recurrence is most frequently found around the perforating vein of the adductor canal (formerly Dodd).
  - In case of large reflux volume, the perforating vein can be surgically interrupted below the fascia surgically, possibly in combination with sclerotherapy (see Sect. 7.12).
  - In case of a thin perforating vein with little reflux, it may be less traumatic to perform a sclerotherapy of the perforating vein under duplex guidance or with endoluminal devices.
- **Persistence of a section of the GSV**: After stripping "from ankle to groin", segments of the GSV may still be found between the fasciae (easily recognised in ultrasound by the "saphenous eye" (see Chaps. 2 and 4)). In these patients, the stripping probe has slipped into a large epifascial vein when pushed through the GSV. If these remains of the saphenous vein are refluxing, classic CHIVA strategy decisions must be used.
- **Reflux from a perforating vein into a subcutaneous venous network**: Multiple small refluxing vessels develop in scar tissue of a perforating vein interruption. Normally a sclerotherapy may be enough as a treatment; alternatively the perforating vein has to be interrupted.
- **Varicose tributaries**: These must be treated in exactly the same way as varicose tributaries in the untreated leg. Nevertheless, it must be borne in mind that the affected veins are often poorly drained, so mini-phlebectomies or sclerotherapies are advisable.

6.16 Getting Started

After learning about CHIVA, sometimes it is difficult to get started. Colleagues of the own team mostly are not convinced that this could work. The patients (and most of all the doctors!) are used to be "ready" after one session, even though often further sclerotherapy sessions are necessary also in patients after venous ablation. They fear that patients will be unsatisfied, if they learn that a second step is to be done. The surprising fact is that patients often are happy when they are told that we are doing the less possible harm, even though this means they have possibly to return for a second little intervention.

A starting difficulty is, as every surgeon knows, that in practice we meet lots of conditions influencing a decision, not included in the images presented in this chapter.

So, it is important to take some time to investigate and document the findings prior to intervention and to be patient with ourselves with these first cases. Routine comes by doing.

6.16.1 General Strategic Decisions

When doctors start using the CHIVA method, they often ask which patients are ideal for their first attempts. These are:

- Young patients with shunt type 5 and a reflux only above knee, where the first step of CHIVA 2 can be applied expecting not to need the second step.
- Patients with expressed varices and shunt type 1 are also ideal, so long as one can resist the temptation to make a lot of incisions on the first day. In these patients, one can get a feeling for vein regeneration after the sole treatment of the junction.
- Multi-morbid patients with high C classes (CEAP) where it is possible only to treat the vessel feeding the skin changes or only the junction—an affordable intervention even in anticoagulated persons under local anaesthesia.

It is important that the first patients are themselves convinced by the CHIVA method. As a second or even third operation is sometimes necessary for a definitive solution during the learning curve, the subject must have patience and cooperate; he is more likely to be motivated if he himself chose the operating method and is convinced that keeping the saphenous trunks is the best option for him.

It must be made very clear to the patient before the intervention starts that the treatment does not end with the first operation. He will have to come for a post-operative examination after 2–3 months, when a complementary operation may be necessary, and he has to know that veins will be visible weeks after intervention. But in nearly all of the cases, he will be able to return to work within little time, and the venous complaints will disappear quickly.

For strategic decisions, it is also advisable to clarify with the patient in advance whether his distress or the cosmetic outcome is more important. If the cosmetic outcome is very important, in cases of shunt type 3 or 5, the tributaries must always be interrupted first and a part removed. If the patient is more concerned about the symptoms, treatment should concentrate on the highest reflux source. If the diameter of the GSV is larger than 10 mm at the thigh or have aneurysmatic dilations in the groin, the SFJ should be operated in the first session, regardless of the shunt type to avoid ascending thrombosis. Operating on the SFJ in the first session in shunt type 3 with a venous ulcer may also be considered. However, the outcomes of shunt type 3 treatment are clearly better when the tributaries are treated first at the CHIVA 2 points.

There are also fearful patients, who by nature prefer CHIVA to stripping. If a patient wants "only a few incisions" per session, this procedure is still possible, but it must be explained to the patient that more sessions may be required in total. In these cases, one should always take the most important step first. In other words, in shunt type 1, the SFJ is always treated first, and in a shunt type 3 or 5, the CHIVA 2 option is the first step.

Even strongly expressed varices, with large calibre and presenting big tributary convolutes, can be treated with CHIVA. However, doctor and patient must both appreciate that the treatment time will be longer than with less strongly expressed varices. That means more appointments and longer examination times per appointment. The risk of superficial vein thrombosis is also higher with strongly expressed varices (see Sect. 6.16.2.1).

6.16.2 Case Examples

6.16.2.1 Large Varicose Veins

A 52-year-old male patient with fears of anaesthesia and absolute negation to undergo stripping, this is the reason why he searched a centre applying CHIVA. Little distress, rarely wearing compression stockings, but fear of progression and thrombosis. This is surely not an optimal case to get started at the first sight, but as the patient is convinced not to want an ablation of the vein, it is a good case to learn what just little gestures can do with large varicose veins:

Findings: incompetent SFJ and 11 mm diameter of the GSV at the proximal thigh. Winding refluxing tributary, filled in the thigh 15 cm below the SFJ (preoperative finding; see Fig. 6.48a, b, blue arrow). Convolute below the knee, filled from this tributary with draining into the distal

GSV. Shunt type 3 with no perforating vein on the GSV at the thigh.

In the first treatment session (28.11.2001), only the SFJ was interrupted to produce a reduction in the calibre of the varicose vein (see Fig. 6.48c).

At the first post-operative examination (15.01.2002) (see Fig. 6.48d), a good reduction in calibre was found with partial thrombosis in the tributary without clinical complaints but also partial flow in the tributaries. The tributary was now interrupted at its junction to the GSV (position of blue arrow in Fig. 6.48a, b), and two stab incisions were made in the occluded convolute below the knee intending to express thrombotic material, which would not be successful. No interruption was performed at the knee site.

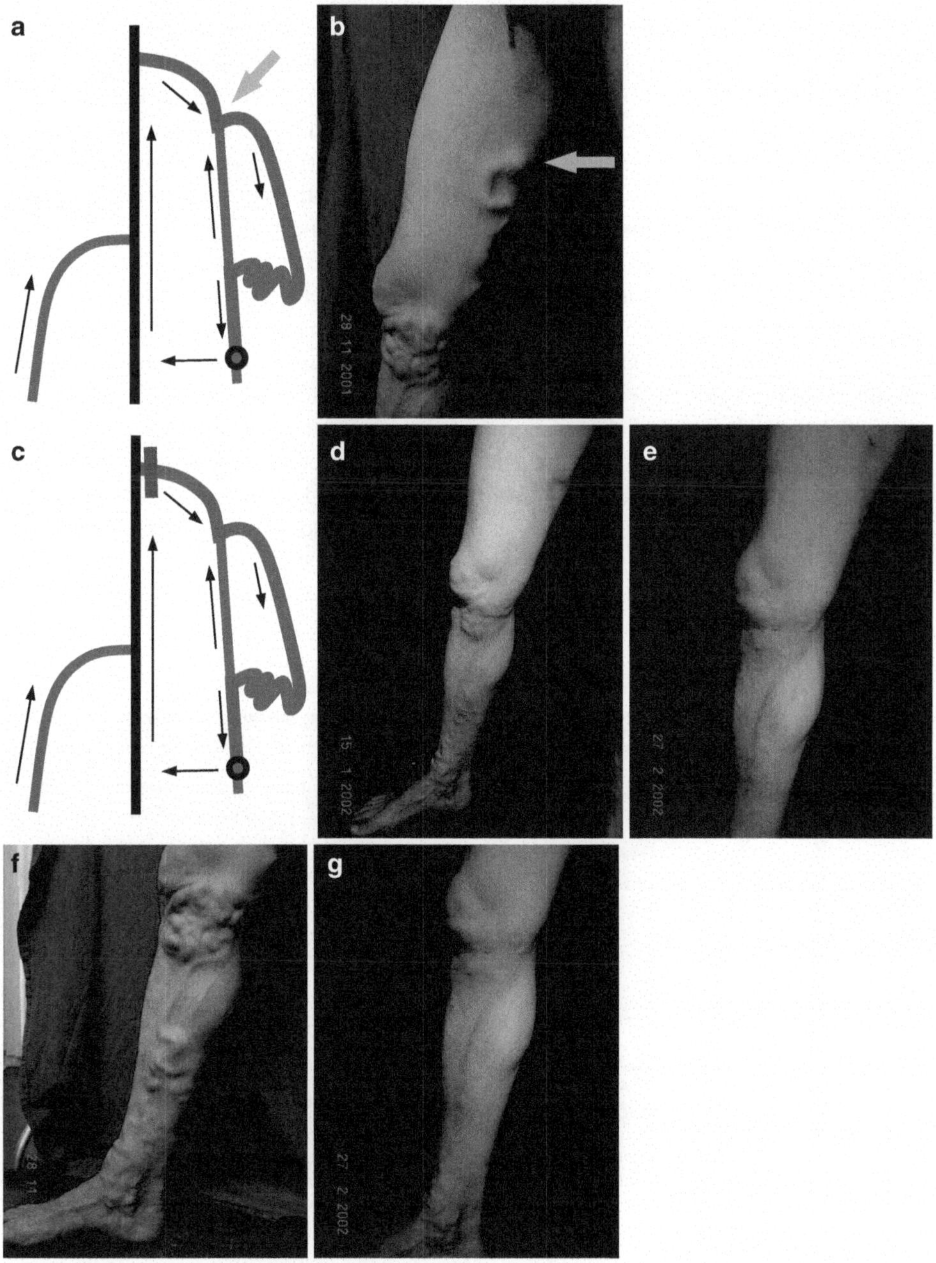

Fig. 6.48 For description of the case, see text. With permission by [10]

In the re examination on 27.02.2002 (see Fig. 6.48e), the patient is completely free of distress. Slight discolouration of the skin along the course of the GSV, which experience tells us, will fade after a couple of months. At both the operation sessions, low molecular heparin in prevention doses was prescribed for 10 days.

Summary: Preoperative situation, detail of the knee and calf before intervention (Fig. 6.48f). Crossotomy at the first session (28.11.2001) and tributary disconnection at the thigh at the second session (15.01.2002). Control 3 months (27.02.2002) after first intervention only discolouration of the skin, no reflux. No clinics. The patient had 2 days loss of work (just the intervention days).

6.16.2.2 Avoiding Difficult Surgery Access

Varicose tributaries are often a cosmetic problem for the patient. Sometimes in case of reflux of SSV with an early drainage through a tributary, the classic intervention would be a crossectomy, stripping of SSV and exhairesis of the tributary. In the situation presented in Fig. 6.49, the indication to such an intervention with the risk of neural lesion is hard to be justified. CHIVA 2 is always a good option in these cases with less surgical risk.

Another option to avoid surgery in the knee crease is to apply endoluminal heating devices to close a short segment of the SSV—although no results have been published so far.

Figure 6.49 shows a not very strongly expressed finding of a shunt type 3 on a SSV with a high and lateral sapheno-popliteal junction. Slight discomfort when working in the squat (the patient was a nursery school teacher). Surgical access to the junction would have meant a large incision and post-operative pain.

CHIVA 2 was applied, which indeed required a relatively large incision (exposure of the SSV junction of the tributary, as it was a CHIVA 2 point). With a mini-phlebectomy, it would have been necessary anyway to make several small incisions—and recurrence would certainly have occurred if the CHIVA 2 point had not been interrupted flush at the SSV level. According to CHIVA therefore, a proximal incision would have been made in any case in this patient, even if treatment was completed with distal mini-phlebectomies.

At the control 2 months later, little rest of varicose veins were seen, and the SSV was competent and stayed at the visit after 1 and 3 years. The remaining findings (Fig. 6.49c) can be treated with sclerotherapy if wished. The discomfort of the patient had completely disappeared.

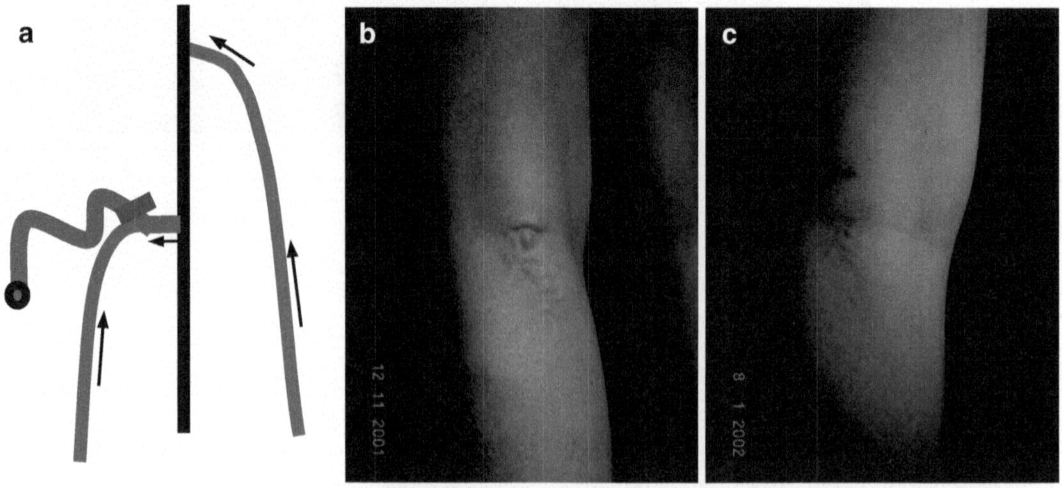

Fig. 6.49 For explanation to the case, see text. With permission by [10]

6.16.2.3 Treatment Involving Refluxing Accessory Anterior Saphenous Vein

The situation of the AASV differs from that of other tributaries. It forms part of an extensive venous network in the front of the thigh, so that in some patients, even if there is no more reflux from the deep veins after the operation, the veins continue to be filled by physiologic draining tributaries and produce cosmetic inconvenience.

In this case, a woman with shunt type 3, incompetent terminal and competent preterminal valve, reflux through SFJ escaping into AASV and after approximately 15 cm subfascial reflux the AASV pierced the fascia becoming clinically evident. Between AASV and GSV, two connecting veins were found, draining refluxing blood into the GSV (blue lines between GSV and AASV in Fig. 6.50a). The interruption of the AASV at its junction with the GSV was the haemodynamic solution of the problem; GSV was found to be antegrade in the follow-up. But the cosmetic bothering tributary would not have reverted properly for it was very large. So, mini-phlebectomies were performed at the level of the blue arrows in Fig. 6.50a, b. The green arrow shows the point, where the tortuous tributary drains into the GSV; below this point, no more phlebectomies were performed. After 5 months (Fig. 6.50c), the vein at knee level (below the green arrow), which had not been extracted, has reduced its calibre; the patient was free of complaints.

The combination of CHIVA at the proximal reflux source with phlebectomy of particularly disturbing sections saves on incisions and produces good outcomes, as long as drained segments are the result. In this case, this was possible thanks to the connections between the AASV and the GSV. It is not good to interrupt the AASV on its course indiscriminately without paying attention to the drainage of the proximal segments—in this case non-drained segments with matting and early recidives will be produced.

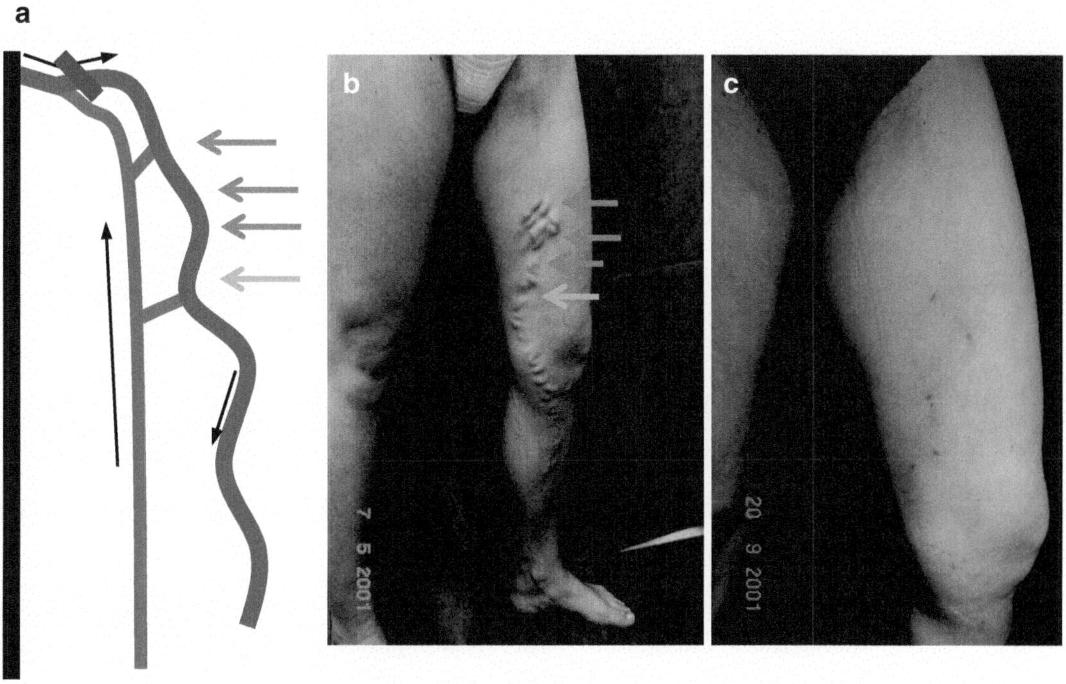

Fig. 6.50 For explanations of the case, see text. With permission by [10]

Last, not least and again, it may be stressed: When starting with the CHIVA strategy: the fewer the incisions, the better the outcome, even if this sometimes means that some sessions are necessary.

Literature

1. Hammersen F, Hesse G. Strukturelle Veränderungen der varikösen Venenwand nach Kompressionsbehandlung. Phlebol Proktol. 1990;19:193–9.
2. Bellmunt-Montoya S, Escribano JM, Dilme J, Martinez-Zapata MJ. CHIVA method for the treatment of chronic venous insufficiency. Cochrane Database Syst Rev. 2012;2:CD009648. https://doi.org/10.1002/14651858.CD009648.
3. Franceschi C, Cappelli M, Ermini S, Gianesini S, Mendoza E, Passariello F, Zamboni P. CHIVA: hemodynamic concept, strategy and results. Int Angiol. 2016;35(1):8–30; Epub 2015 Jun 5.
4. Franceschi C, Zamboni P. Principles of venous haemodynamics. New York: Nova Science; 2010.
5. Franceschi C. Théorie et pratique de la cure Conservatrice et Hémodynamique de l'Insuffisance Veineuse en Ambulatoire. Precy-sous-Thil, France: Editions de l'Armançon; 1988.
6. Padberg FT Jr, Pappas PJ, Araki CT, et al. Hemodynamic and clinical improvement after superficial vein ablation in primary combined venous insufficiency with ulceration. J Vasc Surg. 1997;26:169–71.
7. Mendoza E, Berger V, Zollmann C, Bomhoff M, Amsler F. Kaliberreduktion der V. saphena magna und der V. femoralis communis nach CHIVA. Phlebologie. 2011;40(2):73–8.
8. Mendoza E. Diameter reduction of the great saphenous vein and the common femoral vein after CHIVA long-term results. Phlebologie. 2013;42:65–9.
9. Marshall M, Breu FX. Handbuch der Angiologie. 13. Erg.-Lfg ed. Landsberg: Ecomed; 2005.
10. Mendoza E. Handbuch CHIVA. Arrien GmbH; 2002.
11. Dwerryhouse S, Davies B, Harradine K, Earnshaw JJ. Stripping the long saphenous vein reduces the rate of reoperation for recurrent varicose vein: five-year results of a randomized trial. J Vasc Surg. 1999;29:589–92.
12. Carandina S, Mari C, De Palma M, Marcellino MG, Cisno C, Legnaro A, Liboni A, Zamboni P. Varicose vein stripping vs haemodynamic correction (CHIVA): a long term randomised trial. Eur J Vasc Endovasc Surg. 2008;35(2):230–7.
13. Zamboni GS, Menegatti E, Tacconi G, Palazzo A, Liboni A. Great saphenous varicose vein surgery without saphenofemoral junction disconnection. Br J Surg. 2010;97:820–5.
14. Mendoza E, Amsler F. CHIVA with endoluminal procedures: LASER versus VNUS—treatment of the saphenofemoral junction. Phlebologie. 2017;46:5–12.
15. Mendoza E. The sapheno-femoral junction in ultrasound. Phlebologie. 2014;43:42–5.
16. Stücker M, Moritz R, Altmeyer P, Reich-Schupke S. New concept: different types of insufficiency of the saphenofemoral junction identified by duplex as a chance for a more differentiated therapy of the great saphenous vein. Phlebology. 2013;28:268–74.
17. Zollmann P, Zollmann C, Zollmann P, Veltman J, Kerzig D, Doerler M, Stücker M. Determining the origin of superficial venous reflux in the groin with duplex ultrasound and implications for varicose vein surgery. J Vasc Surg Venous Lymphat Disord. 2017;5(1):82–6.
18. Mendoza E, Stücker M. Duplex-ultrasound assessment of the saphenofemoral junction (Review). Phlebol Rev. 2015;23(3):1–8.
19. Mendoza E. Therapie der Stammvarikose der V. saphena magna—Konsens unter Einbeziehung von Stripping, Verödung, endoluminalen Verfahren und CHIVA als Therapieoptionen. Phlebologie. 2011;40:159–64.
20. Reich-Schupke S, Mendoza E, Dörler M, Stücker M. Frequency of refluxive tributaries of the junction region in the groin in patients with recurrent varicose veins of the thigh. Phlebologie. 2016;45:149–53.

7 CHIVA: Surgical Tips and Tricks

Sergio Gianesini, Roberto Delfrate, Massimo Cappelli, and Erika Mendoza

7.1 Introduction

The general surgical skills and techniques should be known prior to start with CHIVA interventions. General knowledge about disinfection and local anaesthesia techniques are supposed as known in this chapter. Perioperative management, especially heparin administration, is discussed in Chap. 11.

A very cautious treatment has to be given to the saphenous trunks at any moment, avoiding lesions to the venous wall by repeated clamping or squeezing it.

In addition, a perfect cooperation between the ultrasound operator and the surgeon is the cornerstone for success. Both have to understand the CHIVA strategy and have to be used to work together, use the same language and understand the markings on the skin or figures painted in the records of the patient. Interrupting the wrong vein at the surgical site will mostly produce an immediate clinical failure (see Fig. 4.43).

As the veins are left in the leg in CHIVA and are refilled immediately if the flow is not properly interrupted, incorrect operating technique generally becomes apparent immediately after the operation, and certainly in the postoperative examination. With stripping, the varicose vessel is removed, so recurrence only becomes apparent months or years later.

New techniques have been introduced to CHIVA, like the use of a clip in the context of the crossotomy, the interruption of pelvic leak points (see Chap. 8), devalvulation (see Sect. 7.9), sclerotherapy to treat selected tributaries or to improve perforating vein surgery (see Sect. 7.13) or endoluminal techniques to close short segments of the saphenous veins without surgical intervention (see Sect. 7.12).

Surgical gestures in the context of CHIVA are possible in local anaesthesia and on ambulatory basis. Preferences of patients and surgeons are of course to be respected. Some health care systems do not consider venous surgery on ambulatory basis. Thus, the important thing is to apply proper surgical techniques, adapting to the environmental necessities.

S. Gianesini, M.D., Ph.D. (✉)
Vascular Diseases Center, University of Ferrara, Ferrara, Italy

USUHS University, Bethesda, MD, USA

R. Delfrate, M.D.
Responsible Surgery at Casa di Cura Figlie di San Camillo, Cremona, Italy

M. Cappelli, M.D.
Office Surgery, Florence, Italy

E. Mendoza, M.D., Ph.D.
Venenpraxis, Wunstorf, Germany
e-mail: erika.mendoza@t-online.de

P. Zamboni et al. (eds.), *Saphenous Vein-Sparing Strategies in Chronic Venous Disease*,
https://doi.org/10.1007/978-3-319-70638-2_7

7.2 Surgery at the Sapheno-Femoral Junction: Crossotomy

Operating on the sapheno-femoral junction is one of the core surgical skills of the CHIVA method.

The anatomy of the sapheno-femoral junction is extremely variable. It has been explained in Sect. 4.5. Not all the vessels shown in Figs. 7.1 and 7.2 are always present. The diagram only includes important vessels.

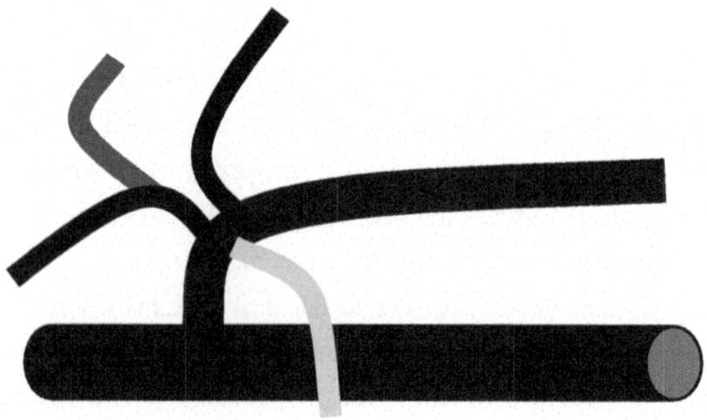

Fig. 7.1 Diagram of the SFJ with the confluence of superficial inguinal veins: Brown—Great saphenous vein, Yellow—Pudendal vein, Green—Epigastric and circumflex iliac veins, Purple—Anterior accessory saphenous vein, Blue—Common femoral vein. With permission by [1]

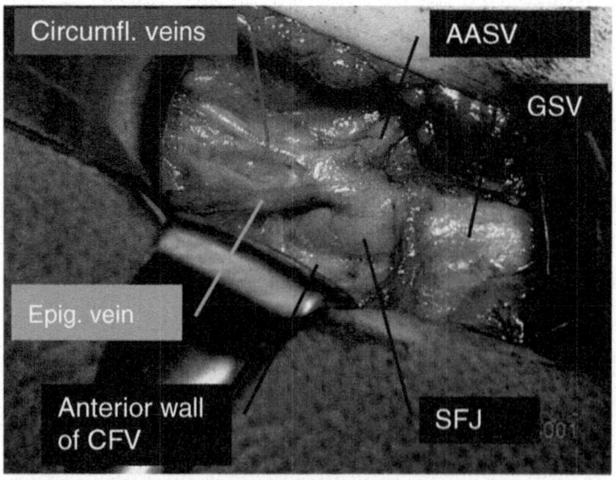

Fig. 7.2 Intraoperative site with exposed sapheno-femoral junction. The deep external pudendal artery crosses the great saphenous vein distal of the sapheno-femoral junction. Followed by: legends on the image, colours analogous to Fig. 7.1. *Epig. vein* epigastric vein, *Circunfl. vein* circumflex iliac vein, *GSV* great saphenous vein, *SFJ* sapheno-femoral junction. With permission by [1]

7.2.1 General Explanations

Using ultrasound preoperatively, the surgeon can discover the exact anatomy of the sapheno-femoral junction in advance, not only to decide the strategy in general but also the features he will find.

The following information is important for the surgeon:

- Height of the sapheno-femoral junction in relation to the groin and its depth below the skin in mm.
- Distance between the confluence of inguinal tributaries veins and the femoral vein.
- How many and which inguinal tributaries are present?
- Which inguinal tributaries are incompetent?
- Does any inguinal tributary flow into the sapheno-femoral junction at the ostium level?
- Are there any perforating veins from the superficial or deep common femoral vein?
- The course of the great saphenous vein under the skin (best drawn with a marker).

The object of treatment of the incompetent sapheno-femoral junction with incompetent terminal valve is to interrupt the recirculation at the highest reflux source. At the same time, a small flow of blood must be maintained in the great saphenous vein to prevent it from becoming occluded by thrombosis. For this reason, the inguinal tributaries must not be interrupted, only the sapheno-femoral junction (see Figs. 7.3 and 7.4). The inguinal tributaries empty into the great saphenous vein and ensure sufficient blood flow to prevent phlebitis. After the operation, this blood flow is redirected to the nearest distal perforating vein (see Fig. 7.5). The crossotomy is different from the distal ligation of the great saphenous vein as depicted in Fig. 7.6, which is considered a technical failure.

From a surgical point of view, leaving the inguinal tributaries untouched is more difficult than a classic crossectomy. The veins must be exposed, and the sutures passed under the inguinal tributaries one by one, until the noose

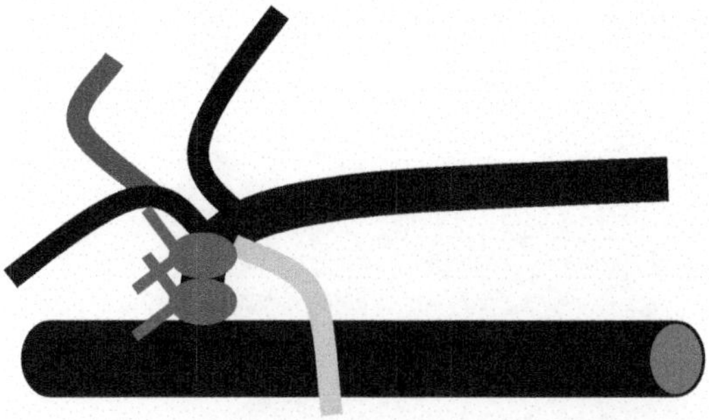

Fig. 7.3 Double ligation of the sapheno-femoral junction central of the confluence of superficial inguinal veins

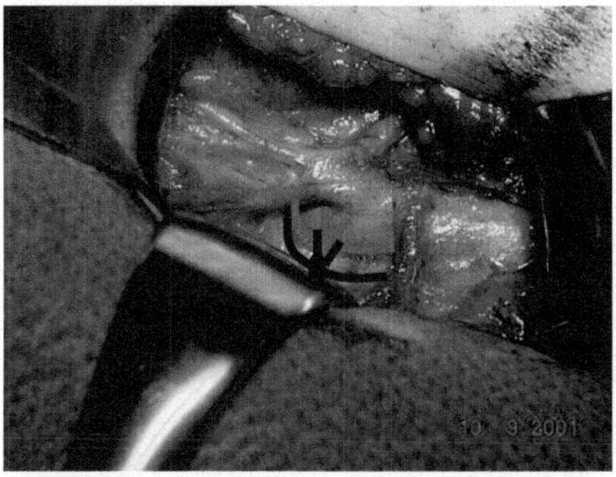

Fig. 7.4 Image as in Fig. 7.2 showing the site of the double ligation. With permission by [1]

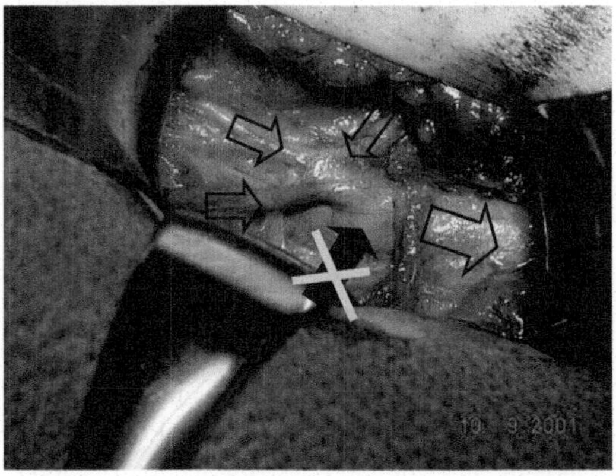

Fig. 7.5 Image as in Fig. 7.2 showing the flow in the great saphenous vein after double ligation at the ostium level: physiological flow from the inguinal tributaries draining into the distal saphenous vein; reflux through the incompetent terminal valve is interrupted. With permission by [1]

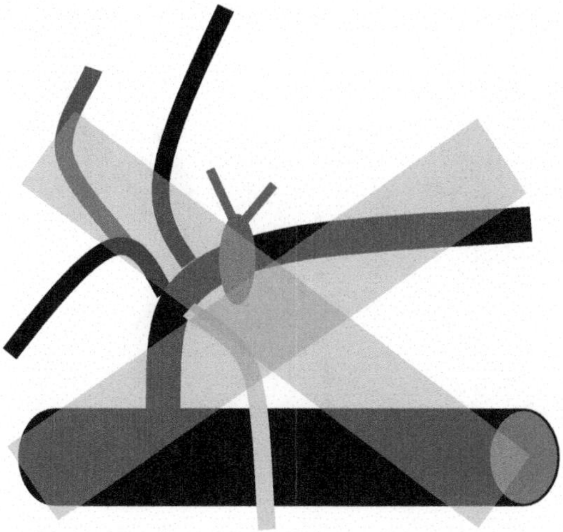

Fig. 7.6 Ligation of the great saphenous vein distal of the confluence of superficial inguinal veins. *Technical error* and not crossotomy according to CHIVA. With permission by [1]

can be drawn tight round the sapheno-femoral junction. Ideally the sapheno-femoral junction should be severed. Sometimes, some of the inguinal tributaries have to be severed into the bargain.

The reflux source in the groin is generally the sapheno-femoral junction. The reflux is N1 → N2, from the deep vein system to the great saphenous vein (shunt type 1 or 3). However, the tributaries of the confluence of superficial inguinal veins may be incompetent as well or instead (pelvic shunt type 4 and 5). These have to be treated by ligation of the pelvic leak point (see Chap. 8).

Even if no incompetence is found in ultrasound, one or more very large veins may appear intraoperatively. After successful ligation of the sapheno-femoral junction, the patient should be asked to perform a Valsalva manoeuvre. If any vein fills more than the rest, it should be severed and excised, to prevent persistence of the recirculation after the intervention.

Figures 7.7, 7.8, 7.9, 7.10 and 7.11 demonstrate the surgical steps of a crossotomy with double ligation of the saphenous vein directly at the ostium level and without disconnection.

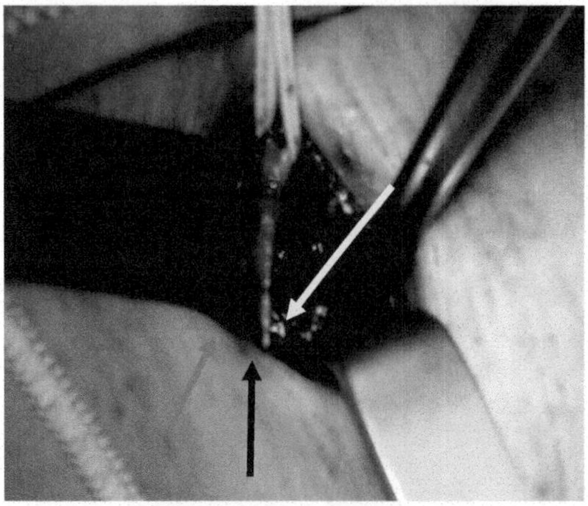

Fig. 7.7 The skin in the right groin was opened with a short incision, and dissection of the junction has been performed. A loop is placed around the great saphenous vein. The green arrow shows the epigastric vein, the black arrow shows the circumflex vein and the beige arrow marks the sapheno-femoral junction (SFJ), below the axis GSV—cranial tributaries (SFJ not clearly visible here)

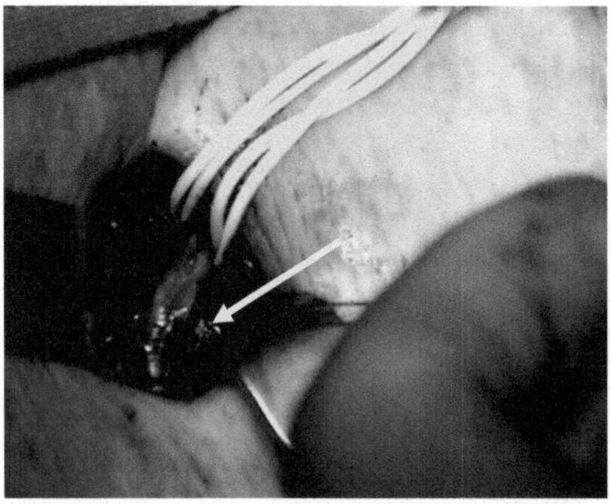

Fig. 7.8 The SFJ tributaries are not severed, but a non-absorbable suture is passed underneath them. The non-absorbable suture has been passed under all the inguinal tributaries. The sapheno-femoral junction is now visible when we pull on the suture (arrow)

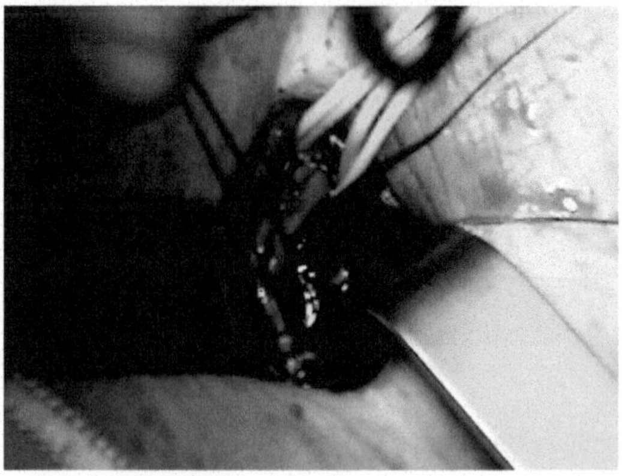

Fig. 7.9 A second non-absorbable suture is passed under the tributaries like the first. By pulling gently on the sutures, we can expose the sapheno-femoral junction

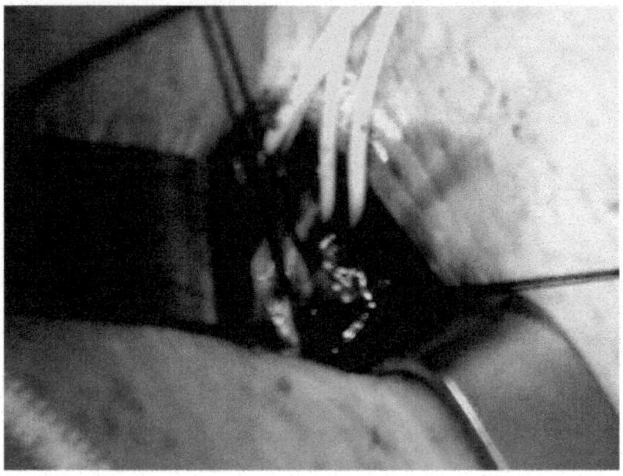

Fig. 7.10 The first knot is tied as close as possible to the common femoral vein, without constricting it. The knot must be pulled very tight to prevent the formation of a filiform lumen afterwards

7.2.2 Technical Notes Concerning the Crossotomy

Crossotomy or sapheno-femoral junction high ligation represents a fundamental step in the treatment of chronic venous disease according to the CHIVA strategy. A small incision is performed at the inguinal crease.

By sharp dissection, the superficial fascia is opened, and the great saphenous vein identified and dissected together with its junctional tributaries (the superficial epigastric vein, superficial external pudendal vein, superficial circumflex iliac vein, anterior and posterior accessory saphenous veins).

The deep external pudendal artery, branch of the femoral artery, often encircles the sapheno-femoral junction. In a cadaveric investi-

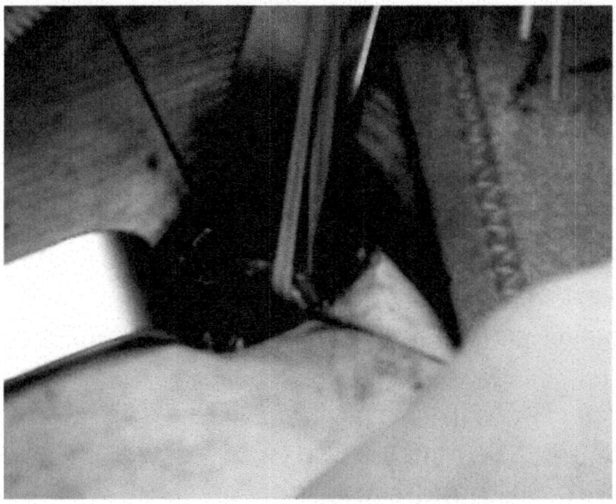

Fig. 7.11 From a different angle, both ligations are in place. A small gap is left between them. Note: Pictures taken by Dr. Michael Martin, intervention performed by Dr. Andreas Hildebrandt during a CHIVA course. All images with permission by [1]

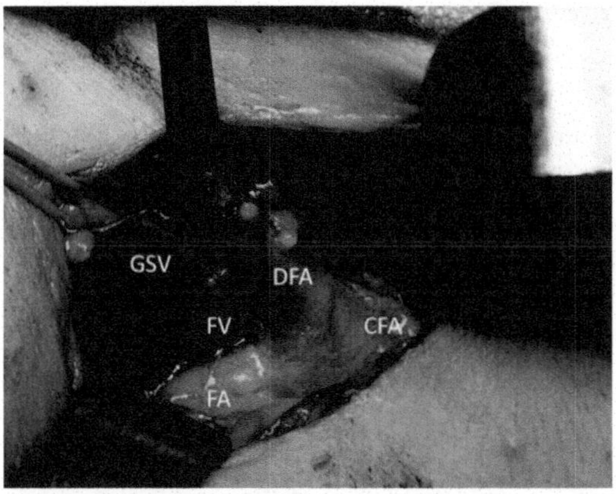

Fig. 7.12 High femoral artery bifurcation with crossing over of the deep femoral artery over the sapheno-femoral junction. *GSV* great saphenous vein, *FV* femoral vein, *CFA* common femoral artery, *DFA* deep femoral artery

gation, its presence was demonstrated in 92% of cases, with a duplication in 46% of patients. Exceptionally, in case of high femoral arterial bifurcation, the profunda femoris artery may cross over the sapheno-femoral junction: a feature that must be taken into consideration in order to avoid damaging the artery. This condition is always visible prior to the intervention during the ultrasound exploration (see Fig. 7.12).

The same anatomical localization of the junction can change quite significantly. According to the investigation of Mirjalili, the centre of the junction is usually located 2.4 + 0.6 cm lateral and 1 + 0.9 cm inferior to the pubic tubercle, the junction is inferior to the pubic tubercle in 90% of cases, while in 10% of cases, it's actually above it [2]. According to the literature, an average of 3.7 tributaries enter the junction in proximity of the terminal and preterminal valves. No significant differences in this anatomic feature are reported related to age or gender [3].

During the dissection of the sapheno-femoral junction, it's highly improbable to encounter nervous structures. The cutaneous innervation of this area is provided by nerves from the crural branch of the genito-crural nerve, but this latter runs far from the junction.

In case of crossotomy, no tributaries should be interrupted. Only refluxing tributaries are interrupted in the same procedure, when closing the SFJ for reflux through the incompetent terminal valve. This will be sorted out preoperatively during the ultrasound exploration or during the intervention as explained above (Valsalva after closure of the knot at the level of the terminal valve).

If there are refluxing tributaries in addition to an incompetent terminal valve, these tributaries are usually ligated by 3/0 or 4/0 absorbable threads. Some authors use to interrupt the tributaries always in the context of the high ligation of the sapheno-femoral junction, but recent evidence shows that avoiding the ligation of the tributaries is associated with a significantly decreased risk of recurrence [4].

In the context of the crossotomy or high ligation, the sapheno-femoral junction can be severed or not. Mostly in case of ambulatory-performed intervention, the surgeons tend to leave the junction interrupted by knots, but not cut, as shown in Figs. 7.10 and 7.11. In case of severing it, after it has been carefully exposed on all its sides, the distal end of the great saphenous vein is ligated by a 2/0 absorbable thread. The closure of the femoral vein can be performed by different techniques: running suture, ligation of the saphenous vein with or without transfixing stich or clip application.

Franceschi and Delfrate [5] have described technical variants including a titanium clip application flush on the femoral with a 2/0 triple non-absorbable braided ligation vs. a 0 monofilament non-absorbable one.

The use of different sutures and sapheno-femoral disconnection techniques remains a still debated topic, also when applying high ligation and stripping. Previous studies demonstrated not significant differences among oversewing the femoral vein with polypropylene sutures and standard transfixion with absorbable suture [6]. No different recurrence rate was reported also when comparing standard SFJ ligation with a running inverting suture on the femoral venotomy [7], while a contradictory outcome was reported by Frings demonstrating a decreased recurrence rate by closing the endothelial stump by a running oversewing [8].

Recently it was demonstrated that limiting the extent of the dissection and applying a titanium clip were associated with a decreased recurrence rate in comparison with traditional ligation in a CHIVA setting [9] (Fig. 7.13). Technically it's always preferable to choose a right-angle titanium clip applicator device versus a linear one. Indeed, the right-angled shape facilitates the clip apposition in case of small surgical accesses.

Once the high ligation has been completed, closure of the fascia and of the skin is performed. Subcuticular sutures can lead also to an aesthetic outcome totally satisfying, and if the incision was kept small, no scars related to the procedure can be detected even shortly after the procedure.

7.3 Surgery in Case of Pelvic Leak Points

Chapter 8 is dedicated to this very complex pathology with diagnostic considerations and surgery skills.

7.4 Surgery at the Sapheno-Popliteal Junction

Operations on the sapheno-popliteal junction are the type of CHIVA operation which has been least investigated. The great variability of the junction (see Sects. 4.6 and 6.7), the readiness with which the small saphenous vein suffers recanalization even when some centimetres are

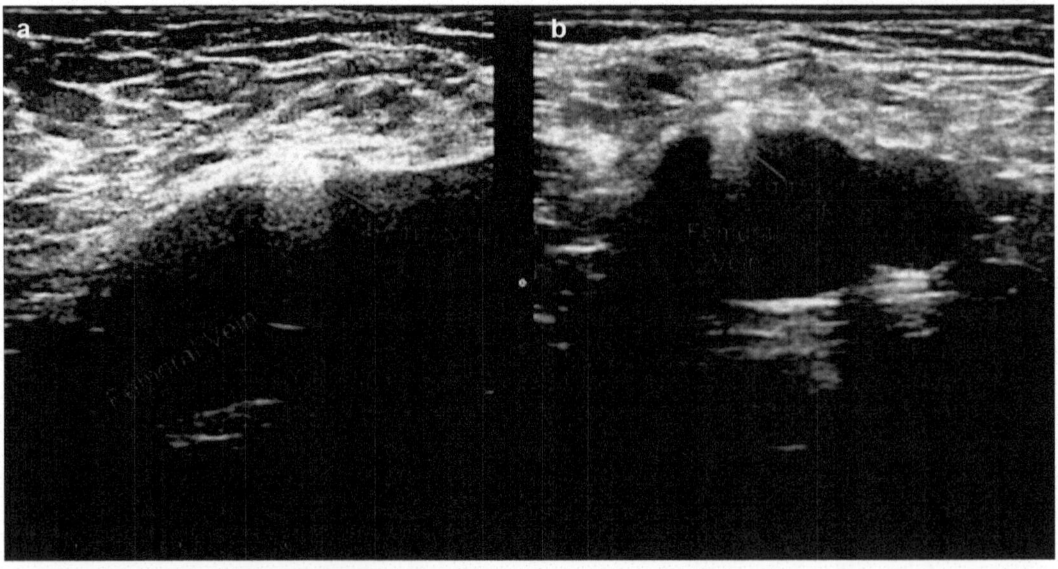

Fig. 7.13 Titanium clip visualization at the postoperative ultrasound longitudinal scan (**a**) and trnsversal scan (**b**). The clip is correctly applied since flush to the femoral vein [9]

removed and the many inflows from muscle veins, which have no valves to separate the deep vein system from the small saphenous vein, make it difficult to standardise procedures.

For these reasons, great care must be taken in the ultrasound examination before operating, to spare the patient complementary operations. The actual operation must be clearly discussed by the ultrasound examiner and the surgeon; resection between the two ligations must be discussed in particular detail.

Duplex examination of the sapheno-popliteal junction must answer the following questions:

- Where is the SPJ? In the upper or lower part of the popliteal region, or to one side?
- Is the reflux source in the Giacomini vein, the SPJ or both? Note: Flow from the vein of Giacomini towards the foot can be physiological; the question here is the duration and the shape of the curve, particularly as compared to the reflux curve in the small saphenous vein.
- How big is the calibre of the vein of Giacomini?
- Do any muscle veins flow into the small saphenous vein distal of the SPJ? (There are no valves to separate the deep vein system from the small saphenous vein, so recirculation may be maintained through these veins despite ligation of the SPJ.)

As with the sapheno-femoral junction, the small saphenous vein must be ligated at the deep leg vein. Unlike the groin, however, in CHIVA, the sapheno-popliteal junction is always severed, and the segment of some centimetres is excised, as there is no confluence of superficial inguinal veins in which the tributaries must be left entirely.

However, this classic interruption directly at the deep leg vein does not always produce the desired outcome. As explained in detail in Sect. 6.7, it may be necessary to interrupt the small saphenous vein below the distal muscle veins (see Fig. 7.14a) or distal of the junction of the Giacomini vein (see Fig. 7.14b). This decision must be taken before the start of the intervention basing on the ultrasound results.

Even after ligation with non-absorbable suture and exhairesis of a segment 2–4 cm long and postoperative control of properly closed vein, after months to years, a new vessel in the fascial

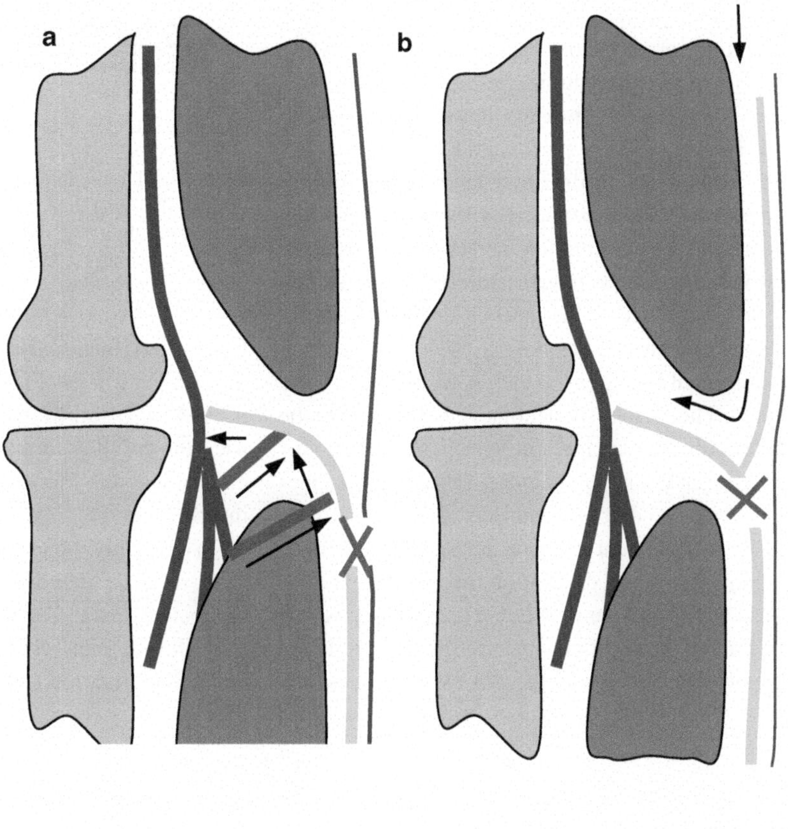

Fig. 7.14 (Legends see Fig. 6.19.) (**a**) Condition after severance of the SSV below the muscle veins. (**b**) Condition after interruption of the SSV below the Giacomini vein. With permission by [1]

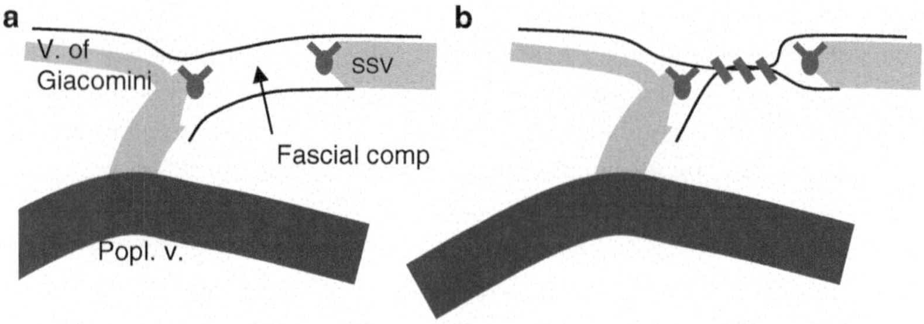

Fig. 7.15 (a) Condition after interruption of the SSV below the Giacomini vein with empty fascial space. (b) Proposed suture closing the fascial space to avoid a neovessel in the empty space. With permission by [1]

compartment with reflux has been observed by the author. In the reoperation, the sutures in the vein walls have been found; the vessel was investigated by histology and no muscle cells found—thus a neovessel was suspected. As the fascial compartment of the small saphenous vein may act as the principal structure triggering neovessels, possibly stitching the fasciae together between the two resection stumps could avoid this problem (see Fig. 7.15).

7.5 Operation for Incompetence of the Anterior Accessory Saphenous Vein

The anterior accessory saphenous vein (AASV) has a special place among leg veins: its distal origin is epifascial, making it an N3 vessel. It receives flow from the distended subcutaneous venous network of the outer leg and the thigh. It pierces the fascia around 10–30 cm distal of the sapheno-femoral junction, and its course over the proximal section is interfascial, like the great and small saphenous veins, and so in this section, it should be classified as N2.

Surgical treatment of the distal segment of the anterior accessory saphenous vein, this means the N3 section, is explained in Sect. 7.10. Criteria for treating an incompetent anterior accessory saphenous vein are discussed in Sect. 6.5.2. Treatment of an incompetent anterior accessory saphenous vein junction will depend on the condition of the great saphenous vein. When a crossotomy is carried out for incompetence of the terminal and preterminal valve, and the AASV is also incompetent, the latter must also be interrupted (see Fig. 7.16a). In case the epigastric vein drains into the AASV, it is best to either interrupt it or close the AASV distal to the junction with the epigastric vein to allow drainage of the epigastric and circumflex vein blood into the deep vein after the intervention.

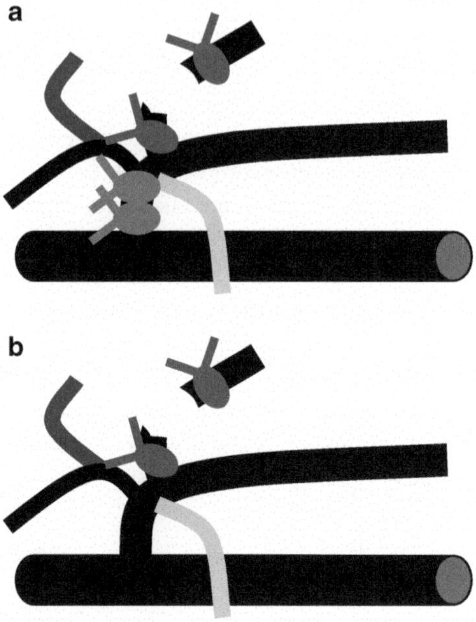

Fig. 7.16 (a) Operation for incompetence of the GSV and the AASV: crossotomy (pink) and in addition (red) ligation and resection of the proximal segment of the AASV. (b) Operation for incompetence of the AASV alone: interruption of the proximal segment of the AASV without touching the GSV. With permission by [1]

In case only the terminal valve is incompetent, with reflux escaping through the AASV, with competent distal GSV, the lateral crossotomy is enough (see Fig. 7.16b). The AASV is exposed, and a flush ligation is performed at its junction to the great saphenous vein with excision of a short segment of the AASV. The sapheno-femoral junction must not be ligated, since in that case, the healthy great saphenous vein would have no drainage. Ligation of the sapheno-femoral junction would cause phlebitis in the healthy great saphenous vein. The incision should be made as far lateral as possible, so that if the great saphenous vein should later become incompetent, the crossectomy will not be hindered unnecessarily by scar tissue.

7.6 Recurrence in the SFJ and SPJ After CHIVA

The first control, some weeks to months after CHIVA, serves to state, if the patient haemodynamics are drained and non-refluxing. A missed flow conversion after CHIVA 2, the consequence of a tactical or technical error (not ligating the correct vein, overseeing a perforating vein), or a procedure planned in two steps will need a second short intervention to finish the treatment. This is not the treatment of a recurrence—but finishing our project.

A recurrence at the junction is meant, when, after the postoperative examination 6 weeks after ligation of the SFJ or SPJ, the junction is found to be closed or antegrade flowing, and there is no longer reflux. The veins have reduced their calibre. After a period of months or years, the patient presents again with varices, and the sapheno-femoral junction perfused in retrograde flow. The patient notices the problem due to the development of new varicose veins or because his old varicose veins are filling again. As mentioned previously, we have unfortunately had to carry out repeat CHIVA operations on these junctions on occasion.

In this case the surgical approach is different from that in recurrence in the SFJ/SPJ after stripping. Either the crossotomy has failed, with a (seldom) recanalization, or a pelvine reflux will fill the distal GSV or through the Giacomini vein the SSV. In case the crossotomy place itself shows a new reflux, and to avoid a new incision in the scar, endoluminal heat or glue could be an alternative to close the saphenous vein. Some devices offer the possibility to apply sclerotherapy through the endoluminal device, so that the feeding tributaries (in case of Giacomini vein reflux or pelvic reflux) could be treated with sclerotherapy through the catheter.

A re-intervention in case of recurrence in the SFJ or SPJ after CHIVA is not so demanding for the surgeon as recurrence after stripping. The great saphenous vein is unmistakably the principal structure helping for orientation.

7.7 Surgical Treatment of the Saphenous Veins

The saphenous vein courses beneath the saphenous fascia, which is the reason why it cannot generally be hooked. Exceptions may be found in thin patients, or occasionally in the lower leg, where the fascia can be opened with a puncture scalpel.

If the great saphenous vein has to be severed, it is necessary to open the fascia and expose the vein. It is also not worth trying to find the great saphenous vein through a point incision. In the region of the great saphenous vein, there is often a parallel vein coursing through the subcutaneous fatty tissue, which may be hooked and exposed through a point incision and mistaken for the great saphenous vein. The diameter may appear rather small, but vasospasms may also be observed in the groin, so this mechanism may produce an analogue effect. The surgeon is pleased to have found the GSV with such a small incision. Unfortunately, the postoperative examination shows that the desired outcome has not been achieved and that the great saphenous vein remains untouched in its compartment.

If it is proposed to ligate the great saphenous vein below a perforating vein or a tributary, this perforator must be identified during exposure, to ensure that the ligation is applied on the distal side.

All ligations of saphenous trunk veins and their tributaries must include severance and excision of a short segment, to prevent the vein from re-establishing continuity in so far as possible. Non-absorbable suture should be used.

7.8 Flush Ligation of the Tributary at the Level of the Saphenous Vein (CHIVA 2 Point)

The first step of the CHIVA 2 procedure is to interrupt recirculation at the CHIVA 2 point, which means at the distal exit point of blood from the saphenous trunk vein (see Sect. 6.4.1).

After a careful marking on the skin, a longitudinal incision is performed. The tributary is hooked and marked with a loop. Then the tributary is followed to meet the saphenous vein. This is exposed and denuded, and the tributary is interrupted directly at the trunk vein, without leaving a stump. The tributary must be interrupted flush with the trunk, so that no stump or "tent" is allowed to form (see Fig. 7.17). The first centimetres of the tributary are then excised.

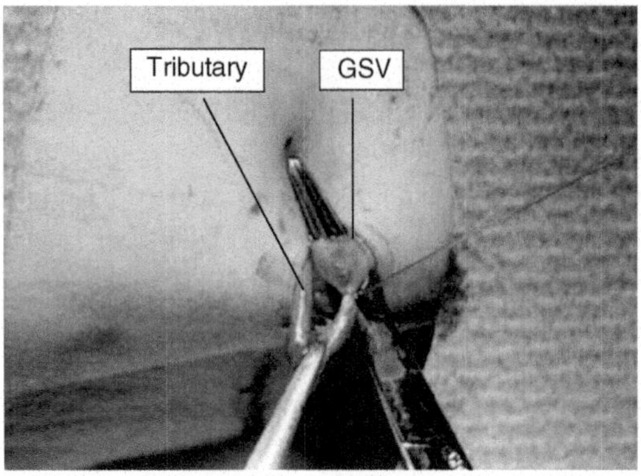

Fig. 7.17 The saphenous vein is exposed after opening the saphenous fascia; a clamp has been passed underneath for better visualisation. The tributary has been flush ligated at the level of the wall of the saphenous vein; the tributary will suffer resection for some centimetres to avoid a recanalization. With permission by [1]

A CHIVA 2 interruption cannot be performed without exposing the saphenous trunk. Hooking the tributary "as close as possible to the great saphenous vein", which is often so tempting, almost always results in the formation of a stump with new varicose veins or matting in the postoperative evolution.

Convolutes or the complete tributary connected with the CHIVA 2 point might be extracted or only some centimetres of the tributary, as to the preference of the surgeon and the patient.

7.9 Devalvulation

As explained in Sect. 6.4.2, sometimes it is helpful to destroy the valves of a segment of the great saphenous vein to achieve a stable, drained situation and to avoid several interventions (CHIVA 2). Prior to the intervention, the diameter of the vein has to be measured to choose the correct size of devalvulator. The devalvulator is introduced into the saphenous vein via the tribu-

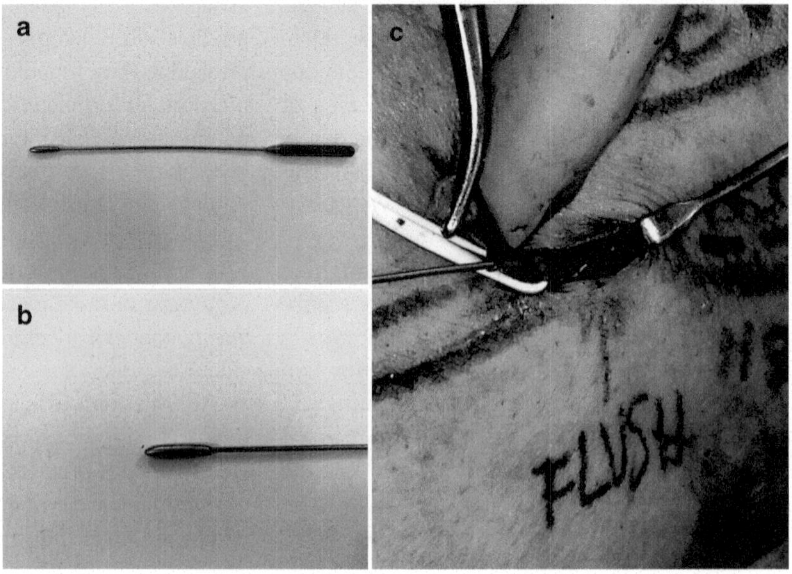

Fig. 7.18 (**a**) Devalvulator. (**b**) Detail of the head of the devalvulator. (**c**) Introduction of the devalvulator via the tributary. A loop has been passed under the proximal, refluxive GSV, the tributary is clamped and the devalvulator is introduced via an incision on the tributary into the distal, competent GSV. Images with permission to be printed by Dr. Roberto Delfrate, Cremona

tary, which will be interrupted in the same session (see Sect. 7.8 and Fig. 7.18). The devalvulator smoothly advances in retrograde fashion through the saphenous vein until being stopped by a competent valve. With a gentle push, the valve is destroyed by pressure; the devalvulator is passed again through the same valve to make sure there is no rest of the valve hindering the passage. This is repeated until all the valves in the segment are treated. At the end of the procedure, the segment is washed with heparin solution, for example, injecting 10 mL sodium heparin 1000 IE/100 mL. Nevertheless, a thrombosis in the first weeks after the intervention in the devalvulated segment is normal. These thrombi resolve in the next months.

Technically, there are two options (see Sect. 6.4.2): one is the devalvulation between two refluxive segments of GSV (type A) and the other the devalvulation between the draining tributary and a perforator (type B).

In case a competent saphenous vein segment between two refluxive tributaries is to be devalvulated (type A), the tributary will be interrupted at the proximal and distal end of the competent segment, and the devalvulator will be introduced at the proximal end until it reaches the distal end (see Fig. 7.19b).

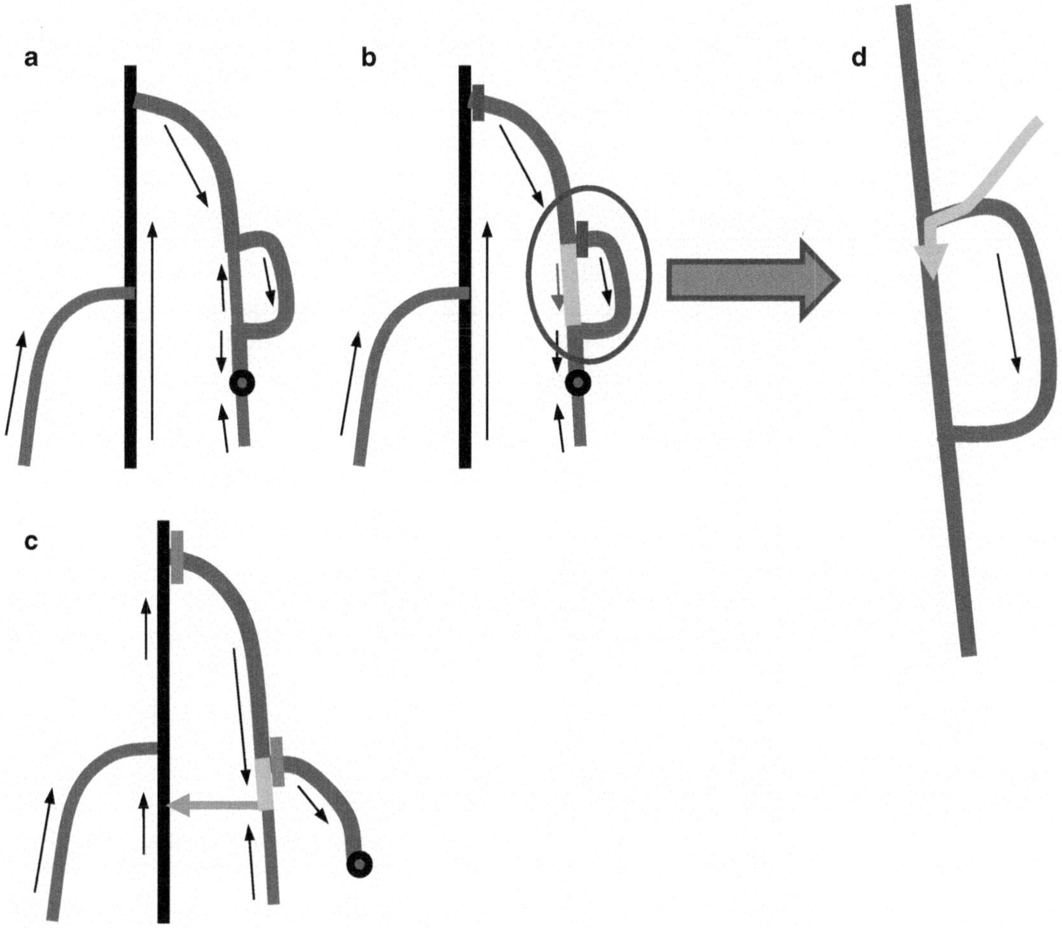

Fig. 7.19 Technical details of devalvulation in Type A: (**a**) GSV with two refluxing segments, separated by an antegrade segment. (**b**) Situation after surgery including devalvulation: after crossotomy and disconnection of the tributary and devalvulation of the antegrade segment (now orange), a drained situation is achieved draining into the distal draining perforator (Type A) (**c**) or into a physiological perforator (Type B). Compare Fig. 6.8. (**d**) Detail of the procedure: the devalvulator (orange) is introduced via the proximal end of the refluxing tributary into the antegrade GSV (compare Fig. 7.18). Copyright: (**a**) With kind permission from [1], the others are new for this book

In case the devalvulation is to be performed between the distal refluxing tributary and the next perforating vein, the progression of the devalvulator is controlled percutaneously until the preoperatively marked point on the skin is reached (see Fig. 7.19c).

7.10 Treatment of Tributaries Apart from a CHIVA 2 Point

Refluxing tributaries often need to be severed where they join the saphenous vein, even if there is no CHIVA 2 point. This is the case of a shunt type 1 + 2: drainage from the GSV via a perforating vein and an additional refluxing tributary. These can be hooked through a small point incision, ligated, severed and 2 cm excised. In this case it is sufficient to operate as close as possible to the trunk; it is not necessary to expose the trunk at the tributary junction, which means, no "flush ligation" has to be performed.

The technique of a point incision and hooking the vein with a hook devoid of sharp borders is also used with all other tributaries. As the vein should not be destroyed, sharp devices should be avoided. An alternative to surgical (often sharp) hooks is found in stainless steel crochet hooks. Absorbable suture can be used in these regions.

Prior to intervention the decision has to be taken together with the patient, if the tributaries will only be interrupted at their origin and to reduce the pressure column or a phlebectomy will be performed. Depending on these decisions, the tributary will be marked on the skin preoperatively in standing position. It is helpful for the surgeon, if based on the ultrasound investigation the points are marked, where the tributary runs next to the skin, as this is not visible in lying position.

7.11 Perforating Veins

Re-entry perforating veins are not interrupted in CHIVA.

If a perforating vein itself is a reflux source, it must be interrupted. The vein is exposed, ligated and severed as normal in traditional surgery. Special care must be taken in CHIVA not to interrupt the saphenous vein, if not part of the strategy, and to close the fascia with non-absorbable suture.

Please note that combining surgery with sclerotherapy (see Sect. 7.12.4.1) can optimize the effects of interruption on perforating veins.

7.12 Sclerotherapy and CHIVA

7.12.1 Introduction to Sclerotherapy

The use of sclerotherapy, an obliterating treatment, matches paradoxically with CHIVA strategy in particular cases, but it must be applied correctly.

The goal of sclerotherapy is to obliterate a vessel, thanks to an endothelium lesion provoked by chemical substances. The exposition of the sub-endothelial collagen provides the conditions for thrombus formation, well fixed to the wall due to the inflammatory process.

7.12.2 Sclerosing Agents and Application

Different sclerosing agents are available, specially detergents and dehydrating substances. Among the dehydrating substances, the following are applied:

- Hypertonic as the saline solution (sodium chloride to 20%)
- Not hypertonic as salicylate and glycerol that interact with the wall by opening the water channels with cellular dehydration of the endothelium

Most often detergents are used in the context of sclerotherapy, specially polidocanol. They attack the cell wall proteins disrupting the membrane of the endothelium. They are divided into anionic and non-anionic:

- Anionic as sodium tetradecyl sulfate (e.g. Trombovar®, Sotradecol®, Tromboject®)
- Not anionic as polidocanol (Aethoxysclerol®, Sclerovein®, Asclera®)

The detergents have the property that they are quickly deactivated when in contact with blood: plasma proteins bind the detergent within seconds. Detergents can be used in two different forms: liquid and foam.

1. *Liquid application*: The substance mixes quickly with blood, so the inactivation is achieved within seconds. This makes it less aggressive as compared to foam and gives it a delimited indication, specially to treat small vessels.
2. *Foam application*: Foam has a high cohesion itself, with the tendency of completely filling the room where it is introduced, displacing the blood. This filling possibility has its limits in large vessels. The contact time with the vein wall is higher for foam than for liquid. The inactivation will only work on the surface of the foam, leaving a higher active time to the sclerosing agent within the foam. This makes the foam more aggressive compared to the liquids that mix with the blood and allows a sclerotherapy of larger vessels than spider or reticular veins.

There are different ways to prepare foam, using different components. The most often used way is the wet foam by Tessari [10] or sometimes dry foam according to Monfreux [11], explained in Fig. 7.20 and in the first part of Table 7.1. In the

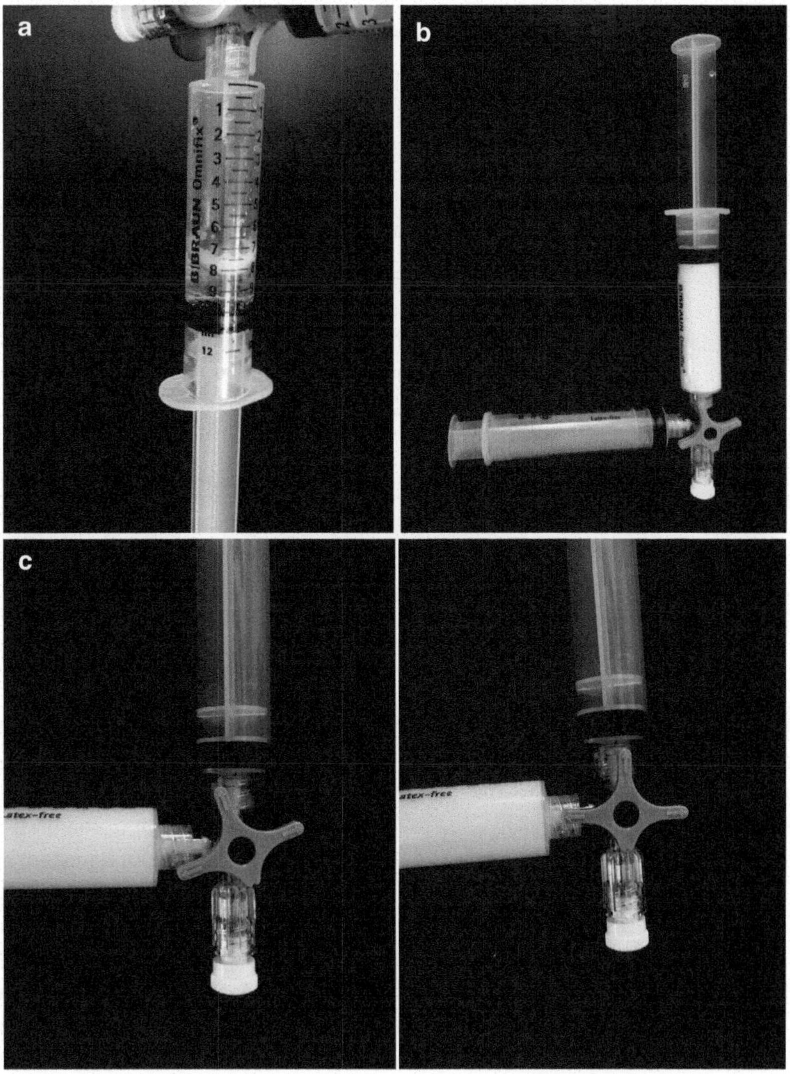

Fig. 7.20 (**a**) To prepare Tessari foam, 2 mL of sclerosing agent is introduced in a 10 mL syringe, added by 8 mL of air. (**b**) This syringe is connected to another empty 10 mL syringe by a three-way stopcock. The content of the syringe is pushed back and forth manually, until a homogeneous foam is achieved. (**c**) The three-way stopcock can be positioned at 90° (left) or slightly turned (right). In this case, the lumen for the foam to pass is less, and the foam will have bubbles of lesser diameter. (**d**) Take a smaller syringe to extract 2–3 mL of foam for an application. (**e**) Never apply more than 3 mL with one injection

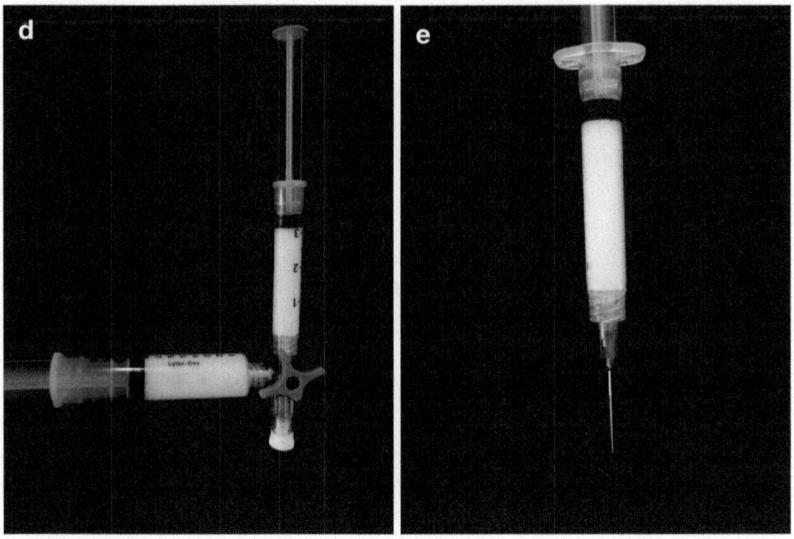

Fig. 7.20 (continued)

Table 7.1 Properties of sclerotherapy foam

	Foam according to Tessari	Dry foam according to Monfreux
Preparation	4 parts of air and 1 part of liquid, according to Tessari's method (see Fig. 7.20)	8 parts of air and 1 part of liquid (this makes 9 mL filling in a 10 mL syringe)
Concentration	All concentrations of sclerosing agent can be used	Only high concentrations of sclerosing agent
Foam stability	Low foam stability, hence action time is reduced with disactivation within some seconds	High stability, hence increased action time
Diffusion inside the vessel	High diffusion in the vessels, as it has a low viscosity with bubbles of different sizes	Low diffusion of the foam because of its high viscosity with small homogeneous bubbles, so the progression is controllable by stopping the application
Application	Extended sclerosing action over a long distance, e.g. long tributaries, saphenous veins (not in CHIVA context)	When powerful action is needed punctually with control of the extension inside the vessel • Recidives of the sapheno-femoral junction after stripping • Closure of a perforator • Closure of the origin of the anterior accessory saphenous vein

author's experience, sometimes a foam with higher consistency is necessary; the way to manufacture it is also explained in the second part of Table 7.1.

7.12.3 Effect of Sclerotherapy on the Vein

In the optimal case, the sclerosing agent provokes an endothelial lesion, which induces a vein wall inflammatory process and a subsequent thrombus formation inside the vessel, well adhered to the vein wall. The end-point of this process is the vein obliteration after thrombus organisation by granulation tissue.

In case of an extensive lesion of the vein wall, involving not only the endothelium but also the external part of the media and the adventitia layer, no granulation tissue will be involved: the vasa vasorum from the adventitia layer will spread into the thrombus and provoke thrombus lysis and early recanalization prior to the formation of fibrous organisation. Still, sometimes after the recanalization of a vein after sclerotherapy, we find a calibre reduction and sometimes not. Eccentric compression reduces the calibre in very superficial vessels and hence possibly the thrombus dimensions.

7.12.4 Sclerotherapy as a Tactic in the CHIVA Strategy

Sclerotherapy as a Tactic in CHIVA Strategy

1. For treating selectively the escape points, N1-N2/N3 are difficult to manage with surgery, unless an extensive surgical procedure with risk of functional damage and not good aesthetic results
   (a) Some perforators
   (b) Sapheno-popliteal junction in some cases
2. Pelvic shunts with low flow
3. Treatment of peculiar shunt II
4. For remodelling the saphenous haemodynamics (1° Step CHIVA 2)
   (a) Small tributaries
   (b) Tortuous tributaries

7.12.4.1 Sclerotherapy in the Context of Perforator Treatment

In the seldom case that a perforator must be disconnected according to CHIVA strategy, one of the main targets is not to leave any stump after treating an escape point, because it would be a source of recurrences.

Perforators show different characteristics that have to be analysed prior to decide how to treat them.

- Which veins are connected? We distinguish
  - Perforators connecting the saphenous vein (N2) with the deep vein (N1). These can be short and without tortuosity—which allows a surgery with little trauma to surrounding structures. These can also be long and tortuous, as it is often the case with perforating veins at the medial aspect of the thigh.
  - Perforators connecting tributaries (N3) with the deep veins (N1).
- Is the perforator mono- or multitroncular?
  - Monotroncular perforator: We can find only one vein connecting the deep and the superficial vein, without branching at the subfascial level.
  - Multitroncular perforator: The perforator branches between the deep and the superficial vein connecting the same or different superficial or deep veins (see Fig. 7.21).

When a perforator is disconnected with a surgical procedure, even if subfascial, often a stump is left (see Fig. 7.21). Therefore, the optimal indications for surgery of perforators without leaving any stump are the following:

1. Short perforators without branching (e.g. Cockett perforators in thin people)
2. A peculiar refluxing multitroncular perforator represented by a perforator of an internal pump collector (vein connecting the posterior tibial vein with a soleus muscular vein) (see Fig. 7.21g)

All the other perforators could be treated with sclerotherapy in addition to surgery or sclerotherapy alone to avoid leaving a stump or other refluxing branches in case of multitroncularity—without provoking the large lesion necessary to do a radical surgery.

Hence the indications of perforator sclerotherapy in CHIVA treatment depend on the length of the subfascial tract and the types of multitroncularity and the superficial vein to which the perforator is connected.

1. Treatment of perforating veins connecting N1–N2

   The first step is the surgical disconnection of the perforator from the saphenous trunk to avoid the extension of the sclerosing action to the saphenous trunk, afterwards introduction of a small catheter in the subfascial perforator and injection of liquid, low-concentrated sclerosing agent. Foam should not be used to avoid longer persistence in the deep vein with subsequent risk of deep vein thrombosis.

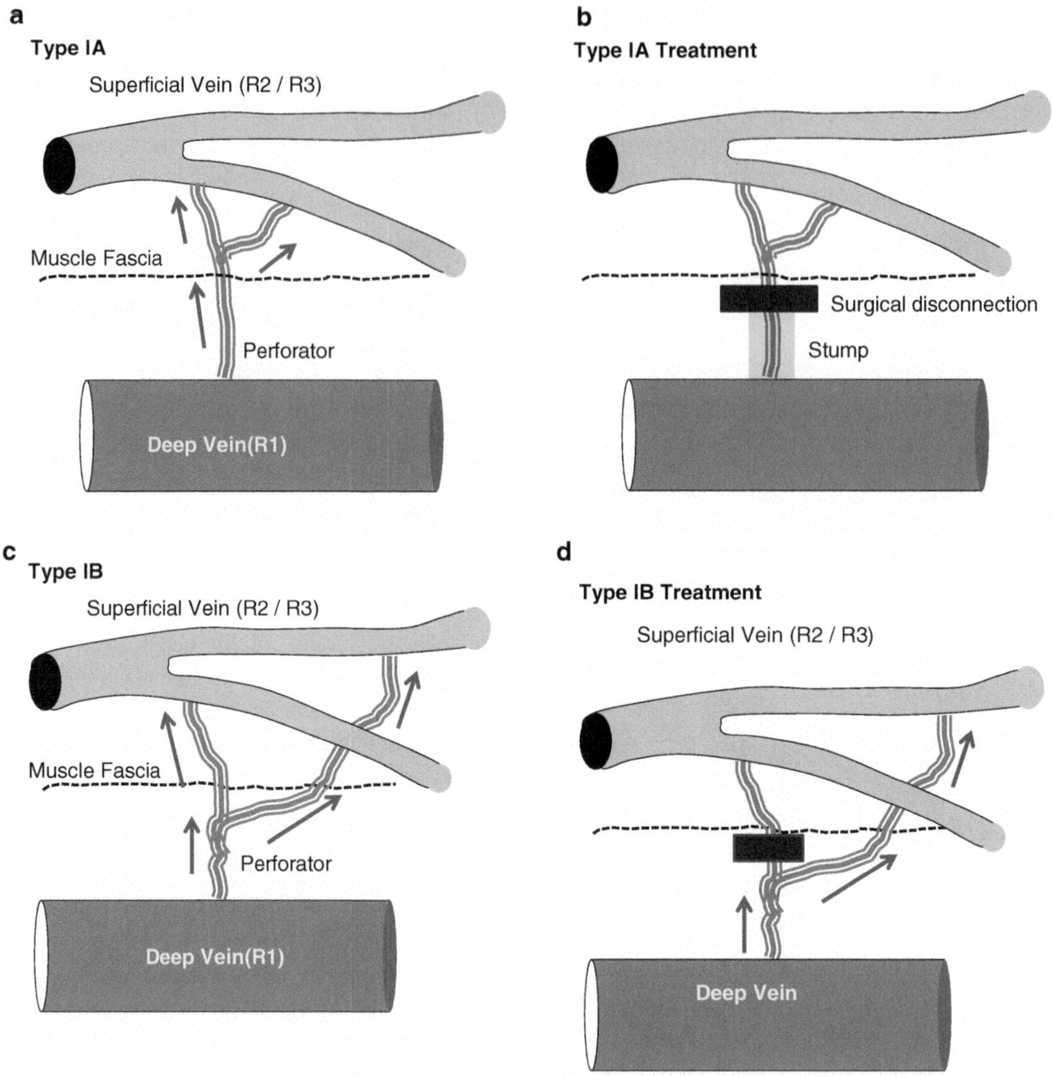

Fig. 7.21 Types of multitroncular perforators and classical treatment errors. (**a**) Type IA: one refluxive perforator connected with the deep vein and branching to feed the same superficial vessel with two arms. In this case, the perforator branches above the fascia; this can also happen below, in the muscular compartment. (**b**) Surgical treatment with stump. Surgical disconnection of the perforator on subfascial level. This leaves a stump between the disconnection point and the deep vein (light green area). (**c**) Type IB: one refluxive perforator connected to the deep vein, division of the refluxing perforator at subfascial level and feeding two different superficial vessels with reflux. (**d**) Interruption of only one of both branches of the perforator. The reflux in vein 2 is interrupted; reflux in vein 1 will persist. The correct way would be to interrupt both parts of the tributary—which would be achieved if the perforator would have been prepared until the connection to the deep vein or if the branching would have been made clear by ultrasound prior to the intervention. (**e**) Type II A: two branches of the refluxing perforator part from one deep vein to feed one superficial vein. (**f**) The subfascial disconnection of the perforator (unitroncular at this level) will lead to a stump with two connections to the deep vein. (**g**) Type IIB: the refluxive perforator connects to a superficial vein, feeding it refluxively (red arrow), but is also connected through another branch to another deep vein, without reflux. This is often the case in refluxive perforators of the inner aspect of the calf. The deep multitroncularity can involve pump collectors (e.g. vessels connecting soleus veins with posterior tibial veins or peroneal veins). (**h**) In this case, the subfascial disconnection of the refluxing perforator results in abolition of the insufficiency point for the superficial vein and in a stable, draining condition for the perforator, which is drained in the same deep compartment into another deep vein. (**i**) Ultrasound example of a multitroncular, subfascial perforating vein. Images (**a**–**h**) prepared by Massimo Cappelli

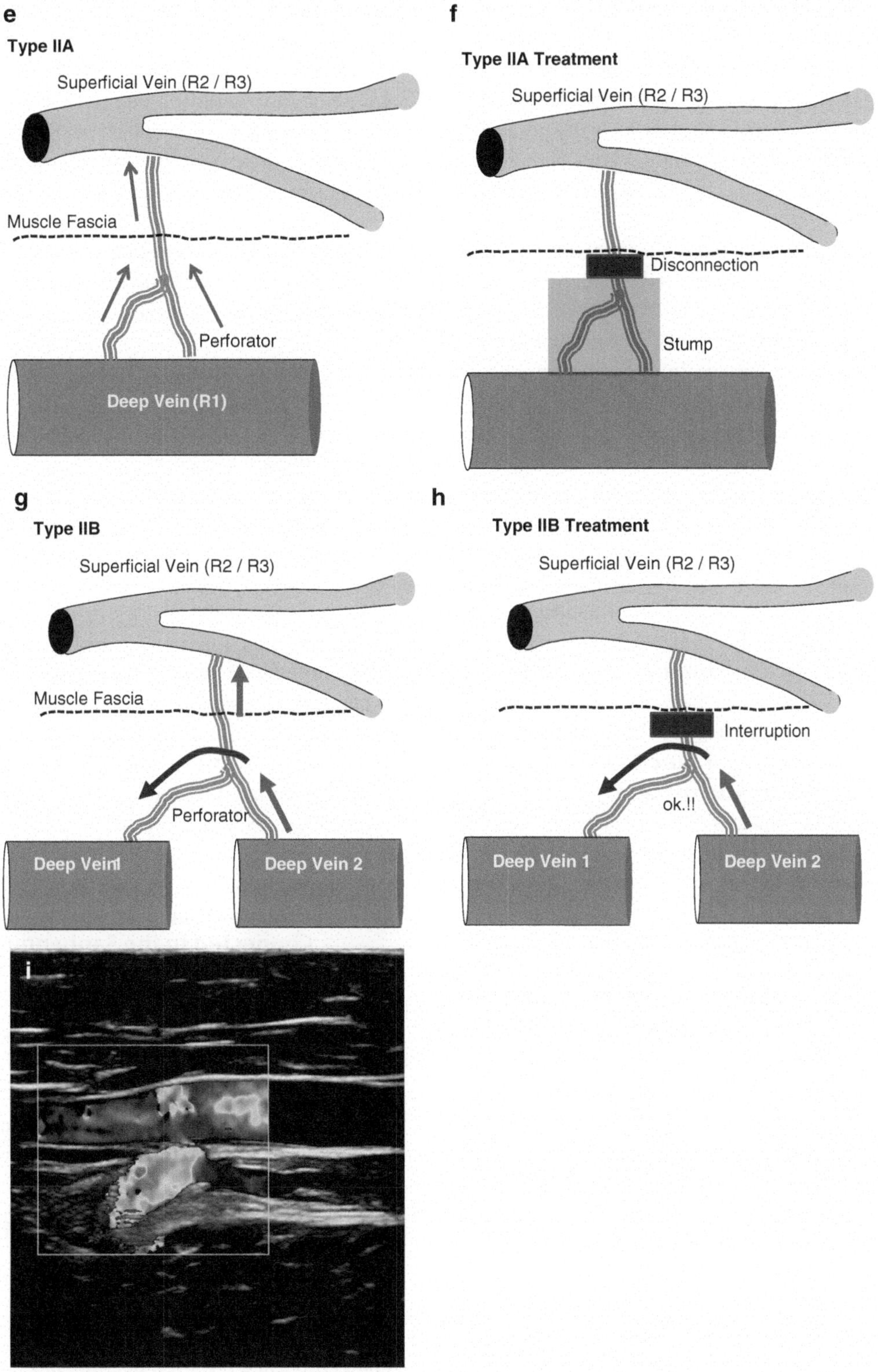

Fig. 7.21 (continued)

Then perform an activation of the calf pump to wash the deep vein and promote the inactivation of the sclerosing agent at this site. In the experience of the author, this method allows a satisfactory closure of the perforator without stump and avoiding large surgery.

2. Perforators connected to a superficial tributary (N1–N3):
   (a) No saphenous vein involved: Usually these perforators and tributaries are not too large and could be treated with foam sclerotherapy in one session without the need of surgery. In case the perforator is large, the surgery combined with sclerotherapy technique could also be applied here (see 1).
   (b) Refluxing perforator fills a tributary, which shortly after joins a saphenous vein. This saphenous vein is incompetent as a result of this perforating vein. Surgical disconnection of the tributary en niveau of the saphenous vein and sclerotherapy of the tributary

7.12.4.2 Treatment of the Sapheno-Popliteal Junction with Sclerotherapy

In case of the sapheno-popliteal junction, we often find the same difficulties to perform a flush ligation at the level of the deep vein (see Sect. 7.4). Some surgeons consider it is not worth it to risk neurological lesions, DVT and bad aesthetic results because of a large incision, just for treating varicose veins.

The consequence is that a lot of stumps are left after surgical treatment with high rate of recurrence, especially if we had a systolic reflux.

The same can happen, when disconnecting the short saphenous vein distally to the first tributary of the junction, which might be the thigh extension of the short saphenous vein or the Giacomini vein. If the tributary is large and well drained, the stump will be washed. In case of a

1. Competent Giacomini vein (the flow is towards the great saphenous vein)
2. Thigh extension of the small saphenous vein with a small calibre compared to the calibre of the saphenous arch

the stump will be poorly washed and could be the source of recurrence.

The sclerotherapy will allow to obliterate the escape point flush with the popliteal vein. The procedure is the same as explained for the saphenous perforator treatment, performing the surgical disconnection first and then applying liquid low-dose sclerotherapy and performing calf movements afterwards for a better washout of the deep vein. This technique impedes the stump formation in the experience of the author.

7.12.4.3 Pelvic Shunts with Low Flow and Sclerotherapy

Pelvic reflux is discussed in Chap. 8, as well as surgical options are presented.

In case of low flow through the pelvic leak points, a sclerotherapy has shown to be helpful to avoid a surgical intervention. To protect the saphenous trunk, either the connection between the refluxive tributary with the saphenous vein should be interrupted first or the saphenous vein must be thoroughly compressed to avoid sclerosing agent dripping inside.

Best indications for sclerotherapy in case of pelvic leak points are the dorsal leak points (gluteal) and the perineal or inguinal points with a long subcutaneous run prior to drain into the saphenous vein.

7.12.4.4 Treatment of Tributaries Connected to the Saphenous Veins

Treatment of tributaries with sclerotherapy at their confluence to the saphenous vein is possible instead of surgery in case of small very superficial vessels or tributaries of the saphenous trunk with a very deep connection to the saphenous vein due to a thick subcutaneous fat layer to avoid large scars:

1. Shunt type 1 + 2 in addition to the treatment of the junction
2. Shunt type 2 where the tributary is the only refluxing segment
3. Shunt type 4 + 2
4. Shunt type 3 and 5 for remodelling the saphenous haemodynamics (1° Step CHIVA 2, see Sect. 6.4.1)

5. Residual visible tributaries after CHIVA
6. Tributary recurrence after CHIVA

This treatment could be performed with sclerotherapy in case the tributary is small or very tortuous. Peripheral vessels should be treated with sclerotherapy without involving the saphenous trunk, applying a digital compression at the junction (reflux outlet) or re-entry level in the saphenous axe. Nevertheless, in the author's experience, the saphenous trunk is involved by the sclerosing action in 11% of the cases after 1 week but with complete recanalization after 3 months, generally with calibre reduction.

On the other hand, a stump of the tributary at the level of the junction with the saphenous trunk should be avoided.

According to different types of vessel connection, straight or tortuous, various compressions and kinds of therapy will be used. Straight junction means that the part of the vessel next to its connection to the saphenous vein is rectilinear; sometimes it runs next to it within the fascial compartment for some cm. It is independent of the fact that the more superficial part of the tributary is tortuous. We find a tortuous junction in case of no straight segment between the tortuous tributary and the saphenous vein (see Fig. 7.22).

Sclerotherapy of a Tributary with a Straight Junction

Refluxive tributaries with a straight junction (see Fig. 7.22a) can be treated under ultrasound control and with compression technique of the

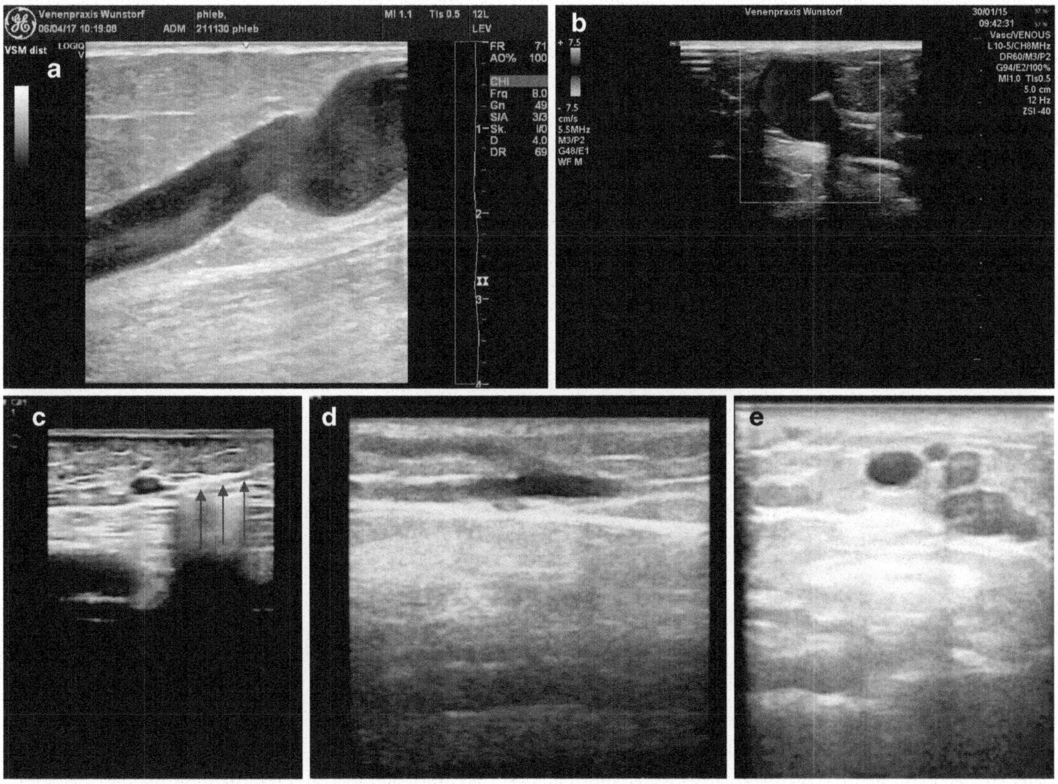

Fig. 7.22 (**a**) Longitudinal section at the medial aspect of the thigh. Straight outlet of a tributary at the junction with the great saphenous vein, the last segment of the vein before joining the saphenous vein is rectilineous. Arrows: delimitation of the fascial compartment. (**b**) Cross section through the medial aspect of the thigh: tortuous outlet of a tributary, the tributary is tortuous until the very point it joins the great saphenous vein (arrow). (**c**) Foam sclerotherapy of the tributary, stopping at the lumen of the GSV. The foam is visible as a white image with ultrasound shadow below it (arrows pointing to the foam are located in the shadow region). (**d**) Result after sclerotherapy of a tributary with straight outlet. Note that the tributary is closed (filled with echogenic material) until the connection to the GSV, which is washed out by higher blood flow. (**e**) Result after sclerotherapy of a tributary with tortuous outlet. The GSV is without intraluminal echoes (black); the tributaries are closed with echogenic contents

saphenous vein at the point of the tributary connection.

1. Compression of the outlet point during injection of liquid agents: The outlet is identified with ultrasound and marked on the skin. Then a compression with a finger is performed at that level during the injection.
2. Specific compression techniques for foam such as bending the probe compressing the outlet level when the foam shows up are currently being investigated using wet foam at low concentration and with air/liquid ratio 4:1 (see Table 7.1)

Sclerotherapy of a Tributary with a Tortuous Junction

In this case, the compression applied at the junction level will involve a large part of the tributary, too, impeding the sclerosing action flush with the saphenous trunk. So, often a stump will be left. This problem can be avoided using dry foam (see Table 7.1). The needle is inserted in the tortuous vein, and 0.5–1 cm^3 of the dry foam manufactured with 2% polidocanol is applied slowly under ultrasound observation of the point where tributary and saphenous vein meet. The high viscosity of the foam allows us to follow its slow progression. As soon as the foam reaches the connection with the saphenous vein, a compression with the US probe at junction level is performed. The injection must be soft and discontinuous, verifying the foam movement towards the junction. Glass syringes are perfect for this purpose.

To increase viscosity, we can add glycerine to the sclerosing agent.

Another way to regulate the progression of the dry foam in the tributary towards the saphenous vein is applying a blood pressure cuff proximally to the injection point. This cuff is filled with 80–90 mmHg before the injection. This stops the flow in the saphenous vein—and in the tributary. After applying foam to the tributary, we deflate the cuff slowly, supervising the foam progression until the junction point from the tributary into the saphenous vein—at this moment we leave the pressure for 2 min to allow an inactivation of the foam by blood proteins, before opening the cuff.

7.12.5 Sclerotherapy Post-CHIVA

Sclerotherapy Post-CHIVA

1. Disconnected vessels from the saphenous trunk when still visible after a while and spider veins correlated
2. Recurrences
   (a) Escape points N1-N2/N3 which are difficult to manage with surgery
   (b) Some perforators
   (c) The stump following the small saphenous vein disconnection in the popliteal area
   (d) Pelvic leak point with low flow
   (e) New refluxing vessels connected with the saphenous trunk
3. Matting post-CHIVA

According to the author's experience, the use of sclerotherapy in post-CHIVA follow-up is applied in around 15% of the cases, but this value is going to grow up in relation to follow-up duration. The recurrence rate is less in case of drained saphenous trunk after therapy (see Sect. 3.5.6).

A total of 2794 previously not treated patients underwent CHIVA intervention on GSV between 1991 and 2013. Of these, 22% were male and 78% female with ages comprised between 16 and 88 years (mean 55 sd 14,1), 51% right legs and 49% left legs. They were evaluated at each follow-up in the office. During the follow-up (minimum 1 year and maximum 22 years, mean 7 years), 415 patients (15% of all the patients) underwent sclerotherapy for the following reasons:

- 134 patients had residual visible tributaries (sclerotherapy of the tributary)
- 25 patients for spider veins (sclerotherapy of the spider vein)
- 20 patients for perforating veins (sclerotherapy of the perforator)
- 9 patients for pelvic reflux (sclerotherapy of the groin tributary)
- 227 patients presented new refluxing saphenous tributaries (sclerotherapy of the tributary)

All patients were controlled 2 weeks after sclerotherapy. In 46 cases (11%), a thrombus extension into the GSV was found, which remitted in all cases after 3 months, leaving a patent GSV [12].

In case of sclerotherapy post-CHIVA in non-disconnected tributaries, the same techniques as explained in Sect. 7.12.4.4 will be applied.

7.12.5.1 Sclerotherapy of Disconnected Vessels

In case of the vessels remaining visible after having been disconnected from the saphenous vein, liquid sclerosing agents with low concentration should be used because the pressure inside the tributary is low, and the liquid can re-enter into the saphenous trunk more distally. In case of a large re-entry connection, a disconnection should be considered, or the saphenous vein should be compressed during the injection (see Sect. 7.12.4.4). Excentric compression should be applied after sclerotherapy.

7.12.5.2 Matting Post-CHIVA

Matting is characterized by an area of red spider veins as an expression of a dilation of the most superficial venous subpapillar network. It can appear after any surgical or sclerotherapeutic procedure. According to clinical experience, we can differentiate two types of matting on the time of appearance.

Early matting appears due to a transmural pressure excess in the dermic subpapillar venous plexus. This happens, if the veins in the leg after the CHIVA procedure have an increased residual pressure. This is the case, if after the therapy, the drainage path for the vessel is not appropriate to its diameter, generating poorly or not drained systems, especially in zones affected by cellulite (cold areas). Another reason is the vasodilation due to an excessive inflammatory reaction after too aggressive sclerotherapy.

Late matting appears after months and is a sign of a progressive valve incompetence of the peripheral vessels without re-entry (higher than third order of division) as a consequence of transmural pressure excess related to hydrostatic pressure increase. Diagnostic with ultrasound should search for tributaries with descending flow into the matting area and treat them with wet foam under ultrasound control with small quantities of wet foam.

7.13 Endoluminal Techniques in the CHIVA Context

Endoluminal heat techniques have become popular and are widely used as alternative to stripping. The most common heat sources are radial *LASER* fibres with 1470 nm and radio frequency. Newer techniques, like application of glue, are starting to claim their rights in the fan of surgical and interventional options.

Little is published concerning endoluminal heat in the CHIVA context [13, 14]; randomized studies are still lacking. Technically it is performed in the same way than under ablative aspects. The difference is the length of the segment to be closed. In case of radio frequency, the heating segment is 6.5 cm (VNUS Closure fast®). At least this length has to be heated. As only one (or in case of enlarged veins, two) segments will be closed, it has to be very sure that enough energy has reached the vein wall. The author applies as much cycles as necessary to have less than 15 W at the display of the device. Usually this is three, seldom four, cycles in the first position. In case of junction diameters above 10 mm, until today two segments have been closed. A new trial in Germany (SOS—save our saphenous) is testing to close only one segment when applying radio frequency. In case of laser, as rule of thumb, a length proportional to the diameter of the junction has been chosen [14]. In the SOS study, also for *LASER*, an extension of 7 cm at the most will be used.

Ideally the tip position is distal to the last draining tributary of the groin. This allows the tributaries to drain into the deep vein, as depicted in Fig. 7.23.

In case of an incompetent terminal valve, the AASV has to be analysed preoperatively. If there is a reflux or a dilated AASV, perhaps this will become incompetent after closing the GSV distal to the terminal valve and tributaries. This has to be explained to the patients. In centres or regions without the possibility to apply pelvic leak point

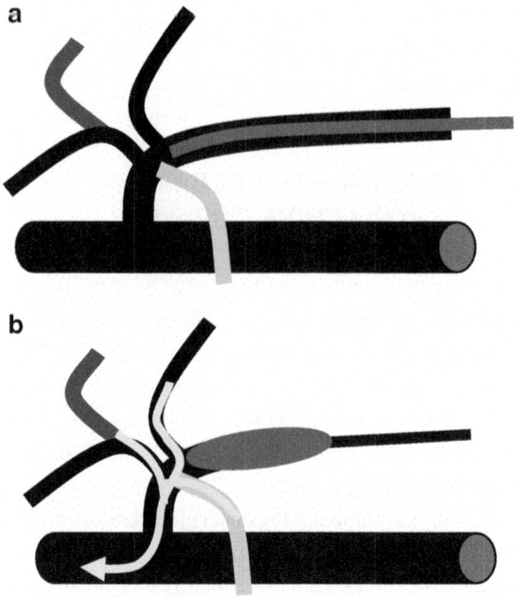

Fig. 7.23 (**a**) Schematic representation of the sapheno-femoral junction (SFJ) (legends compare Fig. 7.1) and tip position (red line) inside the GSV (brown), distal to the tributaries of the SFJ. (**b**) Situation after closure of a short segment of the proximal GSV (heat occlusion: red), distal to the groin tributaries. These are draining into the deep vein via the terminal valve; the distal GSV is thinned

surgery, endoluminal heating is an option to treat patients with competent terminal valve and incompetent preterminal valve and persistent reflux after CHIVA 2. The pelvic reflux is conducted to the deep vein via an antegrade valve and is hindered to fill the distal GSV.

Endoluminal heat has also been applied to close the CHIVA 2 point in rectilineous tributaries (see Fig. 7.22) always paying attention not to destroy the saphenous vein nor to burn the skin. In case of rectilineous refluxing perforating veins, endoluminal heat devices have also been used. Both applications (tributaries and perforators) have not been included in prospective studies, so far.

Glue claims to close the vein independently of the length of the closed segment. If this procedure—after prospective studies to come—could demonstrate its long-time safeness (though a foreign body is introduced inside a vessel), perhaps it would be an option in the context of CHIVA, even to perform the crossotomy between the deep vein and the tributaries, if technically feasible.

Literature

1. Mendoza E. Handbuch CHIVA. Arrien GmbH; 2002.
2. Mirjalili SA, Muirhead JC, Stringer MD. Redefining the surface anatomy of the sapheno-femoral junction in vivo. Clin Anat. 2014;27(6):915–9. https://doi.org/10.1002/ca.22386. Epub 20 Mar 2014.
3. Mühlberger D, Morandini L, Brenner E. Venous valves and major superficial tributary veins near the sapheno-femoral junction. J Vasc Surg. 2009;49(6):1562–9. https://doi.org/10.1016/j.jvs.2009.02.241.
4. Cappelli M, Molino-Lova R, Giangrandi I, Ermini S, Gianesini S. Ligation of the saphenofemoral junction tributaries as risk factor for groin recurrence. J Vasc Surg Venous Lymphat Disord. 2017 Dec 28. pii: S2213-333X(17)30436-5. https://doi.org/10.1016/j.jvsv.2017.09.005.
5. Delfrate R, Bricchi M, Franceschi C, Goldoni M. Multiple ligation of the proximal greater saphenous vein in the CHIVA treatment of primary varicose veins. Veins Lymphat. 2014. https://doi.org/10.4081/vl.2014.1919.
6. Winterborn RJ, Foy C, Heather BP, Earnshaw JJ. Randomised trial of flush sapheno-femoral ligation for primary great saphenous varicose veins. Eur J Vasc Endovasc Surg. 2008;36(4):477–84. https://doi.org/10.1016/j.ejvs.2008.06.022. Epub 20 Aug 2008.
7. Heim D, Negri M, Schlegel U, De Maeseneer M. Resecting the great saphenous stump with endothelial inversion decreases neither neovascularization nor thigh varicosity recurrence. J Vasc Surg. 2008;47(5):1028–32. https://doi.org/10.1016/j.jvs.2007.12.039. Epub 21 Mar 2008.
8. Frings N, Nelle A, Tran P, Fischer R, Krug W. Reduction of neo-reflux after correctly performed ligation of the sapheno-femoral junction. A randomized trial. Eur J Vasc Endovasc Surg. 2004;28(3):246–52.
9. Gianesini S, Menegatti E, Malagoni AM, Occhionorelli S, Zamboni P. Mini-invasive high-tie by clip apposition versus crossectomy by ligature: long-term outcomes and review of the available therapeutic options. Phlebology. 2017;32(4):249–55.
10. Tessari L. Nouvelle technique d'obtention de la scléromousse. Phlébologie. 2000;53:129.
11. Monfreux A. Quelle mousse pour quelles indications? Phlebologie 2013; 66(3):11–18.
12. Mendoza E, Cappelli M. Sclerotherapy technique in CHIVA strategy. Phlebology. 2017;46:5–12.
13. Gianesini S, Menegatti E, Zuolo M, et al. Short endovenous LASER Ablation of the great saphenous vein in a modified CHIVA strategy. Veins Lymphat. 2013;2:e21.
14. Mendoza E, Amsler F. CHIVA with endoluminal procedures: LASER versus VNUS—treatment of the saphenofemoral junction. Phlebologie. 2017;46:5–12.

Minimally Invasive Surgical Treatment of Pelvic Leak Points

8

Roberto Delfrate and Erika Mendoza

8.1 Anatomy of the Pelvic Venous System

The pelvic venous system is a complex venous network of vessels interconnecting parietal and visceral veins and draining extra-pelvic superficial veins as perineal, vulvar, round ligament whose refluxes can extend to the great and small saphenous networks [1–4]. Indeed, the venous pelvic system consists of avalvulated venous trunks (hypogastric, common iliac, caval and renal veins), inconstantly valvulated veins (ovarian veins) generally valvulated parietal veins (gluteal veins, obturator veins inferior gluteal veins) [5] and visceral collectors (internal pudendal vein, uterine vein) connecting vertically and horizontally throughout avalvulated plexuses. This vascular network represents a functional pelvic venous unit, an extremely important bypass path in case of obstructed drainage of a primary venous trunk like the left renal vein (nutcracker syndrome) or even of a common iliac or inferior cava vein. Whilst the right ovarian vein is valvulated, the left one can be without any valve in 50% of cases. The pudendal vein is generally valvulated [6], whilst the uterine vein is generally avalvulated [7–10]. So, a large amount of the pelvic venous system is free of valves. There is no muscle pump applying to the pelvic venous net. Flow is maintained, thanks to the gradient of pressure towards the inferior cava vein and the right heart and breathing suction effect. The presence of valve in the common femoral veins and in the saphenous femoral junctions as well as in the parietal collateral veins of the hypogastric vein (obturator veins, round ligament veins, pudendal veins and also the labial veins) and the spermatic veins with the only exception of the left one is necessary to ensure the correct drainage towards the caval vein and the right heart.

During pregnancy, a valvular damage may occur in consequence of the increase in pelvic blood volume and the vein peripheral resistances and so of the venous transmural pressure. This is caused by the increase of the uterus size, hormonal balance variation with connective tissue compliance variations, as well as the placenta hyperdebit (the placenta works like an arteriovenous fistula). During pregnancy, labial veins and pudendal network connected to the obturatorian and the epigastric veins will have a volume overload followed by restoration after delivery or permanent valvular damage.

The venous valve damage in the presence of a favourable gradient of pressure is the condition necessary to create a refluxing venous path draining towards the legs, either via subcutaneous collaterals or via the tributaries of the

R. Delfrate, M.D. (✉)
Responsible Surgery at Casa di Cura Figlie di San Camillo, Cremona, Italy
e-mail: roberto.delfrate@icloud.com

E. Mendoza, M.D., Ph.D.
Venenpraxis, Wunstorf, Germany
e-mail: erika.mendoza@t-online.de

P. Zamboni et al. (eds.), *Saphenous Vein-Sparing Strategies in Chronic Venous Disease*,
https://doi.org/10.1007/978-3-319-70638-2_8

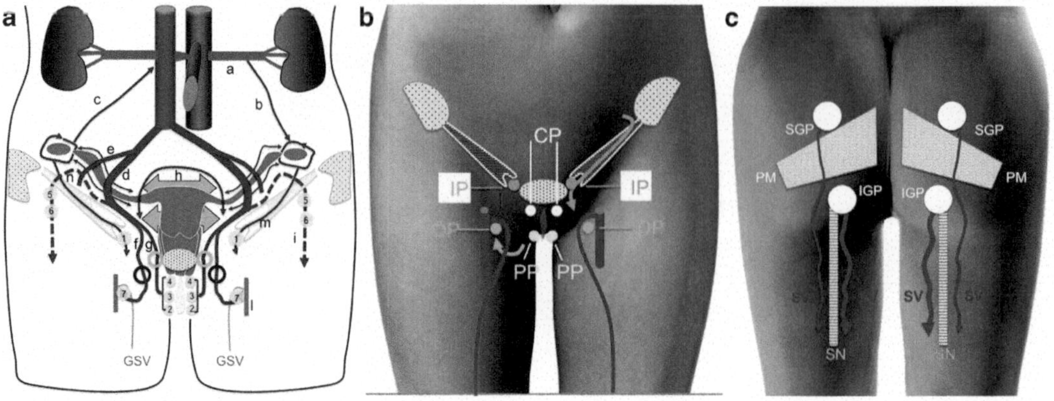

Fig. 8.1 (**a**) a-Left renal vein, b-left ovarian vein, c-right ovarian vein, d-hypogastric vein, e-external iliac vein, f-obturator vein, g-internal pudendal vein, h-pelvic venous plexuses, i-sciatic vein, m-round ligament plexus, n-gluteal veins, green circle Alcock canal and black circle obturator canal, 1-inguinal point, 2-perineal point, 3-intermediate perineal point, 4-clitoridian point, 5-superior gluteal point, 6-inferior gluteal point. (**b**) Pelvic leak points in the ventral part of the body. Ventral vision of a female pelvis with bones (rose) and the inguinal ligaments (white), the common femoral vein (blue, thick) and the saphenous vein (blue thin). IP: Inguinal point, lateral to the mons pubis and at the medial end of the inguinal duct, through which the reflux will be emerging. On the left side of the image is a schematic representation of blood flow. CP: between the mons pubis and the labia, we find the clitoridian point; in analogy in the men, we find this point at the base of the penis. PP: Between the labia and the proximal inner end of the thigh, we find the perineal point (see Fig. 8.9). OP: Obturator point to be found at the sapheno-femoral junction, emerging from medial and dorsal into the SFJ. Flow direction is represented in green. (**c**) Pelvic leak points at the dorsal part of the body—*SGP* superior gluteal point, *PM* piriformis muscle, *IGP* inferior gluteal point, *SV* sciatic vein, *SN* sciatic nerve, sciatic veins representing the refluxing venous path from the gluteal points

sapheno-femoral junction. The consequence might be an involvement of reflux of the lower limb venous system: chronic venous insufficiency and varicose veins of the lower limb of pelvic origin [11–15]. Every refluxing PLP leads to ipsilateral or contralateral varicose veins.

8.2 Diagnostic Approach to the Pelvic Leak Points

To complete a diagnostic investigation of reflux in leg veins, also the pelvic leak points should be investigated with duplex ultrasound, especially in case of competent terminal valve and Valsalva positive reflux in the sapheno-femoral junction or more distally in saphenous vein or tributaries.

8.2.1 General Approach

During the ultrasound exploration of patients with reflux in superficial leg veins, the investigation of pelvic leak points must be performed, when a Valsalva positive reflux is found in any vein. Even when an incompetent terminal valve is responsible for Valsalva positive reflux, an additional inguinal or perineal leak point could be present in addition.

During the exploration of the sapheno-femoral junction, the obturatorian vein is in the focus. The probe can then be moved cranially from the sapheno-femoral junction to explore the inguinal region (I-Point) and medially to it the clitoridian point (C-Point) (see Fig. 8.1b). Perineal points are best found starting at the inner aspect of the proximal thigh and moving cranially, softly to avoid a compression of the very superficial veins. In case of difficulty of the patient separating the legs, the explored leg can be put, the foot on an elevated platform to give the probe space. Afterwards the patient is asked to turn around to investigate the posterior aspect of the thigh using the sciatic nerve as a B-mode mark and investigating reflux signs next systematically with a Valsalva test (see Fig. 8.2).

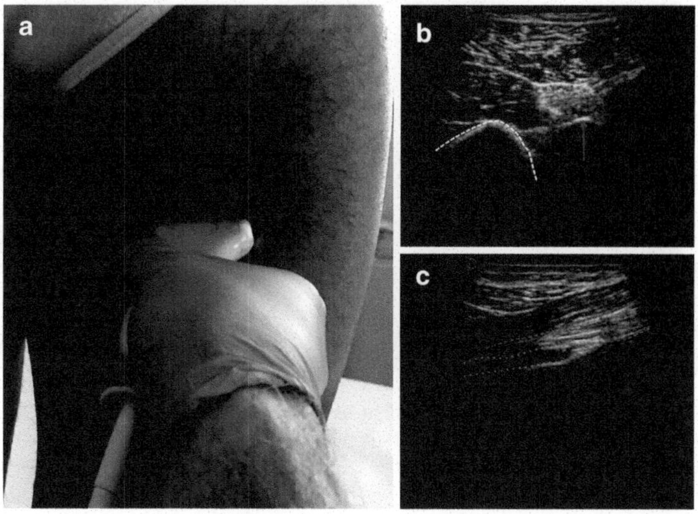

Fig. 8.2 (**a**) Photo of the back of a leg with the position of the probe on the skin. (**b**) B-mode ultrasound of the sciatic nerve as landmark for the evaluation of pelvic leak points; transversal image blue arrow, sciatic vein; red dashed line, the sciatic nerve; white dashed line, the bone. (**c**) Longitudinal image of the sciatic nerve between the red dashed lines and the vein between the blue dashed lines

A linear probe (7.5–12 MHz) is used first, but a convex or micro-convex one (5 MHz) may be necessary in overweight patients. It's important that the patient properly performs the Valsalva test. A simple way is to ask the patient to blow into a straw that was closed at one end (Cremona Manoeuvre, see Sect. 3.2.2) [16, 17].

A short outward flow of less than 1 s through leakage points shortly after a provocation manoeuvre is normal; it represents the natural drainage pathway for these vessels. A long-lasting flow after a provocation manoeuvre or permanent during Valsalva is demonstrative of a pathologic situation with pelvic reflux.

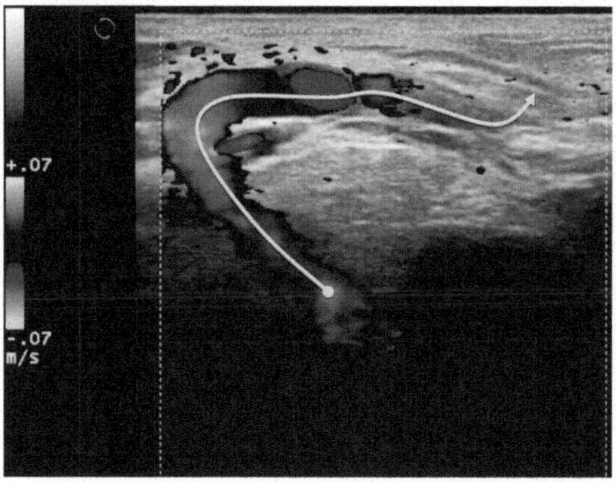

Fig. 8.3 Spontaneous inguinal point reflux in a patient in standing position without any breath variation. The probe is positioned over the right inguinal ligament in transverse position, showing the flow through the inner ring (yellow arrow) running from the deep network into the inguinal canal

8.2.2 Spontaneous Flow Through a Pelvic Leak Point

If a spontaneous reflux on any of the pelvic leak points is detectable with the patients in upright position, a pelvic hypertension must be suspected, and it must be investigated, if a pelvic leak does represent the escape point of an open bypassing shunt (see Sect. 3.7.3) (see Fig. 8.3). This would be the case, if there is any obstruction in the deep venous system forcing the blood to find a bypass through the pelvic network, the network serving as a drainage for other vessels, as happens in the pelvic congestion syndrome. When finding a permanent flow in upright position through a PLP, examination is continued with the patient lying down on the bed. If the spontaneous reverse flow continues also in recumbent position, the existence of an open vicarious shunt due to pelvic venous hyperpressure is highly likely. In this case, the PLP must be preserved, and further abdominal haemodynamic and chemistry investigations are needed (left renal vein evaluation, left ovarian or

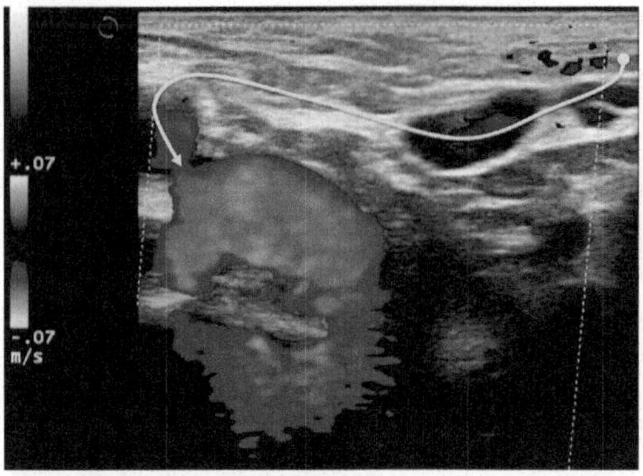

Fig. 8.4 Image of the same patient as in Fig. 8.3 in recumbent position. The reflux has stopped and an inward flow is detectable (yellow arrow)

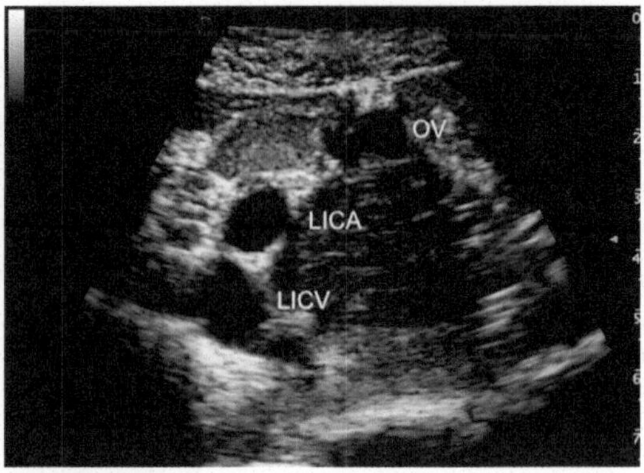

Fig. 8.5 Typical image of an enlarged left ovarian vein, next and laterally to the left iliac common artery (LICA) and left iliac common vein (LICV), best found in a transverse image performed with a 5 MHz probe positioned between the anterior and superior iliac spine and the xifo-pubic line on the skin

spermatic vein pressure evaluation, urine tests to detect microscopic haematuria and proteinuria). If the PLP reflux disappears in the lying position, the mini-invasive surgical treatment of the escape point may be possible, because of a deep draining path existence, but not before ensuring that there is another deep draining path (Fig. 8.4). This is best done with further duplex investigation of the abdomen or second-level investigations (see Chap. 5).

8.2.3 Pole Test to Evaluate the Pressure in the Left Ovarian Vein

In any case the haemodynamic evaluation of the flow in the left ovarian vein is useful to sort out pelvic congestion syndrome. The left ovarian vein is easy to identify with a convex probe in transverse view and laterally to the left iliac vessels, without any necessity of full bladder and in longitudinal (Fig. 8.5).

We find a permanent flow in case of pelvic congestion syndrome—breath modulation of the flow is a favourable prognostic sign, whilst on the contrary, continuous reflux without any modulation isn't. Venous pressure is an important clinical parameter. It can be estimated by checking flow variations in the left ovarian vein. This is achieved by changing the bed inclination angle as encoded by the Pole test [18, 19]. The Pole test method considers the flow hydrostatic pressure resistance induced by elevation of a checked point of a vessel, searching for the flow stop. When ovarian reflux stops, the height (in centimetres) from the point checked of the ovarian vein and the horizontal line passing through the heart is converted in mmHg; this value represents the venous ovarian pressure. Assuming the density of blood to be 1.055 g/cm^3 and that of mercury 13.54 g/cm^3, the pressure unit, 1 cm blood above the heart, is equal to 0.78 mmHg (10 mm × 1.055/13.54 = 0.78 mmHg).

8.3 General Considerations to the Treatment of Pelvic Leak Points

Thanks to Claude Franceschi pelvic leak point ultrasound identification and anatomical description [1–3], a minimally invasive strategy of treatment of varicose veins fed by pelvic reflux can be performed. The surgical procedure is minimally invasive under local anaesthesia. Pelvic endovascular treatment remains only necessary in case of pelvic congestion syndrome in women.

Perineal and inguinal points account for 97% of all PLPs treated in women. The favourable feature of perineal and inguinal point but even clitoridian point is the well-defined anatomical position easy to reach with a mini-invasive surgical dissection. Their depth ranges from 3 mm for the perineal point to 30 mm for the inguinal point. The treatment is possible under local anaesthesia and needs a perfect B-mode preoperative skin marking using a 10–18 MHz linear probe. To detect the flow, the pulse repetition frequency (PRF) is set between 0.75 and 1 KHz, suitable for detecting low-speed flow, even less than 10 cm/s. Skin marking is performed in the operation field without further changes of position of the patient.

Local anaesthesia consists of a mixture of lidocaine (2%) and ropivacaine (7.5 mg/mL), and a mild sedation may be useful. The author recommends finishing the surgical procedure with a rifampicin solution washing inside the wound, without systemic antibiotic therapy. Perineal skin incisions are closed with cyanoacrylate glue, without any need of plasters. Discharge is possible few hours after the intervention. The treatment is completed with daily elastic stockings for 4 weeks and low-molecular-weight heparin in prophylactic dose for 10 days.

8.4 Complications of Surgery of Pelvic Leak Point

In the author's experience of 366 PLP-treated patients, no deep vein thrombosis, pulmonary thromboembolism or deaths were observed, nor any bruises, subcutaneous inguinal or perineal haemorrhage, neuralgia, wound infection or superficial phlebitis, except one immediate postoperative inguinal bleeding after the treatment of the inguinal point.

On the contrary, endovascular procedures are more invasive and might provoke serious complications [20]. A main venous access is needed, including subclavian, brachial, femoral or transjugular approaches. The patient and the staff are exposed to radiation. Complications due to deep venous puncture as well as to embolization like haematoma, pneumothorax, closure of nontarget vessels, coils migrations, pulmonary embolism and stroke had been described [19].

8.5 The Female Inguinal Leak Point (IP)

The IPs represent the 36% of all the pelvic leak points treated by the author in women. The inguinal point (IP) is the superficial ring of the inguinal canal crossed by the mons veneris veins which connects to the uterine round ligament vein. The latter is a venous plexus running across the inguinal canal close to the round ligament, crossing the deep ring of the inguinal canal to reach the ovarian, fallopian and uterine plexuses. The IP is located just above and medially to common femoral vein (see Fig. 8.6).

Using a linear probe 7.5–12 MHz starting from the femoral junction, the IP is detectable tilting the probe upward focussing on the inguinal canal. The superficial ring of the inguinal canal is clearly detectable as an interruption of the oblique external muscle fascia. Once a skin marking has been done, it's easy to recognise with the tip of a finger the superficial ring of the inguinal canal laterally to the pubic tubercle (see Fig. 8.6).

The surgical procedure is possible with a little skin incision after an accurate mapping marking the I-Point on the skin (see Fig. 8.7). In case of incontinence of the terminal valve and added reflux from the ipsilateral IP, the skin marking considers both the escape points, and the skin incision can be done between both.

Dissection of the I-Point: Once the skin has been engraved and the surface layer of the subcutaneous tissue dissected, the subcutaneous fascia appears. This fascia should not be confused with the oblique internal muscular fascia, which is deeper, white and shiny. The finger-tip is helpful to search the superficial ring of the inguinal canal. Once the content coming out the superficial ring is detected (Fig. 8.8a), the genitocrural nerve must be distinguished from the vascular bundle (Fig. 8.8b). The nerve is isolated as well as the venous plexus of the round

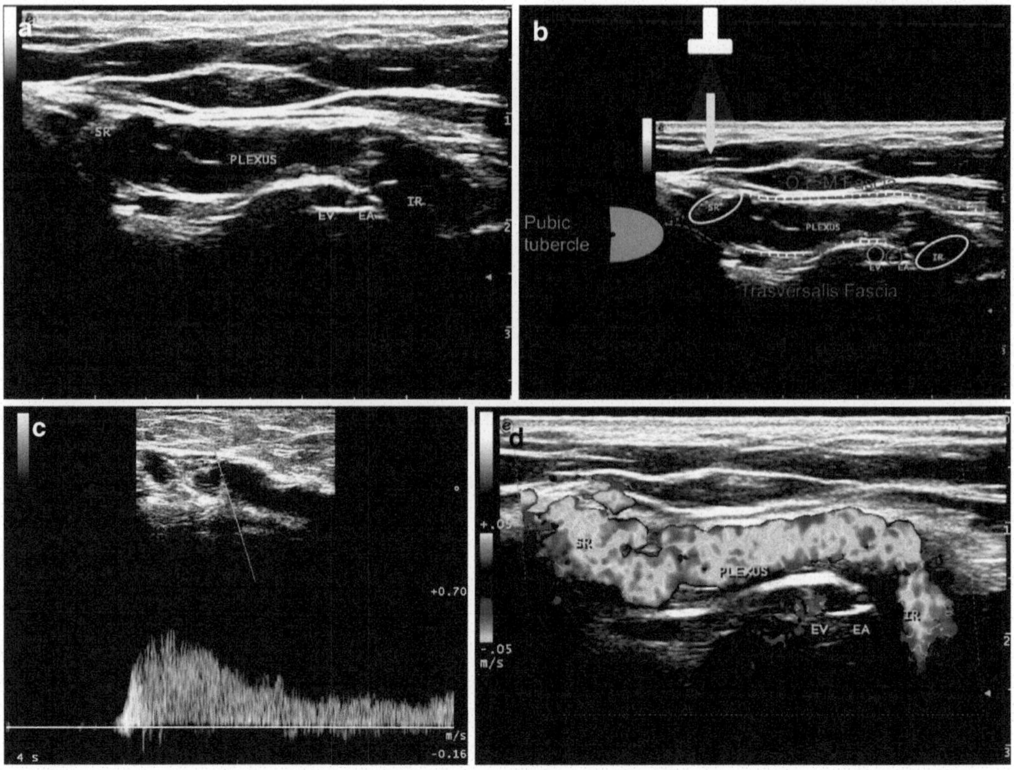

Fig. 8.6 (**a**) B-mode appearance of the left inguinal canal, the probe is transversely on the inguinal fold. The venous plexus of the round ligament has a hypo-echogenic appearance with hyper-echogenic lines inside (PLEXUS). The superficial ring (SR) and the internal ring (IR) of the canal are visible, as the inferior epigastric vein (EV) and epigastric artery (EA). Immediately above and below the round ligament, the hyper-echogenic lines corresponding to the oblique muscle fascia and the fascia transversalis are visible. Medially there is the un-echogenic image of the pubis. (**b**) Same image as (**a**) with schematic description of the anatomy with the probe position to mark the incision in the preoperative mapping (white inverted T with yellow arrow). Medially we find the tuberculum pubis (orange) and the superficial ring of the inguinal canal (yellow ring at the left, underneath the arrow). This is the inguinal point (IP), where the fascia of the oblique external muscle is discontinued and we no longer see it as a white line in the image, marked with OEM fascia in the image and red dotted line. The vein "plexus" runs between this fascia and the fascia transversals, the deeper white line (red dotted), and its lateral end is the yellow circle "IR" marking the internal ring of the inguinal canal. (**c**) Pulsed wave Doppler measuring in the venous plexus running through the inguinal canal, at the same site than images (**a**) and (**b**). Reflux demonstration during the Valsalva test. (**d**) Same image as (**a**) and (**b**) with colour-coded duplex under Valsalva manoeuvre. The flow emerges through the inner ring, runs medially through the inguinal canal and becomes superficial at the superficial ring

ligament, the latter surrounded with a silicone loop as to avoid injuries to the nerve. The venous plexus is cleaned and ligated with non-absorbable braided coated suture (Fig. 8.8c) before being severed (Fig. 8.8d). Then the stumps are sutured with a transfixed polypropylene stitch, the deeper folded up into the inguinal canal and sutured to oblique external muscle fascia (Fig. 8.8e) so that the proximal stump is not in front of the distal one. The polypropylene stitch prevents bleeding from the stump, whilst folding the proximal stump is useful to avoid recurrence due to neovessels going from one stump to the other. Proximal or

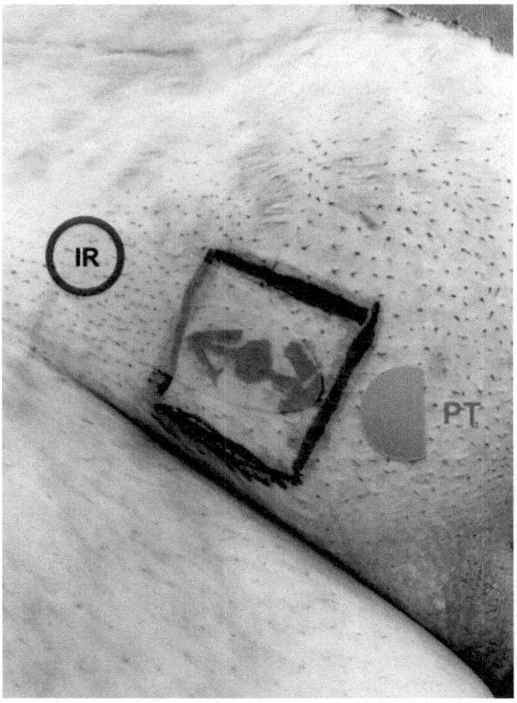

Fig. 8.7 Image of the right groin crease with preoperative mapping on the skin with the exact position of the superficial ring with a point; the arrows show the direction of the incision and of the inguinal canal. *IR* internal ring, *PT* pubic tubercle

distal ligation without ligation at the very IP level has shown to fail either immediately or after a time due to the large anastomoses in this region (see Fig. 8.1). Only once in the experience of the author, in an overweight patient, the oblique external muscle had to be opened to reach the venous plexus inside the inguinal canal. Usually this extension of the incision is not necessary so to reduce postoperative discomfort.

8.6 The Perineal Leak Point (PP)

The posterior perineal points (PPs) represented 61% of all the female PLPs treated by the author. The perineal point (PP) is the superficial perineal fascia hole crossed by the posterior labial vein. The draining order is as follows: the superficial perineal veins (epifascial) drain into the vulvar venous plexus and then into the perineal vein. The latter crosses the deep transverse perineal muscle to connect with the internal pudendal vein.

The PP, one for each side, is located posterolaterally to the labia majora about 1 cm anteriorly with respect to the origin of the frenulum labia minora (see Fig. 8.9). The perineal escape point can be responsible for ipsilateral or contralateral varicose veins. The diameter of the posterior labial vein crossing the vulvar facial hole ranges from 1.8 to 3 mm. Variations in the localisation of the perineal point are possible: the intermediate perineal point (IPP) is located about 1 cm anteriorly to the PP, but even a position in the middle between the anterior and posterior commissure is possible, as well as one single posterior labial vein (see Fig. 8.9). If more than one escape point is present, they can be treated through one incision, but only a very accurate preoperative marking can help to identify them. In ultrasound both perineal points can be represented in one image applying the transducer perpendicular to the labia (see Fig. 8.9a).

Surgical dissection of the P-Point: The patient is in gynaecological position. After preoperative marking of the point on the skin under ultrasound guidance, accurate preparation of the operative field with a clear sterile drape on the skin (see Fig. 8.10a). The surgical procedure starts with a little skin incision of 10 mm length (see Fig. 8.10b). Dissection of the collaterals joining into the posterior labial veins and ligation of the posterior labial vein with a 3 zero non-absorbable braided coated suture before being severed (see Fig. 8.10c). The labial vein is gently pulled and dissected to highlight the vulvar fascia hole (see Fig. 8.10d) and is then ligated at the vulvar fascia hole level (see Fig. 8.10e). The last mandatory surgical manoeuvre is the closure of the vulvar fascia hole with a six zero polypropylene stitch, so to definitively separate to different venous compartments: the subcutaneous and the vulva

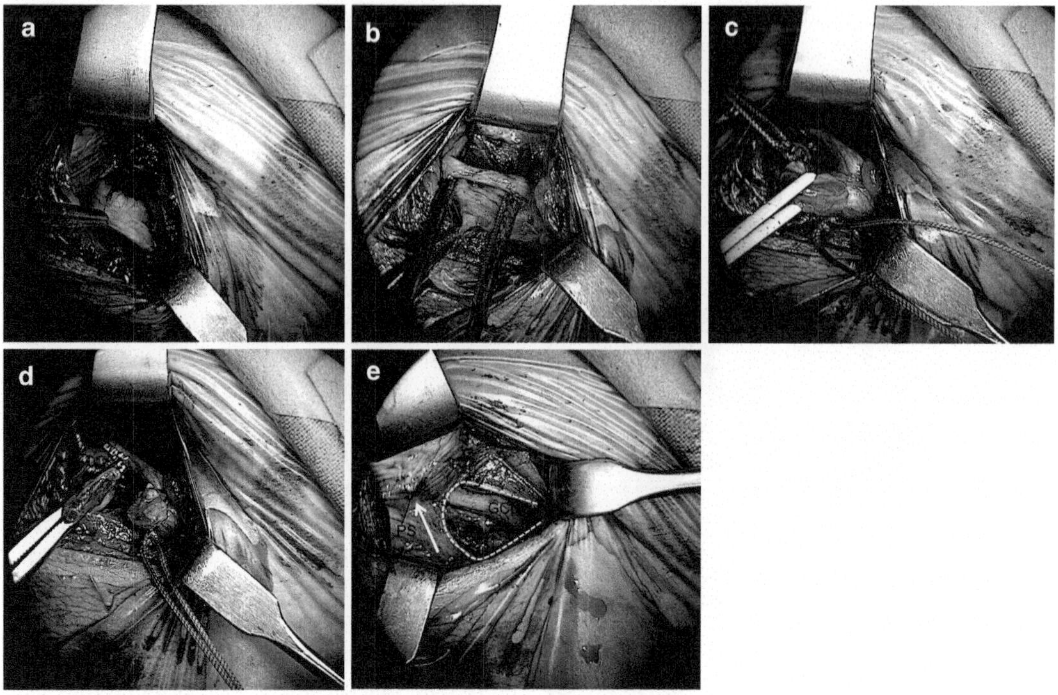

Fig. 8.8 (**a**) Deep down the oblique external muscle fascia, it can be detected as the round venous plexus together with the genitocrural nerve and connective tissue arising from the subcutaneous ring. (**b**) The genitocrural nerve has been isolated. (**c**) Ligation of the round ligament veins with non-absorbable braided overcoated suture. (**d**) The stump emerging the superficial ring is folded up and fixed to the fascia with a transfixing suture (PS, polypropylene stitch). The genitocrural nerve is visible in the upper part of the surgical field. (**e**) The surgical procedure is finished. The genitocrural nerve has been spared. The white line highlights the superficial ring of the inguinal canal without any visible vein. On the left, the transfixed polypropylene stitch fixing the proximal plexus stump is visible (arrow)

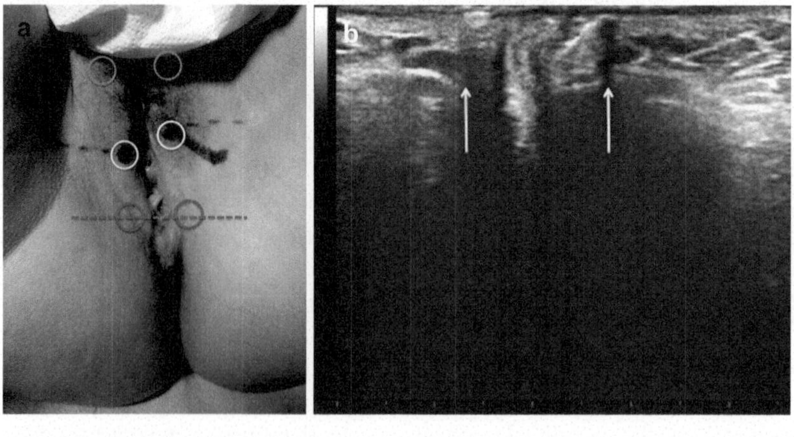

Fig. 8.9 (**a**) This image shows the position of the PP (red ring), the CP (blue ring) and the intermediate PP (white ring). The red dotted line shows the position of the transducer used to create the image shown in (**b**). (**b**) B-mode representation of the PP at both sides of the labia (see red dotted line in **a**). The white arrows show the fascia holes: P-Points

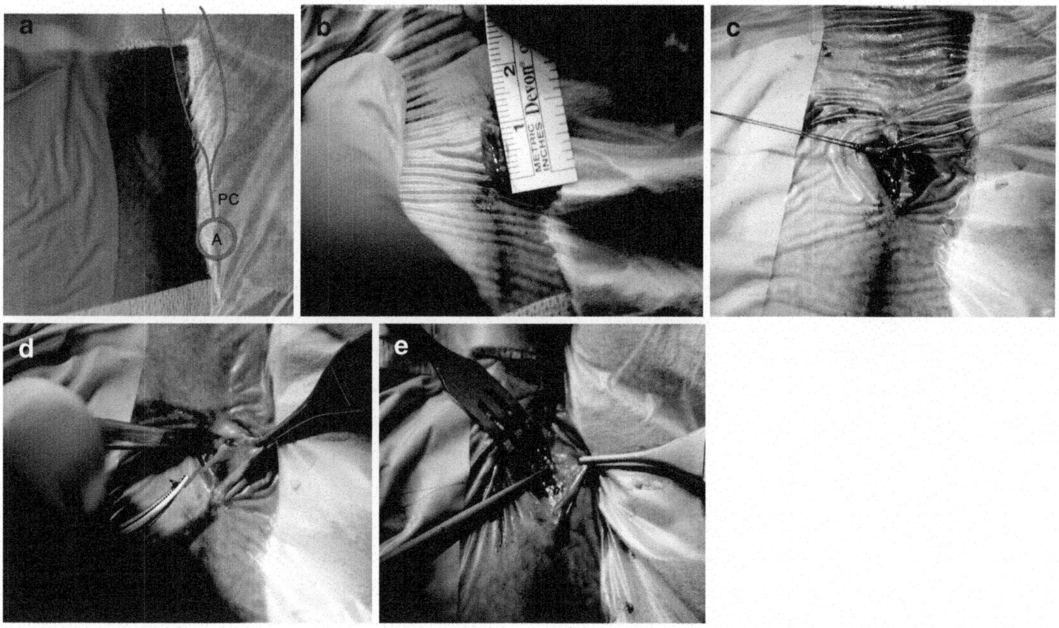

Fig. 8.10 (**a**) Appearance of the operative field. A clear sterile drape is on the skin. The black marker on the skin represents the PP. The horizontal and the longitudinal black lines are the skin markers drawn in the first step of the marking procedure. The red lines highlight the anatomical structure of the region, particularly the posterior commissure (PC) and anus (A). (**b**) 10 mm length skin incision and gentle dissection, paying attention to fine nervous branches of the pudendal nerve: minimally invasive surgery. (**c**) The posterior labial vein is ligated with a 3 zero non-absorbable braided coated suture before being cut. (**d**) Gentle posterior labial vein traction to highlight the vulvar fascia hole. (**e**) Ligation of the posterior labial vein at the vulva fascia hole level paying attention to avoid pudendal nervous branch ligation, and closure of the fascia hole with a six zero polypropylene stitch. The forceps thin tips at the suture level

plexuses. The operative field is washed with a rifampicin solution, the subcutaneous tissue sutured and the skin repaired with a cyanoacrylate surgical glue.

8.7 The Clitoridian Point (CP)

The clitoris is a complex structure attached to the mons pubis and labia and ventrally to the urethra and vagina. It's composed by an erectile body, composed of a pair of bulbs, and the glans that represents the most superficial part of it. The glans is a non-erectile structure well provided of nervous fibres, and for this reason, a surgical dissection at this level can be dangerous and should not be recommended. Alternatively, a sclerotherapy could be considered.

The venous path of the clitoris represents a connection between the deep venous system of the internal pudendal vein and the external pudendal vein, the former communicating with the hypogastric vein and the latter with the saphenous femoral junction. The veins of the external layers usually drain into the great saphenous veins, whilst the venous flow of the body and glans normally runs into the internal pudendal vein. There is an extensive venous communication between the clitoris veins and the subcutaneous mons veneris venous path.

The clitoris leak point (CP) (see Figs. 8.1b and 8.9a) is the anastomotic plexus between the bulbar vein and the superficial dorsal clitoris vein through which the flow reaches the external pudendal vein and runs into the great saphenous vein (see Fig. 8.11).

8.8 Male Pelvic Leak Points

Pelvic escape points can also be detected in men. These are the inguinal point (male IP), which is different from a female inguinal point, and a second point located medially from the root of the penis called the C-Point (male CP), sharing the same name as that used for females in the analogous position. These escape points may be the cause of ipsilateral as well as contralateral varicose veins and are generally the consequence of the increased venous pressure in the pampiniform plexus in case of varicocele.

8.8.1 Male Inguinal Point (IP)

The veins of the superficial and deep penile venous plexuses surrounding the urethra and penis connect the right and left pampiniform plexuses and so do the scrotal veins [2]. The pampiniform plexus consists of an anterior and a posterior group of veins, with the deferent duct between them. The anterior group, surrounding the spermatic artery in the inguinal canal, drains into the renal vein on the left and the inferior cava vein on the right side. The posterior group of veins drains the epididymis head and body, mainly into the epigastric inferior vein, and is detectable with the echo-duplex scan in the terminal third of the spermatic cord in the subcutaneous tissue which goes through the subcutaneous fascia, joining the saphenous femoral junction.

Through these veins, a reflux coming from the spermatic veins can be transmitted to the saphenofemoral junction. In other cases, a collector running from the medial segment of the pampiniform plexus and going through the subcutaneous fascia runs into collaterals of the anterior or great saphenous vein, bypassing the saphenous femoral junction.

The subcutaneous fascia hole is considered the male I-Point and is always detectable medially and above the sapheno-femoral junction and valve, near the pubis in the inguinal region (see Fig. 8.12).

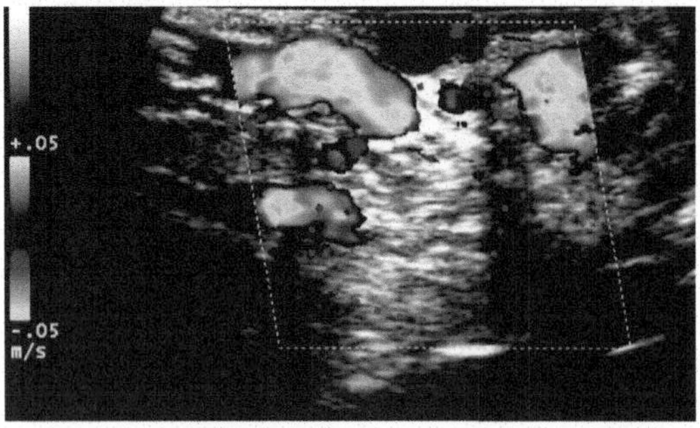

Fig. 8.11 The clitoris is the hyper-echogenic and irregular image in the centre (dashed blue line). CP reflux during the Valsalva manoeuvre

8.8.2 Male "C" Point

The scrotum is composed of different layers: the skin, the subcutaneous tissue, the dartos and a thin layer of subcutaneous tissue with vessels immediately below the dartos. The dartos of both

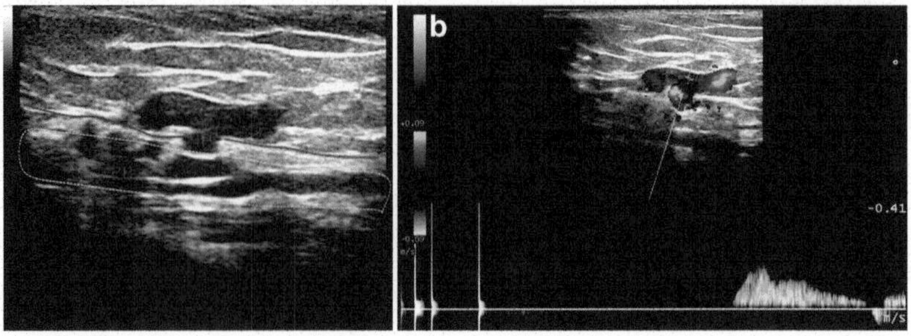

Fig. 8.12 (**a**) B-mode in cross section above the saphenofemoral junction. The red line highlights the subcutaneous fascia. The fascia hole crossed by the venous collector (IP) and the pampiniform plexus (PP) below the subcutaneous fascia can be clearly seen. (**b**) Reflux from the pampiniform plexus through the IP to a tributary, which will feed the GSV

sides merges in the middle into the scrotal septum: the lower part of the scrotal septum joins the vaginal tunic in the scrotal ligament. Scrotal veins form a single venous path communicating with the subcutaneous veins of the lower part of the abdominal wall, the perineal region, the penis and the venous plexus draining the didymus and the epididymis. Thanks to the veins crossing through the scrotal septum, communication between the paths of the two scrotal veins is possible. The venous flow of the scrotal veins normally runs into the pudendal external vein to reach the great saphenous vein but can also drain directly into the femoral vein. The veins of the posterior part of the scrotum drain into the internal pudendal vein, and through it the flow reaches the hypogastric vein. For these anatomical reasons, a venous reflux even in males can be transmitted from one side to the other. Therefore, a reflux from the spermatic plexus of one side can create ipsilateral as well as contralateral varicose veins of the lower limbs.

In the penis, there is a superficial network and a deep venous network. The subcutaneous penile venous path drains mainly the skin and the subcutaneous tissue, and the flow normally runs into the subcutaneous dorsal veins of the penis. This vein drains into the subcutaneous plexus of the inferior part of the abdominal wall, and then the flow runs into the saphenous femoral junction. The veins of the inferior part of the superficial layer of the penis drain into the scrotal veins. The deep venous penis network drains the glans, the two corpora cavernosa and the corpus spongiosum. The flow of the deep path runs into the deep dorsal vein, normally valvulated, and through it to the pudendal vein, which represents one of the origins of the hypogastric vein. The superficial and deep paths widely communicate first through the glans and the foreskin veins and second through the veins located at the symphysis pubis level.

Furthermore, venous collectors run into the subcutaneous tissue, crossing a well-defined hole of the subcutaneous fascia, coming from the deep venous network of the penis. Through these collectors, a reflux from the deep penile venous path can be transmitted in the subcutaneous tissue of the pubic region. If there is a reflux through this fascia hole, it represents a further pelvic male leak point like the female CP: the male C-Point. It can be easily detected with a duplex scan next to the root of the penis, and minimally invasive surgical treatment is possible under local anaesthesia, thanks to a refined B-mode preoperative marking.

8.9 Obturator Leak Point

The obturator vein drains the muscles of the upper-medial segment of the thighs. Anterior and posterior muscular collectors run together into the main obturator vein trunk. The obturator vein passes through the obturator canal and runs into the hypogastric vein. The existence of anastomoses with the epigastric inferior veins and the pudendal external vein is well known [3, 6, 7, 9]. An anterior muscular circumflex collector is sometimes detectable. It runs below the muscular pectineus fascia lying on the pectineus muscle and normally drains medially into the common femoral vein at the sapheno-femoral junction level: either into the common femoral vein itself or into the junction—centrally to the terminal valve or between the terminal and preterminal valve. The confluence of this collector into the saphenous femoral junction is the so-called obturator point (see Fig. 8.13).

It represents an important anastomotic venous path between the common femoral vein and the hypogastric vein as well as the pudendal external vein. This muscular venous collector is quite distinguishable from the external pudendal vein; in fact, the latter runs superficially whilst the first is located below a muscular fascia (see Fig. 8.14).

In case of pelvic reflux and anastomosis with the obturatorian vein, this path can just drain into the common femoral vein independently of the superficial venous system, or it ends in the sapheno-femoral junction (see Fig. 8.13). This pathway is possible in male and female population.

Depending on the competence of the terminal and preterminal valve, the blood from the obturatorian vein leak could just feed the common

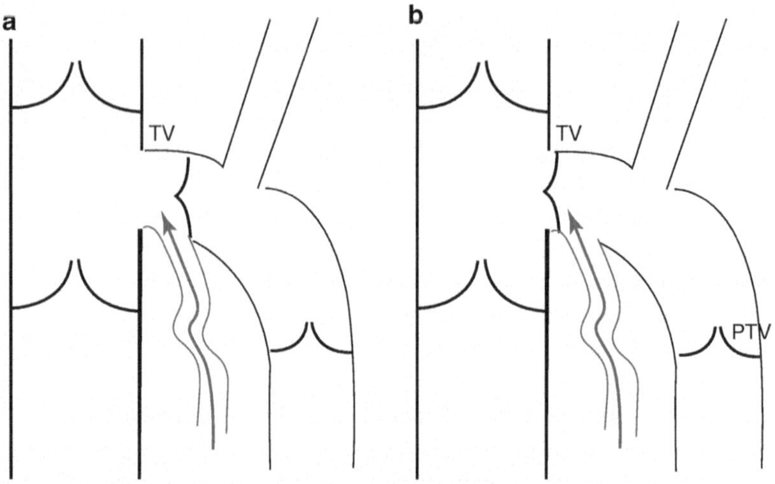

Fig. 8.13 (**a**) The circumflex muscular medial collector (red) drains into the sapheno-femoral confluence from medially, between the common femoral vein and the terminal valve (TV) of the great saphenous vein. (**b**) The circumflex muscular medial collector (red) drains into the saphenous vein arch, between the terminal (TV) and preterminal valve (PTV)

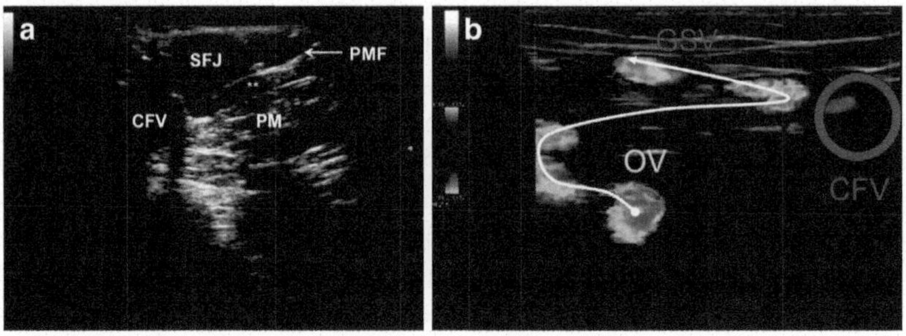

Fig. 8.14 (**a**) Cross section of the left groin region in B-mode: image of a circumflex muscular medial collector (**). It represents an anterior origin of the obturator vein. The collector runs below the pectineus muscular fascia (PMF), on the pectineus muscle (PM), and reaches the sapheno-femoral junction draining on the saphenous side of the terminal valve. (**b**) Valsalva manoeuvre. Reflux from the circumflex medial collector into the SFJ

femoral vein via the circumflex muscular medial collector or be the leakage point for a venous insufficiency in the leg.

The anterior muscular circumflex collector can be ligated if necessary opening the pectineus muscle fascia, under B-mode preoperative marking or even intraoperative control without any saphenous femoral junction dissection. In addition, different strategies are possible: OP ligation during saphenous femoral disconnection for an associated terminal valve incompetence or simple saphenous high ligation immediately below the superior collaterals of the junction. Endovenous laser treatment is a further possible therapeutic technique as encoded by the CHIVA laser strategy.

8.10 Gluteal Leak Points

Gluteal leak points are seldom found in relation to varicose veins of lower limbs.

The inferior gluteal vein (sciatic vein) is a large valvulated parietal collector that represents one of the origins of hypogastric vein. One of the main collateral branches of the inferior gluteal vein is the sciatic vein running together with the sciatic nerve, and thanks to collaterals it is connected to the superior gluteal vein and to the common femoral vein through the femoral circumflex medial vein, the terminal segment of the deep femoral vein representing an important venous bypass path in case of iliac obstruction or stenosis. Two different escape points can be detected: the inferior gluteal point (IGP) and the superior gluteal point (SGP) (see Fig. 8.1c). Anatomically the inferior one is located below the lower margin of the piriformis muscle exactly at the ileotrochanteric line level, whilst the superior gluteal point (SGP) is located at the superior margin of the piriformis muscle. The sciatic vein can be found immediately below the margin of the piriformis muscle with the colour-coded duplex ultrasound, checking low-speed flow about 12 cm/s. The sciatic vein is also detectable posteriorly at the thigh by focussing the hyper-echogenic image of the sciatic nerve and checking the flow during the Valsalva manoeuvre in veins surrounding the nerve. From here the vein might be followed cranially to find the origin in the superior or inferior leak point and distally to find the drainage path.

The author has never treated a gluteal escape point with surgery. To access the leak point, a big surgical procedure would be necessary. So, peripheral disconnections could be one option to treat them, or ultrasound-guided sclerotherapy could be another therapeutic option, though it requires a very experienced operator, considering that veins lie close to the sciatic nerve.

Literature

1. Franceschi C, Bahnini A. Points de fuite pelviens viscéraux et varices des membres inférieurs. Phlébologie. 2004;57:37–42.
2. Franceschi C, Bahnini A. Treatment of lower extremity venous insufficiency due to pelvic leak points in women. Ann Vasc Surg. 2005;19:284–8.
3. Franceschi C. Anatomie fonctionnelle et diagnostic des points de fuite bulboclitoridiens chez la femme (point C). J Mal Vasc. 2008;33:42.
4. Pernkopf. Atlas of topographical and applied human anatomy. 1964. Vol. II, p. 222–3.
5. Lockhart LD, Hamilton GF. Fyfe Fv. Italian edition. Azzali G., Casa Editrice Ambriosana; 1973. p. 674.
6. Chiarugi G, Bucciante L. Istituzioni di anatomia dell'uomo. 11th ed. In: Vallardi F, editor. 1975. Vol. 2, p. 675–93. Vol. 3, p. 729–36.
7. Rouviere H. Anatomie humaine Masson édit. 1959. Vol. II, p. 731–2, 737–8.
8. Lechter A, Lopez G, Martinez C, Camacho J. Anatomy of the gonadal veins: a reappraisal. Surgery. 1991;109:735–9.
9. Lepage PA, Villavicencio JL, Gomez RE, Sheridan MN, Rich NM. The valvular anatomy of the iliac venous system ands its clinical implications. JVS. 1991;14(5):678–83.
10. Dixon JA, Mitchell WA. Venographic and surgical observations in vulvar varicose veins. Surg Gynecol Obstet. 1979;131:458–64.
11. Franceschi C, et al. CHIVA: hemodynamic concept, strategy and results. Int Angiol. 2016;35(1):8–30.
12. Franceschi C. Theorie et practique de la Cure Conservatrice et Hemodynamique de l'Insuffisance Veineuse en Ambulatoire. Precy-sous-Thil, France: Edition de l'Armançon; 1988.
13. Franceschi C, Zamboni P. Principles of venous haemodynamics. New York: Nova Science Publishers; 2010.
14. Delfrate R. Manuale di emodinamica venosa degli arti inferiori. Fantigrafica; 2010. ISBN 9788890496837.
15. Delfrate R. A new diagnostic approach to varicose veins: haemodynamic evaluation and treatment. Lorenadioni Publisher; 2014.
16. Delfrate R. Nuovo approccio diagnostic alle vene varicose. In: Dioni L, editor. 2014. p. 64.
17. Delfrate R, Bricchi M, Franceschi C, Goldoni M. Multiple ligation of the proximal greater saphenous vein in the CHIVA treatment of primary varicose veins. Veins Lymphat. 2014;3:19–21.
18. Paraskevas N, Ayari R, Malikov S. 'Pole test' measurements in critical leg ischaemia. Eur J Vasc Endovasc Surg. 2006;31:253–7.
19. Pahlsson HI, Wahlberg E, Olofsson P, Swedenborg J. The toe pole test for evaluation of arterial insufficiency in diabetic patients. Eur J Vasc Endovasc Surg. 1999;18:133–7.
20. Lopez AJ. Female pelvic vein embolization: indications, techniques and outcomes. Cardiovasc Intervent Radiol. 2015;38:806–20.

9 Haemodynamic Management of Deep Venous Insufficiency

Sergio Gianesini, Erika Mendoza, and Paolo Zamboni

9.1 Introduction

Femoral vein (FV) duplication is a higher prevalent anatomical variant than what generally thought [1, 2]. In primary and post-thrombotic reflux patterns, the duplication feeds a closed circuit with one incompetent vessel constituting the leaking point and with the other conduit representing the antegrade draining route. The described pattern offers the opportunity of suppressing the deep venous reflux by means of a surgical closure of the leaking point, using haemodynamic principles to restore a physiological venous drainage.

S. Gianesini, M.D., Ph.D.
Vascular Diseases Center, University of Ferrara, Ferrara, Italy

USUHS University, Bethesda, MD, USA

E. Mendoza, M.D., Ph.D.
Venenpraxis, Wunstorf, Germany
e-mail: erika.mendoza@t-online.de

P. Zamboni, M.D. (✉)
School of Vascular Surgery and Vascular Diseases Center, University of Ferrara, Ferrara, Italy

Unit of Translational Surgery, AOU Ferrara, Ferrara, Italy
e-mail: zmp@unife.it

9.2 Applied Deep Venous Anatomy

Lower limb deep venous anatomy plays a major role in venous return, thanks to the interaction with the muscle masses creating the so-called calf venous pump [3]. Indeed, while the venous return in a supine position is mainly triggered by the pressure gradient created by the cardiac pump and by the thoraco-abdominal aspiration, in the standing position, the venous drainage counteracts the force of gravity by activating the lower limb muscle, thus squeezing the veins and propelling the blood.

It is interesting to notice that four-legged animals do not possess a calf pump mechanism: an evidence of the role of the gravitational force and of the synergistic action of lower limb veins and muscles. The interconnection among the deep and the superficial venous system is functionally separated by the two fascial layers: the deep and superficial fascia. While the first is a strong membrane with little elasticity, the latter is softer and provides less support to the saphenous system which lies in between the same two fascial structures (see Sect. 2.2).

The deep venous system below the knee is constituted by the anterior and posterior tibial veins, the peroneal and popliteal veins (see Fig. 2.1) [4]. The anterior tibial vein is the continuation of the venae concomitantes of the dorsalis pedis artery, and it drains the anterior part of the lower limb. It

P. Zamboni et al. (eds.), *Saphenous Vein-Sparing Strategies in Chronic Venous Disease*,
https://doi.org/10.1007/978-3-319-70638-2_9

runs just above the interosseous membrane between the tibia and the fibula.

The posterior tibial vein generates at the confluence of the medial and lateral plantar veins below the medial malleolus, and it drains the posterior lower part of the leg together with the plantar surface of the foot. This vein runs behind the tibia and joins the popliteal vein at the posterior knee.

The peroneal vein drains the lateral part of the lower leg while ascending along the posteromedial side of the fibula and joins the posterior tibial vein in the upper third of the lower leg. The anterior and posterior tibial veins unite together forming the tibio-peroneal trunk which then generates the popliteal vein at the lower aspect of the posterior knee.

The popliteal vein than ascends along the anteromedial part of the thigh, medial to the artery in the lower knee, superficial to the artery at the posterior knee and lateral to it above the knee. At the adductor hiatus, the popliteal vein becomes the femoral vein. The term superficial femoral vein is no longer in use considering the potential misunderstanding as the vein is deep [5].

In the lower part, the femoral vein is lateral to the artery, in the middle third behind and in the upper portion medially. The deep femoral vein joins the femoral vein running along the deep femoral artery, so forming the common femoral vein which is located medially to the common femoral artery. Once the common femoral vein has passed underneath the inguinal ligament, it becomes the external iliac vein.

From a structural point of view, the deep veins are thin walled and have little smooth muscle. They are present also as sinuses collecting significant amount of blood volume, such as in the soleal (draining into the posterior tibial vein) and gastrocnemius (draining into the popliteal vein) muscles. Deep veins are subfascial and are imbedded inside the muscle masses, and they play a fundamental role in venous return, particularly during standing.

Indeed, the cardiac and thoraco-abdominal pumps are insufficient in the generation of the pressure gradient that drives the venous blood back to the heart against the force of gravity. Together with the valvular apparatus and the muscle masses, the deep veins constitute the so-called peripheral heart: a main actor in venous drainage regulation. Like in the heart, the venous blood is collected in the deep venous network and then propelled by the muscles through a valvular apparatus towards against the force of gravity.

The deep veins receive the full transmission of the energy generated by the systolic contraction thanks to their anatomical location just inside the muscle masses. Thanks to the valvular apparatus the blood is propelled in one direction.

The most superficial network is solicited by a smaller pressure gradient because of its localization above the muscular fascia. Subsequently, an energy gradient differential is generated between the deep and superficial system, so favouring the drainage from the most superficial towards the deepest compartment, from the distal to the proximal parts. In case of valvular failure, a deep venous reflux can originate, presenting different possible networks of pathological drainage.

9.3 Rationale for the Haemodynamic Management and Clinical Scenario

Literature is clearly showing how descriptive anatomy must take into consideration the extremely frequent variations in the course and number of lower limb veins [6]. In particular, duplication of deep veins has been found in 42% of popliteal veins and in 31% of femoral veins (see Fig. 9.1).

The duplicated vessel has been called accessory femoral vein. It was found to be medial to the femoral vein in 46% of cases while lateral in 49% of patients. The remaining 5% of cases were triplications. The average length of the duplicated femoral vein was reported to be in between 6 and 15 cm. No correlation among gender, age and duplication was found, while the presence of a duplication on one leg was strongly associated with the presence of a duplication in the contralateral limb [7].

The same vessel duplication predisposes a network potentially developing a reflux through a closed circuit (Fig. 9.2).

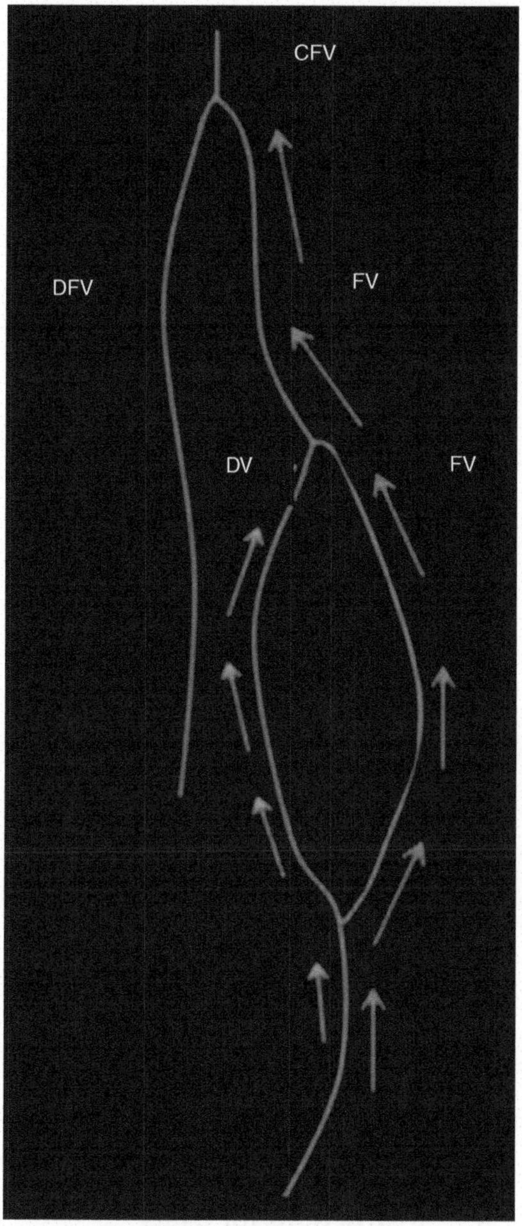

Fig. 9.1 Duplication (DV) of the femoral vein (FV). *DFV* deep femoral vein, *CFV* common femoral vein (With permission from [8])

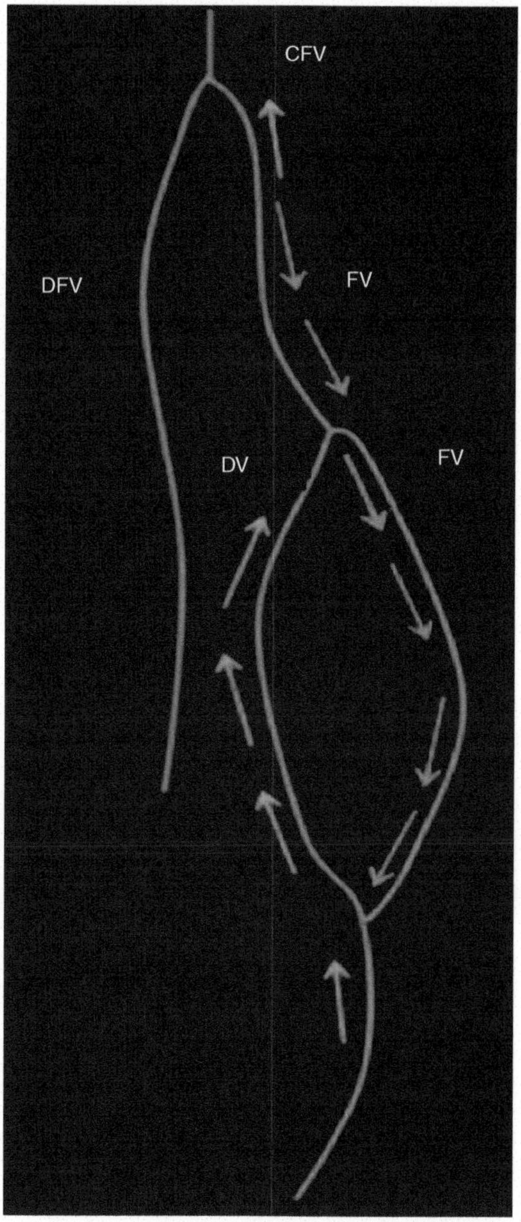

Fig. 9.2 Closed refluxing network generated by the incompetence at the confluence among the femoral vein (FV) and its duplication (DV). *CFV* common femoral vein, *DFV* deep femoral vein (With permission from [8])

As previously described in Sect. 3.7.1, dedicated to the superficial system, a reflux generated inside a closed circuit (closed shunt) can be suppressed by adequately changing the pressure gradient through a selective ligation of the leaking point.

In the case described in Fig. 9.2, for example, a simple titanium clip apposition at the confluence among the femoral vein and its duplication can restore the venous drainage by creating a favourable pressure gradient, thanks to the suppression of the leaking point (Fig. 9.3).

Published data show the feasibility and effectiveness of the technique [8].

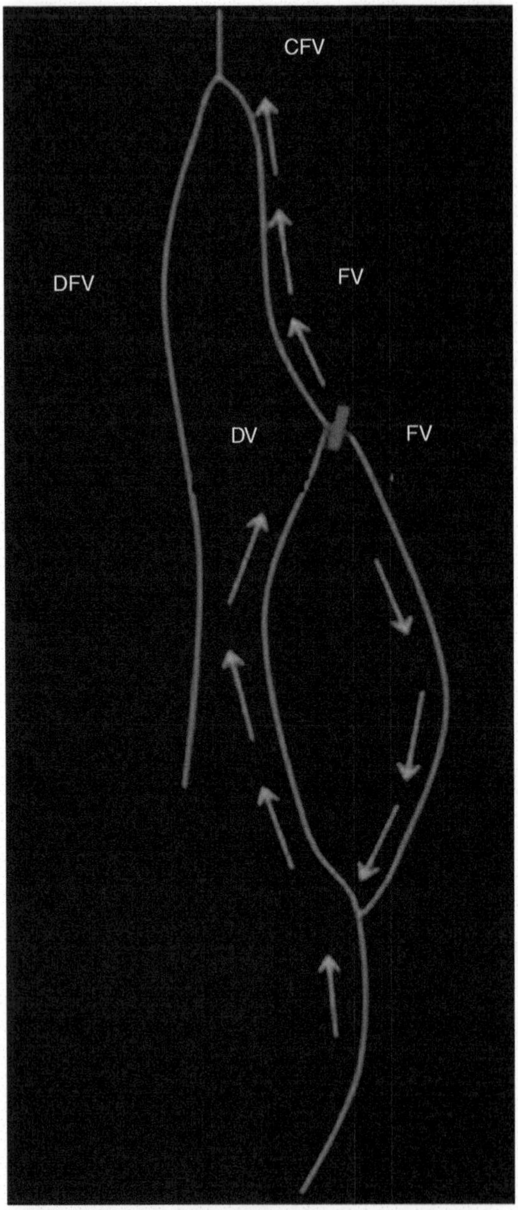

Fig. 9.3 Suppression of the leaking point by titanium clip apposition (red line). Breaking the close circuit established by the femoral vein (FV) duplication (DV) leads to the reflux suppression. *DFV* deep femoral vein, *CFV* common femoral vein (With permission from [8])

As initially postulated back in the early twentieth century by Linton and Bauer, femoral ligation seems to be not only safe but even effective in deep venous reflux control [9].

The frequent presence of deep venous duplication creates an anatomical premise for suppressing refluxes that are originated by closed circuits while maintaining the upward flow in the competent segment. Lower limbs' deep venous system constitutes one of the most fascinating but challenging topic in the vascular disease field.

Despite the high frequency of venous reflux occurrence, the related pathophysiology is still lacking of a clear interpretation [10–14].

Nowadays, therapeutic options such as valvuloplasty, transpositions and translocations are utilized in a limited number of cases and just in highly specialized centres [15, 16].

The feasibility and performance of a haemodynamic approach to deep venous insufficiency allow a potential widening of the indication to treatment, thanks to both the venous duplication frequency and the surgical easy feasibility. As it was demonstrated in case of haemodynamic restoration in the superficial venous insufficiency, the suppression of the leaking point of a closed refluxing circuit reduces the ambulatory venous pressure and improves the plethysmographic parameters [17].

The same haemodynamic improvement follows also in the deep venous system. An active muscle pump action is required to generate the post-operative retrograde draining flow. For this reason, this haemodynamic procedure is suggested just in the case of not bedridden patients, who have previously failed conservative measure and with a severe deep reflux affecting the possible ulcer healing.

9.4 Instructions for Users

9.4.1 Preoperative Diagnostics

The ultrasound assessment in colour identifies a deep venous reflux along a duplicated vein, with the leaking point at the vessels bifurcation (Fig. 9.4).

A magnetic resonance venography (MRV) protocol can be customized in order to detect the

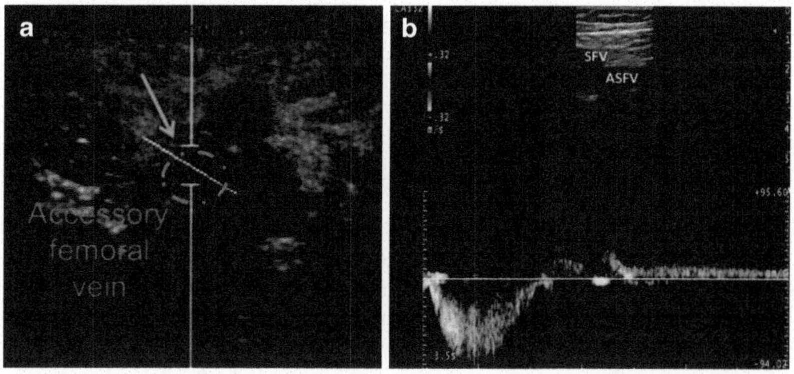

Fig. 9.4 (**a**) Duplicated femoral vein (orange dotted line, accessory femoral vein) at the confluence with the femoral vein. (**b**) Reflux documentation with the ultrasound in PW mode (With permission from [8])

slow flow of the deep venous system, providing further evidence of this anatomical bifurcation.

9.4.2 Surgical Technique

The patient lies supine with a leg flexed at the knee and in abduction (frog-legged), in order to facilitate the access to the medial side of the thigh.

Under local anaesthesia and after an accurate preoperative echo-guided mapping, a longitudinal incision is performed along the medial aspect of the upper thigh over the anterior border of the sartorius muscle, and dissection between sartorius and the medial edge of the vastus medialis muscle is performed to expose the femoral vein, the duplicated (accessory femoral) vein and the femoral artery. The vessels are isolated and controlled, mobilizing the femoral artery additionally in order to get a better exposure of the femoral venous bifurcation. A titanium clip (large size) is flush applied at the confluence among the femoral vein and its duplication (Fig. 9.5).

The dissection layers are closed by running 3–0 absorbable sutures, while the skin by a subcuticular 4–0 absorbable monofilament.

Neither antibiotics nor LMWH prophylaxis is considered mandatory. Only in post-thrombotic cases an anticoagulation therapy is suggested because of increased deep venous thrombosis risk.

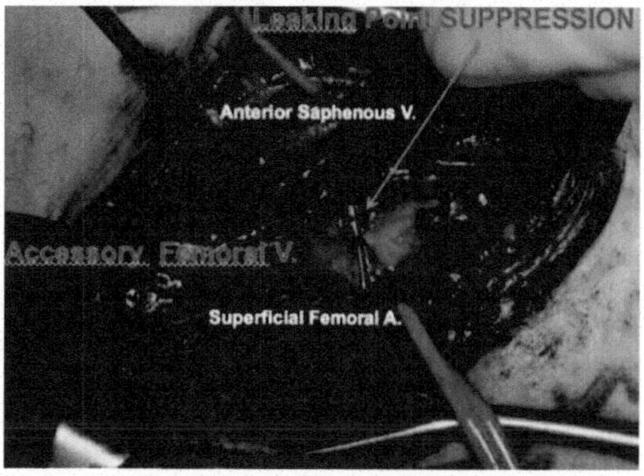

Fig. 9.5 Titanium clip application at the duplicated femoral vein confluence with the femoral vein

9.5 Haemodynamic Management of Deep Venous Insufficiency at the Calf

The same rationale as described in Fig. 9.3 can be applied to a selective reflux situation at the calf. The most often observed situations are:

- Refluxing muscle veins with connection to the distal small saphenous vein. The treatment is to interrupt the muscle vein at its junction with the popliteal vein in the popliteal fossa (see Fig. 9.6a).
- Refluxing posterior tibial vein with connection to the distal great saphenous vein. The

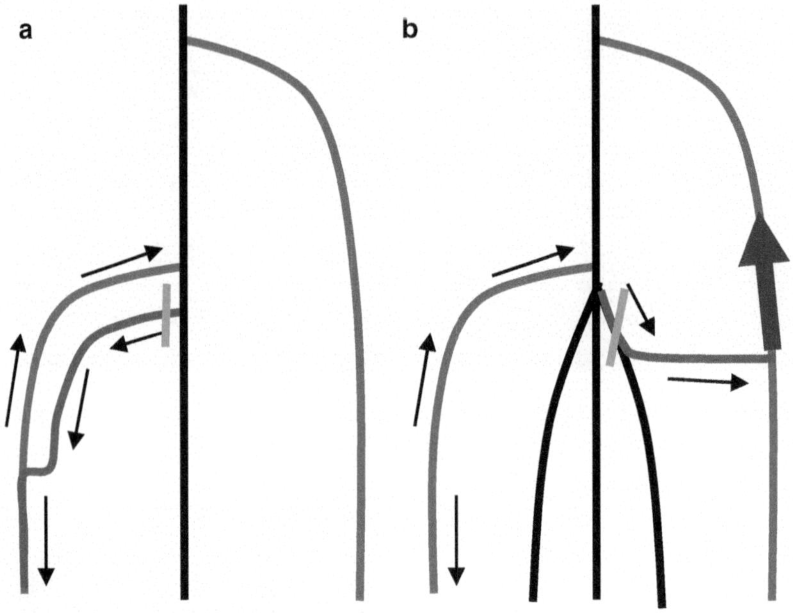

Fig. 9.6 (**a**) Reflux via a muscle vein, joining the distal small saphenous vein (compare Fig. 4.31). The treatment is to interrupt the refluxing muscle vein (red) at its junction with the popliteal vein in the popliteal fossa (green line). (**b**) Reflux in the posterior tibial vein, filling the great saphenous vein via a paratibial perforator (Boyd). The deep reflux is drained via an antegrade but overloaded GSV (violet arrow) (compare Fig. 4.34). The treatment is to interrupt the posterior tibial vein at the junction with the popliteal vein

treatment is to interrupt the posterior tibial vein at its junction with the popliteal vein in the popliteal fossa (see Fig. 9.6b).

The surgical access in both cases is the same as to perform an interruption of the sapheno-popliteal junction. In the hands of an experienced surgeon, the intervention is safe.

Literature

1. Casella IB, Presti C, Yamazaki Y, Vassoler AA, Furuya LA, Sabbag CD. A duplex scan-based morphologic study of the femoral vein: incidence and patterns of duplication. Vasc Med. 2010;15:197–203.
2. Dona E, Fletcher JP, Hughes TM, Saker K, Batiste P, Ramanathan I. Duplicated popliteal and superficial femoral veins: incidence and potential significance. Aust N Z J Surg. 2000;70:438–40.
3. Goldman MP. Anatomy and pathophysiology of varicose veins. J Dermatol Surg Oncol. 1989;15:138–45.
4. Meissner M. Lower extremity venous anatomy. Semin Intervent Radiol. 2005;22(3):147–56.
5. Caggiati A, Bergan JJ, Gloviczki P, Eklof B, Allegra C, Partsch H, et al. Nomenclature of the veins of the lower limb: extensions, refinements, and clinical application. J Vasc Surg. 2005;41:719–24.
6. Park EA, Chung JW, Lee W, Yin YH, Ha J, Kim SJ, Park JH. Three-dimensional evaluation of the anatomic variations of the femoral vein and popliteal vein in relation to the accompanying artery by using CT venography. Korean J Radiol. 2011;12(3):327–40. https://doi.org/10.3348/kjr.2011.12.3.327. Epub 2011 Apr 25
7. Quinlan DJ, Alikhan R, Gishen P, Sidhu PS. Variations in lower limb venous anatomy: implications for US diagnosis of deep vein thrombosis. Radiology. 2003;228(2):443–8. Epub 2003 Jun 23
8. Zamboni P, Gianesini S. Surgical technique for deep venous reflux suppression in femoral vein duplication. EJVES Short Rep. 2016;30:10–12.
9. Glasser ST. Ligation of the femoral vein for chronic occlusive arterial disease. A review of one hundred and eighteen ligations. Arch Surg. 1945;50:56–62.
10. Labropoulos N, Tassiopoulos AK, Kang SS, Mansour MA, Littooy FN, Baker WH. Prevalence of deep venous reflux in patients with primary superficial vein incompetence. J Vasc Surg. 2000;32:663–8.
11. Robertson LA, Evans CJ, Lee AJ, Allan PL, Ruckley CV, Fowkes FG. Incidence and risk factors for venous

reflux in the general population: Edinburgh vein study. Eur J Vasc Endovasc Surg. 2014;48:208–14.
12. Meissner MH, Manzo RA, Bergelin RO, Markel A, Strandness DE Jr. Deep venous insufficiency: the relationship between lysis and subsequent reflux. J Vasc Surg. 1993;18:596–605.
13. Meissner MH, Moneta G, Burnand K, Gloviczki P, Lohr JM, Lurie F, et al. The hemodynamics and diagnosis of venous disease. J Vasc Surg. 2007;46 Suppl S:4S–24S.
14. Meissner MH. Pathophysiology of varicose veins and chronic venous insufficiency. In: Comprehensive vascular and endovascular surgery. Edinburgh: Mosby; 2009. p. 729–48.
15. Lurie F, Kistner R, Perrin M, Raju S, Neglen P, Maleti O. Invasive treatment of deep venous disease. A UIP consensus. Int Angiol. 2010;29(3):199–204.
16. Goel RR, Abidia A, Hardy SC. Surgery for deep venous incompetence. Cochrane Database Syst Rev. 2015;2:CD001097.
17. Zamboni P. Reflux elimination without any ablation or disconnection of the saphenous vein: a hemodynamic model for venous surgery. Eur J Vasc Endovasc Surg. 2001;21(4):361–9.

CHIVA: Results from Literature

10

Erika Mendoza and Erica Menegatti

10.1 First Non-randomized Series

10.1.1 Four-Year Follow-Up of CHIVA Patients [1]

Three hundred and fifty-seven patients were operated using CHIVA and monitored for 4 years. They were not compared with another group. In 94% of the patients, by the end of the study, the GSV was perfused throughout its whole length (i.e. not closed by superficial vein thrombosis). Eleven percent of the patients suffered recurrence of their varicose veins. Light reflection rheography showed significant improvements immediately after the operation and after 6 months in comparison with preoperative values.

10.1.2 Comparison Between Stripping and CHIVA [2, 3, 4]

Cappelli et al. investigated 148 patients treated by CHIVA with mean follow-up of 3 years. Then they compared their own results with the three great stripping series from the literature [5–7].

E. Mendoza, M.D., Ph.D.
Venenpraxis, Wunstorf, Germany
e-mail: erika.mendoza@t-online.de

E. Menegatti, Ph.D. (✉)
Vascular Diseases Center, University of Ferrara, Ferrara, Italy
e-mail: mngrce@unife.it

The evaluation criteria were chosen on the basis of three published stripping series (the "Hobbs criteria") so that the groups would be comparable. The Hobbs criteria were established in 1974 as follows: the different clinical parameters must be evaluated by the patient or by the investigator in three groups—excellent, better and the same or worse [5] (Table 10.1).

Maeso et al. monitored 90 CHIVA patients prospectively for 3 years after CHIVA and compared them with 85 of his own historical stripping patients, with patients from the literature (see above) and with Cappelli's patients. In the Vall d'Hebron University Clinic in Barcelona, stripping was abandoned completely in favour of

Table 10.1 Hobbs classification

Objective evaluation		Points
Class 1	No visible or palpable varicose veins	1
Class 2	Little number of visible and palpable veins with diameter less than 5 mm	2
Class 3	Residual or new veins with diameter over 5 mm	3
Class 4	Incompetent saphenous veins or perforators	4
Subjective evaluation		
Class 1	No complaints	1
Class 2	Little functional or cosmetic complaints but clear improvement	2
Class 3	Improvement but still functional and cosmetic complaints	3
Class 4	Disease without changes or worse	4

P. Zamboni et al. (eds.), *Saphenous Vein-Sparing Strategies in Chronic Venous Disease*,
https://doi.org/10.1007/978-3-319-70638-2_10

the CHIVA method in 1995, so no prospective comparison of the two methods was possible.

In both groups, CHIVA produced significantly better outcomes than in the three stripping groups from the literature ($p < 0.001$).

The comparison between the two CHIVA groups—Cappelli and Maeso—produced no significant differences nor did a comparison between their own stripping patients and the stripping groups from the literature.

The most important results from the comparison of their own CHIVA patients with their own stripping patients, and those from the literature used for comparison in Maeso's study (Barcelona), are given in Tables 10.2, 10.3, 10.4 and 10.5.

Table 10.2 Comparison of objective and subjective Hobbs criteria in the Maeso Group own CHIVA vs. own historical stripping (every item differs significantly with $p < 0.05$)

Group	Item	Excellent (no varices)	Better (fewer varices)	The same or worse
CHIVA group	Presence of varicose veins after 3 years	51 (56.7%)	38 (42.2%)	1 (1.1%)
Stripping group		46 (54.1%)	26 (30.6%)	13 (15.3%)
CHIVA group	Clinical symptoms	60 (66.6%)	29 (32.2%)	1 (1.1%)
Stripping group		24 (28.2%)	43 (50.6%)	18 (21.2%)
CHIVA group	Subjective cosmetic satisfaction	52 (57.6%)	35 (38.9%)	3 (3.3%)
Stripping group		43 (50.6%)	38 (32.9%)	14 (16.5%)

Table 10.3 Comparison of neurological disturbances and the visible spider vein between the own CHIVA and the own stripping groups, Maeso (all comparisons are significantly different with $p < 0.05$)

		Present	Absent
CHIVA group	Neurological disturbances after 3 years	1 (1.1%)	89 (98.9%)
Stripping group		16 (18.8%)	69 (81.2%)
CHIVA group	Spider veins after 3 years	8 (8.9%)	82 (91.1%)
Stripping group		33 (659%)	29 (34.1%)

Table 10.4 Comparison of the presence of varicose veins after 3 years between own CHIVA patients with published stripping series ($p < 0.05$)

Hobbs criteria	Excellent (no varices)	Better (fewer varices)	The same or worse
Taulaniemi	55 (44%)	64 (50%)	7 (6%)
Hobbs	98 (39%)	127 (51%)	25 (10%)
Einarsson	34 (55%)	21 (35%)	6 (10%)
CHIVA group	51 (57%)	38 (42%)	1 (1%)

10.1.3 Reflux Elimination Without Any Ablation or Disconnection of the Saphenous Vein [8]

The aim of this prospective study was to investigate the possibility of the haemodynamic suppression of reflux in the greater saphenous vein without any high ligation and/or stripping procedure. The authors investigated 40 patients affected by primary chronic venous insufficiency of all clinical classes, with demonstrated duplex incompetence both of the sapheno-femoral junction and the great saphenous vein trunk, with the re-entry perforator located on a great saphenous vein tributary. Air plethysmographic parameters and duplex scanning were performed both preoperatively and 1 and 6 months later, respectively. Duplex investigation demonstrated both a forward flow and reflux disappearance in the GSV in 100% and 85% of the cases after 1 and 6 months, respectively. The air plethysmographic parameters are shown in Table 10.6.

This early investigation did not discriminate between cases with competent or incompetent terminal valve and had a short follow-up (Compare Sect. 10.3.1).

10.1.4 Postoperative Thrombosis in Great Saphenous Vein [9]

Pintos et al. investigated 165 patients after CHIVA treatment in their hospital. They compared the postoperative superficial vein thrombosis found in the GSV after so-called drained CHIVA (101 patients, CHIVA 1 or 2) and undrained CHIVA (64 patients, CHIVA 1 + 2).

Table 10.5 Summary of the first non-randomized studies between 1998 and 2001

Author	Type	Number of patients	Follow-up	Results
Zamboni	Prospective, no comparison	357	4 years	Drained great saphenous vein in 94% after 4 years Recidives after 4 years (11%) Air plethysmography: Significant improvement immediately and after 6 months as compared to preoperatively
Cappelli	Prospective and compared to literature	148	3 years	Significantly better results in the CHIVA group as compared to the published stripping data after 3 years with $p < 0.001$ concerning symptoms, subjective and cosmetic improvement and objective presence of visible varicose veins
Maeso	Prospective and compared to literature and to own treated stripping patients	90 (vs. 85 own stripping patients)	3 years	Significantly better results in the CHIVA group compared to own stripping patients concerning symptoms, subjective and cosmetic improvement and objective presence of visible varicose veins with $p < 0.05$ after 3 years
All	Not randomized	595		

Table 10.6 Venous volume, venous filling index and residual volume fraction improvement assessed, respectively, by means of air plethysmography preoperatively, as well as at 1 and 6 months after the surgical procedure

Plethysmographic parameter	Pre-op	1-month follow-up	6-month follow-up	*P*
Venous volume (VV) mL	150 ± 9	119 ± 6	114 ± 7	<0.0001
Venous filling index (VFI) mL	5 ± 0.5	2 ± 0.2	2 ± 0.2	<0.0001
Residual volume fraction (RVF) mL	42 ± 3	30 ± 2	30 ± 2	<0.0001

This work was presented on the Spanish Congress of Angiology and Phlebology 2001, Valladolid.

One hundred and one patients (61%) were treated either with CHIVA 1 or 2; 64 patients (39%) were treated with a non-drained method under CHIVA 1 + 2 (simultaneous closure of the sapheno-femoral junction and the CHIVA 2 point with Shunt Type 3).

The overall mean preoperative diameter of the GSV was 0.78 cm (0.28–1.70 cm). All the patients received subcutaneous low-molecular-weight heparin in a prophylactic dose for 15 days after the operation. They wore class 2 compression stockings for 6 weeks.

All legs were examined by duplex ultrasound 1, 3 and 6 months after the intervention.

The incidence of superficial vein thrombosis of the GSV in the drained CHIVA group was 9 patients (9%) and in the undrained CHIVA group 25 patients (38%). The difference between the incidences of superficial vein thrombosis in the two groups was statistically significant ($p < 0.001$). This shows that the relatively high incidence of superficial vein thrombosis from early publications on CHIVA was negatively influenced by the use of the CHIVA 1 + 2 procedure. If the CHIVA 1 + 2 procedure is not used, the incidence of superficial vein thrombosis falls clearly.

The diameter of the GSV at the proximal thigh correlated with superficial vein thrombosis as follows: In the group with drained CHIVA, patients with superficial vein thrombosis presented a mean GSV diameter of 1.03 cm ± 0.19. In patients without superficial vein thrombosis, the preoperative mean diameter at the proximal thigh was 0.89 cm ± 0.36. The difference was statistically significant ($p < 0.001$).

In the undrained CHIVA group, patients with superficial vein thrombosis presented a mean GSV diameter of 0.89 cm ± 0.19, while the mean diameter in the group without superficial vein thrombosis was 0.91 cm ± 0.29; the difference was not significant.

If the patients are divided into those who suffered discomfort due to their superficial vein thrombosis and those who did not, the mean GSV diameter in the group with discomfort was 1.04 cm ± 0.29, and in superficial vein thrombosis patients without discomfort, it was 0.78 cm ± 0.31. The difference was statistically significant ($p < 0.001$).

It was calculated that above 0.85 cm, the risk of superficial vein thrombosis in the GSV is significantly higher, meaning that the relative risk of superficial vein thrombosis after CHIVA is three times higher for patients with a GSV diameter greater than 0.85 cm at the proximal thigh than it is when the diameter is less than 0.85 cm. The number of patients suffering discomfort was also significantly higher among patients with a diameter greater than 0.85 cm.

10.1.5 Evolution of CHIVA 2 Treatment on Shunt Type 3 [10]

José María Escribano and the team from the Vall d'Hebrón University in Barcelona published an investigation about the results of CHIVA in two steps in case of Shunt Type 3.

Fifty-eight patients were analysed during 3 years after performing the first step of "CHIVA 2" in the case of Shunt Type 3 with draining tributary below the knee. The diameter of the GSV reduced significantly, though 51 of the patients had reflux recurrence after 6 months and 53 after 3 years. In all the patients, a re-entry perforator was found, so that Shunt Type 3 was changed into Shunt Type 1. Forty-six patients underwent high ligation of the sapheno-femoral junction in the 3 years of the investigation (crossotomy). 89.9% of the patients had a clinical cure situation according to the Hobbs criteria and 10% an improvement (see Table 10.1) at the moment of the reflux reappeared, and still 79% were classified as "cured" at the moment of the crossotomy.

The conclusion is that the recurrence rate after the first step of CHIVA in Shunt Type 3 in case of great saphenous vein reflux above and below the knee is high.

Comments of the authors: Personal experience is not that always a perforator takes the drainage but mostly a new tributary, making the management much more difficult than found in this study (see Sect. 6.4.1). Possibly the fact that the refluxive segment of the GSV was long (above and below the knee) could explain this different evolution. Zamboni et al. [11] demonstrated 29% of permanent competence of GSV for 3 years after CHIVA 2 in Shunt Type 3 in a group with above-knee and above- and below-knee reflux situation.

10.2 Randomized Studies

10.2.1 Ulcer Healing: CHIVA vs. Compression [12]

This prospective randomized study compared CHIVA with the use of compression in the treatment of venous ulcers with incompetence of the superficial leg veins (C6 in the CEAP classification). Twenty-four legs in 24 patients were treated with compression, if necessary after antibiotic treatment; in suppurating wounds, the bandage (hydrocolloid) was changed every 3–5 days during the first month and every 7 days thereafter. Non-suppurating wounds were first covered with a zinc oxide bandage. The CHIVA group included 23 legs on 21 patients. Sixteen legs with Shunt Type 1 were treated with crossectomy, and with further interruptions, seven legs with Shunt Type 3 were treated with the CHIVA 2 procedure.

The study evaluated:

- Healing progress based on the area of the ulcer
- The venous function of the leg based on air plethysmography before treatment and 6 months and 3 years after treatment
- Quality of life based on the SF-36 questionnaire before treatment and 6 months after treatment

Apart from the clinical evaluation, a duplex ultrasound was performed every 6 months for a total of 3 years. The results are presented in Table 10.7.

Preoperative air plethysmography presented no differences between the two groups. These

Table 10.7 Comparison of ulcer healing with compression or with CHIVA

	Compression	CHIVA
Healing success rate	96%	100%
Healing time ($p < 0.005$)	61 ± 11 days	29 ± 4 days
Speed of healing ($p < 0.02$)	1.66 ± 0.4 mm²/day	2.86 ± 0.3 mm²/day
Recurrence of ulcer ($p < 0.05$)	9 cases (38%)	2 cases (9%)[a]

[a]Both these patients needed the second step of CHIVA 2 treatment (crossotomy), which was not carried out during the investigation period, i.e. they continued to present reflux from the deep leg vein into the affected saphenous vein

values did not alter significantly in the compression group, whereas in the CHIVA group, all the values, including the ejection fraction, were significantly improved after 6 months.

There was no preoperative difference in the quality of life index. All eight areas presented significant improvements in the CHIVA group ($p < 0.001$). In the compression group, only four parameters were improved ($p < 0.05$). Comparison between the two groups 6 months after the start of treatment presented significantly better results in four parameters ($p < 0.05$).

10.2.2 Varicose Vein Stripping vs. Haemodynamic Correction (CHIVA): A Long-Term Randomized Trial [13]

This randomized comparative trial was aimed to compare the long-term results of stripping vs. CHIVA in the treatment of superficial venous incompetence. The study enrolment followed CONSORT requirements. One hundred and eighty consecutive patients were screened by clinical examination, including CEAP clinical classification, and duplex ultrasonography undertaken by physicians experienced in the management of venous disease. Thirty patients were excluded according to the exclusion criteria, while 150 patients were randomized into two groups, 75 were treated with saphenous stripping and 75 with CHIVA. All limbs were examined by three independent assessors who had not been involved in previous surgical decision-making and operative procedures. The assigned score to each limb was in accordance to the method reported by Hobbs. The results are presented in Table 10.8 and the recurrence analysis in Table 10.9.

Table 10.8 Results of CHIVA vs. stripping, Carandina

	CHIVA	Stripping	Sign. level
Duration of hospital stay	0.5 day	2 days	$p < 0.0001$
Mean value of subjective Hobbs score	1.65	1.8	n.s.
Mean value of objective Hobbs score	1.9	2.2	$p < 0.038$
Recidive rate after 10 years	18%	35%	$p < 0.038$

Table 10.9 Duplex analysis of the recurrences identified five different haemodynamic patterns of recurrence

	CHIVA	Stripping	Sign. level
Type 1: Sapheno-femoral recurrence	2.9%	5.5%	n.s
Type 2: Reflux coming from the pelvis	1.4%	3.7%	n.s.
Type 3: Evidence of incompetent perforator	0%	7.4%	n.s.
Type 4: Reflux from the proximal saphenous vein to a varicose tributary	18%	0%	$p < 0.01$
Type 5: Recurrence from varicose veins greater than 5 mm without connection to the deep veins	8%	22%	$p < 0.01$

The relative risk of recurrence in the stripping group is doubled at 10 years compared to CHIVA (OR 2.2; 95% CI 1e 5, $p < 0.04$).

No significant differences were found between the two techniques at 3 years. During the period 3–10 years, the different recurrence rates in the two groups become apparent and significant.

10.2.3 Randomized Comparison Stripping vs. CHIVA [14]

Iborra and her team published in 2006 (Spanish) a prospective randomized investigation with 100 legs treated either with CHIVA or stripping with a follow-up of 9 years; the study was presented at the European Venous Forum in 2006. Sixty-two women and 38 men with median age 49 were selected following the Spanish guidelines for varicose vein treatment (symptomatic varicose veins with saphenous reflux) but also large varicose veins without symptoms. Patients should not have a history of venous interventions or thrombosis nor overweight or age over 70 years.

After confirming inclusion and exclusion criteria, 100 patients of the waiting list (Bellvitge University Hospital) were randomized, 49 into the stripping group (above and below knee) and 51 into the CHIVA group. No differences concerning age, sex, weight and CEAP between the groups were found. All patients were investigated with duplex ultrasound. After intervention, they received the same dose of heparin (prophylactic) and were investigated 1 week after intervention and then after 1, 3 and 6 months and yearly for 5 years with questionnaires and ultrasound.

All patients with stripping were admitted to the hospital (44 spinal and 5 general anaesthesia). In the CHIVA group, 9 patients stayed for one night; the rest was treated on ambulatory base (6 spinal, 3 general, 42 local anaesthesia) (Table 10.10).

The mean inability of work time in the stripping group was 19.25 days, in the CHIVA group 8.04 days ($p < 0.001$).

In neither group, severe complications were found. Eleven patients in the stripping group complained because of neural lesions at the ankle, five still at the control after 6 months and one permanently after 5 years. In the CHIVA group, four patients suffered symptomatic superficial vein thrombosis; sonographically this condition was found in 11 legs. In all cases after 12 months, the vein was recanalized and the GSV calibre reduced.

Patients with recidives and asking for a redo intervention were immediately treated (five patients each group) (Table 10.11).

The results after 5 years are represented in Table 10.12. Apart from a slight better result in the CHIVA strain concerning the absence of visible varicose veins, the results were similar after 5 years.

10.2.4 Varicose Vein Surgery: Stripping vs. CHIVA Methods—A Randomized Controlled Trial [15]

The objective of this study was to compare the efficacy of the CHIVA method for the treatment of varicose veins with respect to the standard treatment of stripping. The study design was open-label, randomized controlled trial, in which 501 adult patients with primary varicose veins were included. They were treated in a single centre. The patients were assigned randomly to CHIVA procedure (experimental group $n = 167$) or stripping with clinic marking (control group 1, $n = 167$) and stripping with duplex marking

Table 10.10 Complaints after 1 week [14]

	Stripping		CHIVA		Sign. level	
Indoor activities with restrictions	7	33	0	3	0.005	<0.001
Indoor activities without restrictions	17		2		<0.001	
Outdoor activities with restrictions	9		1		0.007	
Normal outdoor activities without restrictions	12	15	29	48	0.001	<0.001
Normal activities, returned to work	3		19		<0.001	
	48		51			
Mean inability of work time	19.25 days		8.04 days		<0.001	

Table 10.11 Anaesthesia, complications and treated recidives

Anaesthesia	Stripping	CHIVA
Local	0	42
Spinal	44	6
General	5	3
Complications		
Neural lesion after 1 week	11	0
Neural lesion after 6 months	6	0
Neural lesion after 5 years	1	0
Symptomatic superficial vein thrombosis	0	4
Redo interventions	5	5

Table 10.12 Results (Hobbs) after 5 years, Iborra

Symptoms	Stripping	CHIVA	*p*
Asymptomatic	20	27	0.219
Better	25	20	0.225
No changes	1	2	1.000
Worse	1	0	0.490
Cosmetics—Subjective evaluation (patient)			
Success	43	46	0.712
Better but not optimum	3	2	0.674
Not happy	1	1	1.000
Cosmetics—Objective evaluation (staff)			
No visible varicose veins	10	16	0.210
Visible varicose veins <5 mm	20	19	0.760
Varicose veins of >5 mm at the thigh or calf	9	12	0.527
Varicose veins of >5 mm at the thigh and calf	8	2	0.048
Lost to follow-up	2	2	n.s.
All	47	49	

(control group 2, $n = 167$). The outcome measure was clinical recurrence within 5 years, assessed clinically by previously trained independent observers. Duplex ultrasonography was also used to assess recurrences and causes. The results are summarized in Table 10.13. The study was financed by the Spanish Ministry of Health.

The odds ratio between the stripping with clinic marking and CHIVA groups, of recurrence at 5 years of follow-up, was 2.64 (95% confidence interval [CI], 1.76–3.97; $P < 0.001$). The odds ratio of recurrence at 5 years of follow-up, between the stripping with duplex marking and CHIVA group, was 2.01 (95% CI, 1.34–3.00; $p < 0.001$).

The conclusion was that CHIVA had less side effects and less recidives after 5 years than both stripping groups. No statistical differences between both stripping groups (with and without duplex marking) were found.

10.2.5 Cochrane Review: Bellmunt-Montoya S, CHIVA Method for the Treatment of Chronic Venous Insufficiency (2013–2015) [16]

This is an update of the review first published in 2013 aimed to compare the efficacy and safety of the CHIVA method with alternative therapeutic techniques to treat varicose veins. Randomized controlled trials (RCTs) were included to compare the CHIVA method versus any other treatments. Two review authors independently selected and evaluated the studies [12–15]. One review author extracted data and performed the

Table 10.13 Results Parés 5 years: Group 1 stripping without duplex, group 2 stripping with duplex and group 3 CHIVA

Results	Group 1 stripping	Group 2 stripping	Group 3 CHIVA	Sign. level
Mean days of work inability	20.77 days	17.56 days	5.3 days	$p < 0.001$
New veins visible in ultrasound after 5 years	67.1%	60.5%	35%	$P < 0.001$
Clinically visible veins and bad result after the Hobbs criteria after 5 years	47%	43.5%	26.8%	$p < 0.001$

quantitative analysis. The risk ratio (RR), the mean difference (MD), the number of people needed to treat for an additional beneficial outcome (NNTB) and the number of people needed to treat for an additional harmful outcome (NNTH), with 95% confidence intervals, were calculated.

The primary endpoint, clinical recurrence, pooled between studies over a follow-up of 3–10 years, showed more favourable results for the CHIVA method than for vein stripping (721 people; RR 0.63; 95% CI 0.51–0.78; I2 = 0%, NNTB 6; 95% CI 4–10) or compression dressings (47 people; RR 0.23; 95% CI 0.06–0.96; NNTB 3; 95% CI 2–17). Only one study reported data on quality of life (presented graphically), and these results significantly favoured the CHIVA method.

The vein stripping group had a higher risk of side effects than the CHIVA group; specifically, the RR for bruising was 0.63 (95% CI 0.53–0.76; NNTH 4; 95% CI 3–6), and the RR for nerve damage was 0.05 (95% CI 0.01–0.38; I2 = 0%; NNTH 12; 95% CI 9–20). There were no statistically significant differences between groups regarding the incidence of limb infection and superficial vein thrombosis.

10.3 Recent Non-randomized Series

10.3.1 Great Saphenous Varicose Vein Surgery Without Sapheno-Femoral Junction Disconnection [11]

This case-control study was designed to determine whether preoperative duplex imaging could predict the outcome of varicose vein surgery without sapheno-femoral junction (SFJ) disconnection. The duplex protocol included a reflux elimination test (RET, see Sect. 3.8.9) and assessment of the competence of the terminal valve of the femoral vein. Patients with negative reflux elimination test (those with draining perforators on the saphenous vein) were excluded.

One hundred patients with chronic venous disease who had a positive reflux elimination test result and an incompetent terminal valve (Shunt 5) were compared with 100 patients matched for age, sex, CEAP clinical class and diseases duration but who had a positive reflux elimination test result and a competent terminal valve (Shunt 3). All patients underwent ligation and proximal avulsion of the incompetent tributaries from the great saphenous vein trunk without sapheno-femoral junction disconnection or any intervention on the saphenous vein. Clinical and duplex follow-up lasted for 3 years and included Hobbs clinical score.

The objective assessment (Hobbs clinical score) and subjective symptom score after 3 years are detailed in Table 10.14 while duplex assessment after 1 and 3 years in Table 10.15.

Recurrence rate after 3 years was significantly different depending on the competence or not the terminal valve. With competent terminal valve (Shunt Type 5), the recurrence rate was 3% at the sapheno-femoral junction, compared with 71% in case of incompetent terminal valve (Shunt Type 3) after 3 years.

10.3.2 Calibre Reduction of Saphenous and Deep Veins After CHIVA [17, 18]

The diameters of the great saphenous vein (GSV) and the common femoral vein (CFV) seem to give a hint about the severity of venous illness. Inspired by the question of Prof. Hach in 2002,

Table 10.14 Results of Hobbs clinical score subdivided in the two different groups after 3 years

	Objective assessment			Subjective assessment		
	Class A	Class B	Class C + D	Class A	Class B	Class C + D
Incompetent terminal valve	4 (4.0)	25 (25.0)	71 (71.0)	3 (3.0)	23 (23.0)	74 (74.0)
Competent terminal valve	85 (85.0)	15 (15.0)	0 (0)	86 (86.0)	14 (14.0)	0 (0)

Table 10.15 Duplex assessment of reflux in the great saphenous vein after 1 and 3 years

	One-year follow-up				Three-year follow-up			
	Incompetent terminal valve	Competent terminal valve	Odds ratio	*P*	Incompetent terminal valve	Competent terminal valve	Odds ratio	*P*
Recurrence sapheno-femoral junction	58 (58.0)	2 (2.0)	67.7 (15.8–290.1)	<0.0001	71 (71.0)	3 (3.0)	9·2 (23.2–270.2)	<0.0001
Recurrence from new incompetent tributary	4 (4.0)	5 (5.0)	1.2 (0.4–3.7)	0.783	7 (7.0)	6 (6.0)	1.2 (0.4–3.7)	0.783
Recurrence at site of tributary ligation	4 (4.0)	4 (4.0)	1.0 (0.2–4.1)	1.000	4 (4.0)	5 (5.0)	0.8 (0.2–3.0)	1.000
Overall great saphenous vein recurrence	66 (66.0)	11 (11.0)	17.5 (8.0–37.9)	<0.0001	82 (82.0)	14 (14.0)	31.5 (14.4–68.6)	<0.0001

who asked if the femoral vein would not suffer an overload after CHIVA, this study was designed. Hach postulated that the tributary blood (N3) draining through the saphenous vein (GSV, N2) into the deep vein (N1) usually through the sapheno-femoral junction could overload the femoral vein. Usually it would never circulate through the femoral vein. But after the crossotomy in the context of CHIVA, this blood will flow retrogradely and drain through a thigh or calf perforator. Thus, the femoral vein and the common femoral vein (CFV) distal to the sapheno-femoral junction would be overloaded with it after the treatment. The aim of this study was to discover long-term effects of CHIVA on diameters of the CFV.

Patients underwent drained interventions (CHIVA 2 in one or two steps, depending on the evolution or crossectomy) (Note that in Germany the crossotomy is not reimbursed; thus a crossectomy has to be performed.) In the first step, the evolution of diameters of GSV at the proximal thigh and the diameter of the CFV was measured [19]: In a prospective multicentre study, 557 legs of 458 patients were scanned with ultrasound preoperatively measuring the diameter of the common femoral vein distal to the sapheno-femoral junction, as well as the diameter of the great saphenous vein 10–15 cm distal to the groin in standing position. Three hundred and eighty-three patients with 470 treated legs (84.4%) returned to follow-up between 8 and 25 weeks after surgery for a duplex examination. Diameters of the great saphenous vein and common femoral vein were compared pre- and postoperatively. The diameter of the great saphenous vein changed from 6.1 mm preoperatively to 4.5 mm postoperatively in the female group and from 6.8 to 5.1 mm in the male group. The diameter of the common femoral vein changed from 14.0 mm preoperatively to 13.7 mm postoperatively in the female group and from 16.5 to 16.1 mm postoperatively in the male group, all these results being statistically highly significant.

In the second investigation [17], the long-term effect on the diameter was controlled after 5 years in 43 patients included in the first trial. Clinical class (CEAP) and refilling time were compared to preoperative values and values after 8 weeks. The patients were evaluated 5.36 years after CHIVA intervention. The diameter of the CFV and the diameter of GSV were reduced significantly also over 5 years (see Table 10.16). The C class was reduced from 2.77 ± 0.81 preoperatively to

Table 10.16 Evolution of diameters of the common femoral vein (CFV) and great saphenous vein (GSV) at the proximal thigh

	Prior to intervention	After 8 weeks	After 5 years
Diameter CFV	15.4 ± 2.9	15.1 ± 2.3	14.2 ± 2.6
Diameter GSV	7.0 ± 2.0	5.0 ± 1.5	4.4 ± 1.4

1.72 ± 1.10 after 5 years ($p = 0.007$). Refilling time in photoplethysmography was prolonged from 15.24 ± 6.18 s to 21.61 ± 9.2 s preoperatively after 5 years ($p = 0.022$).

The authors concluded that not only on a short-term but also a long-term result the treatment with CHIVA reduced the diameter of the CFV and GSV as well as the C class of CEAP and improved the refilling time.

10.3.3 Role of Surgical Technique (Stripping vs. CHIVA) and Surgeon's Experience on the Outcome of CHIVA [20]

This study was a retrospective analysis comparing the outcome after stripping versus CHIVA (5-year follow-up) in two periods of time: The first group concerned the patients treated in the years 1995–2000 after learning about CHIVA, the second the patients treated between 2001 and 2005 after the team was trained in the method. The outcome measurement was performed with Hobbs criteria, including cure with no visible varices and failure in case of varices of more than 0.5 cm diameter.

In the first period, 223 patients underwent stripping and 88 CHIVA. A cure was achieved in 30.9% after stripping and 12.6% after CHIVA ($p < 0.05$); a failure was found in 47.5% of stripping and 67% of CHIVA patients ($p < 0.05$).

In the second period, 186 patients were treated with stripping and 208 with CHIVA. The cure rate in the stripping group remained constant at 29.5% and changed in the CHIVA group to 44.2% ($p < 0.05$). 46.7% of stripping patients were classified as failure and 30.2% in the CHIVA group ($p < 0.05$). 1.6% in the stripping group had permanent neural damage compared with none in the CHIVA group.

In the second observational period, the results reach the level of other publications. The authors conclude that significant training and adequate experience of vascular surgery and ultrasound mapping are required to perform CHIVA successfully. Achieving good results with this method is much more challenging than with traditional stripping.

10.3.4 Multiple Ligation of the Proximal Greater Saphenous Vein in the CHIVA Treatment of Primary Varicose Veins [21]

To determine whether a crossotomy is necessary or a ligation could be performed instead for safety reasons on ambulatory patients, 199 legs underwent follow-up after sapheno-femoral interruption in the CHIVA context with three different techniques. Common to all techniques was a titanium clip (10 mm long and 1 mm thick) placed flush with the femoral vein in order to prevent the presence of a residual saphenous stump:

- Group 1: ($N = 61$) Crossotomy (with interruption of the sapheno-femoral junction, follow-up 29 months)
- Group 2: ($N = 82$) Triple saphenous flush ligation (TSFL) was performed with a No. 2 non-absorbable braided coated suture (follow-up 14 months)
- Group 3: ($N = 56$) Triple polypropylene ligation (TPL) with No. 0 polypropylene (follow-up 12 months)

In the first two groups, the rate of new reflux with Valsalva at the SFJ Level was 6.1%; in the second (shorter follow-up!), the reflux rate at the SFJ under Valsalva was 4.9%, showing no statistical difference to group 1. In group 3, a recanalization rate of 37.5% was found after 1 year; the difference between groups 3 and 1, as well as group 2, was highly significant with $p < 0.001$.

10.3.5 Hemodynamic Classification and CHIVA Treatment of Varicose Veins in Lower Extremities (VVLE) [22]

Prospective comparison of 150 patients with varicose veins is divided into three groups: one with high ligation and stripping, one with high ligation and LASER of the saphenous vein and one with CHIVA, with follow-up of 18 months. This work was supported by the Scientific Program of Medicine and Health in Zhejiang Province: 2014KYB263.

No differences in CEAP or shunt types between both groups were found. The surgery time was less in the CHIVA group compared to the other two groups ($p < 0.05$), and the incision length was less in the LASER and CHIVA group compared to the surgery group ($p < 0.05$).

Results and complications are depicted in Table 10.17.

The article concludes that CHIVA produces less cost and is less invasive and has lesser complication, with a better cure rate and lesser recidives, though a learning curve has to be considered.

Table 10.17 Comparison between the results after stripping, LASER and CHIVA after 18 months

Groups	Traditional surgery	High ligation and LASER	CHIVA
Total number	50	50	50
Cure	25 (50%) $p < 0.05$ vs. LASER group, $p < 0.01$ vs. CHIVA group	32 (64%)	41 (82%)
Recurrence	5 (10%) $p < 0.05$ vs. CHIVA group	32 (64%)	2 (4%)
Superficial vein thrombosis	4 (8%)	3 (6%)	1 (2%)
Ecchymosis	4 (8%)	3 (6%)	1 (2%)
Numbness	6 (12%)	5 (10%)	0
Phlegmon	5 (10%)	4 (8%)	1 (2%)

10.3.6 CHIVA: A Prospective Study of a Vein Sparing Technique for the Management of Varicose Vein Disease [23]

This is a prospective study assessing the rate of recurrence of venous reflux with CHIVA. The authors evaluated 150 primary procedures with clinical and duplex ultrasound examinations pre- and postoperatively. Patients were followed at <3-month and >1-year post-op. Postoperative duplex assessment of reflux was performed in supine position; the intervention at the sapheno-femoral junction site consisted in double ligation with 2–0 silk at 2 cm of the sapheno-femoral junction (this means distal to the confluence of epigastric veins).

Recurrence was defined as reflux in the great saphenous vein at the thigh on duplex examination (Table 10.18).

There was no documented recurrence at the early follow-up. To date, 58 legs have completed the late follow-up, and reflux was found in duplex ultrasound in 5 legs resulting in a recurrence rate of 8.6%, 95% CI (2.4%, 19%). None of these patients had clinical complaints. The authors concluded that the recurrence rate using the

Table 10.18 Outcomes at <3-month and >1-year follow-up

	Male $N = 38$ (25%)	Female $N = 112$ (75%)	Total $N = 150$ (100%)
Outcome at early follow-up			
Recurrence	0 (0%)	0 (0%)	0 (0%)
No recurrence	38 (25%)	112–75%	150 (100%)
Bruising	0 (0%)	2 (3%)	2 (3%)
Superficial thrombophlebitis	1 (2%)	2 (3%)	2 (3%)
Outcome at 1-year follow-up			
Recurrence	1 (2%)	4 (7%)	5 (9%)
No recurrence	14 (24%)	39 (67%)	53 (91%)

CHIVA method compared favourably with vein ablation techniques. High patient satisfaction, low complication rate and low cost encourage to pursue further study using this technique.

10.3.7 Endoluminal Treatment of Great Saphenous Vein in the CHIVA Context [24]

In its description, the CHIVA strategy was performed with surgical techniques [22]. After the introduction of endoluminal heat techniques, this first approach had the aim to compare LASER and radiofrequency applied over short segments closing the saphenous junction in the CHIVA context. One hundred and four patients were investigated before and 3–6 months after the treatment of the great saphenous vein (GSV) with CHIVA strategy using endoluminal heat techniques to close the groin segment (75 patients with VNUS ClosureFast or 29 patients with LASER [1470 nm, Intros radial]).

A significant reduction of diameters of GSV at the proximal thigh and VFC, as well as a reduction of clinical scores, was found (see Table 10.19). These results are comparable to those achieved after surgical crossectomy (see Table 10.16). The author concludes that it seems to be possible to apply endoluminal heat techniques in the context of the CHIVA strategy. No difference could be found between both techniques, LASER and VNUS ClosureFast.

10.4 Further Publications

10.4.1 German CHIVA Group Consensus: How to Treat Veins When Stripping, CHIVA Endoluminal Treatments and Foam Sclerotherapy Are Available? [18]

In 2010 on a meeting of the German Society of CHIVA, a consensus was developed about how to treat a great saphenous vein insufficiency depending on type of shunt and length of reflux having the options to apply ablative strategies (stripping, endoluminal heating or foam sclerotherapy) or CHIVA to find a consensus for treatment of the refluxive great saphenous vein (GSV) [12].

Nineteen participants (14 surgeons, 4 of them are vascular surgeons, 4 internists, 1 dermatologist and 1 general practitioner, the latter 6 cooperating in their office with surgeons) presented different forms of reflux in GSV and different patient situations (age, obesity, multimorbidity). They gave their votes to "therapy is possible", "is useful" or "is optimum". In the first two options, more than one could be mentioned; optimum could only be given to one treatment option. All participants were familiar with all methods, but only 13 participants used foam sclerotherapy regularly.

All methods were considered as possible in all situations of refluxive GSV. Stripping, endoluminal heating procedures and CHIVA had mentions

Table 10.19 Diameter of the common femoral vein (D CFV) and great saphenous vein (D GSV) at the proximal thigh and clinics prior to intervention (pre) and evolution after CHIVA with endoluminal heat devices (post)

	VNUS pre	VNUS post	*p*	LASER pre	LASER post	*p*	All pre	All post	*p*
	Mean ± SD	Mean ± SD	*N* = 75	Mean ± SD	Mean ± SD	*N* = 29	Mean ± SD	Mean ± SD	
D CFV	15.1 ± 2.3	14.6 ± 2.2	0.001	15.5 ± 2.5	15.2 ± 2.1	0.347	15.1 ± 2.5	14.7 ± 2.3	0.000
D GSV	6.5 ± 1.7	3.7 ± 1.1	0.000	6.6 ± 1.6	3.9 ± 1.3	0.000	6.5 ± 1.9	4.1 ± 1.5	0.000
VCSS	5.4 ± 2.8	2.1 ± 1.7	0.000	6.3 ± 4.0	2.5 ± 2.8	0.000	5.6 ± 3.3	2.0 ± 2.0	0.000
C (CEAP)	3.2 ± 1.0	2.1 ± 1.0	0.000	3.4 ± 1.1	2.1 ± 1.4	0.000	3.1 ± 1.0	2.1 ± 1.3	0.000
PPG	20.6 ± 11.1	30.1 ± 10.7	0.000	19.4 ± 10.6	24.6 ± 7.5	0.072	20 ± 10.8	28.8 ± 10.1	0.000

PPG refilling time after photoplethysmography

as useful in more than 50% of all cases, foam slightly less. Stripping is more often mentioned as above- and below-knee refluxes, foam in shorter refluxes (only above knee) and thinner veins. Stripping, CHIVA and endoluminal procedures were mentioned in 30% of cases, foam in 10%. In the category "optimum," foam had 5% of mentions, especially in cases of short reflux, thin veins and obese patients. Stripping was found optimum in 6% of cases: postphlebitic GSV and large GSV with refluxes above and below knee. Endoluminal techniques had 33% of mentions as optimum, especially in case of large veins and in all cases of obese patients. CHIVA was mentioned as optimum in 56% of cases. A special indication is the reflux only above knee with no re-entry to the deep vein from GSV and generally in case of short refluxes independently of diameter and in long refluxes in a thin GSV.

Venous sparing options were mentioned to be optimum solution for the patient in 56% of the cases. The surprising conclusion was that the only procedure reimbursed by health insurances (stripping) by that time was no longer seen as optimal treatment option. The consensus result has an obvious bias, as all the voters were members of the Society of CHIVA and familiar with CHIVA—but they were also familiar with the other techniques. On private bases, endoluminal techniques receive higher reimbursement than CHIVA, and still the votes were favourable to CHIVA. Further discussions and trials have to be completed to find the optimal treatment option for each reflux situation.

Literature

1. Zamboni P, Marcellino MG, Cappelli M, Feo CV, Bresadola V, Vasquez G, Liboni A. Saphenous vein sparing surgery: principles, techniques and results. J Cardiovasc Surg. 1998;39:151–62.
2. Maeso J, Juan J, Escribano J, Allegue NM, Di Matteo A, Gonzalez E, Matas M. Comparison of clinical outcome of stripping and CHIVA for treatment of varicose veins in the lower extremities. Ann Vasc Surg. 2001;15:661–5.
3. Cappelli M, Molino Lova R, Ermini S, Turchi A, Bono G, Bahnini A, Franceschi C. Ambulatory conservative hemodynamic management of varicose veins: critical analysis of results at 3 years. Ann Vasc Surg. 2000;14:376–84.
4. Cappelli M, Molino Lova R, Ermini S, Turchi A, Bono G, Franceschi C. Comparison between the CHIVA cure and stripping in the treatment of varicose veins of the legs: follow-up of 3 years. J Mal Vasc. 1996;21:40–6. French
5. Hobbs JT. Surgery and sclerotherapy in the treatment of varicose veins. Arch Surg. 1974;109:793–6.
6. Taulaniemi E. On the treatment of varices. Acta Chir Scand. 1963;125:429–32.
7. Einarsson E, Eklöf B, Neglén P. Sclerotherapy or surgery as treatment for varicose veins: a prospective randomized study. Phlebology. 1993;8:22–6.
8. Zamboni P, Cisno C, Marchetti F, Quaglio D, Mazza P, Liboni A. Reflux elimination without any ablation or disconnection of the saphenous vein. A haemodynamic model for venous surgery. Eur J Vasc Endovasc Surg. 2001;21:361–9.
9. Pintos T, Senin E, Ramos R, Rodrıguez E, Martınez Perez M. Trombosis de safena interna post-CHIVA. Incidencia, factores condicionantes y repercusiones clınicas. Presented at the XLVII National Congress of the Spanish Society of Angiology and Vascular Surgery, Valladolid; 2001.
10. Escribano JM, Juan J, Bofill R, Maeso J, Rodríguez-Mori A, Matas M. Durability of reflux-elimination by a minimal invasive CHIVA procedure on patients with varicose veins. A 3-year prospective case study. Eur J Vasc Endovasc Surg. 2003;25:159–63.
11. Zamboni P, Gianesini S, Menegatti E, Tacconi G, Palazzo A, Liboni A. Great saphenous varicose vein surgery without saphenofemoral junction disconnection. Br J Surg. 2010;97(6):820–5. https://doi.org/10.1002/bjs.7022.
12. Zamboni P, Cisno C, Marchetti F, Mazza P, Fogato L, Carandina S, De Palma M, Liboni A. Minimally invasive surgical management of primary venous ulcers vs. compression treatment: a randomized clinical trial. Eur J Vasc Endovasc Surg. 2003;25(4):313–8. Erratum in: Eur J Vasc Endovasc Surg 2003;26(3):337–8
13. Carandina S, Mari C, De Palma M, Marcellino MG, Cisno C, Legnaro A, Liboni A, Zamboni P. Varicose vein stripping vs. haemodynamic correction (CHIVA): a long term randomised trial. Eur J Vasc Endovasc Surg. 2008;35:230–7.
14. Iborra-Ortega E, Barjau-Urrea E, Vila-Coll R, Ballón-Carazas H, Cairols-Castellote MA. Estudio comparativo de dos técnicas quirúrgicas en el tratamiento de las varices de las extremidades inferiores: resultados tras cinco años de seguimiento. Angiologia. 2006;58(6):459–68.
15. Parés JO, Juan J, Tellez R, Mata A, Moreno C, Quer FX, Suarez D, Codony I, Roca J. Varicose vein sur-

gery: stripping versus the CHIVA method: a randomized controlled trial. Ann Surg. 2010;251:624–31.
16. Bellmunt-Montoya S, Escribano JM, Dilme J, Martinez-Zapata MJ. CHIVA method for the treatment of chronic venous insufficiency. Cochrane Database Syst Rev. 2013 Jul 3:CD009648. https://doi.org/10.1002/14651858.CD009648.pub2. Review. Update in: Cochrane Database Syst Rev. 2015:CD009648
17. Mendoza E. Diameter reduction of the great saphenous vein and the common femoral vein after CHIVA long-term results. Phlebologie. 2013;42:65–9.
18. Mendoza E. Treatment of great saphenous vein reflux – consensus considering stripping, foam-sclerotherapy, endoluminal techniques and CHIVA as options (German:Therapie der Stammvarikose der V. saphena magna - Konsens unter Einbeziehung von stripping, Verödung, endoluminalen Verfahren und CHIVA als Therapieoptionen). Phlebologie. 2011;40:159–64.
19. Mendoza E, Berger V, Zollmann C, Bomhoff M, Amsler F. (Calibre reduction of great saphenous vein and common femoral vein after CHIVA) Kaliberreduktion der V. saphena magna und der V. femoralis communis nach CHIVA. Phlebologie. 2011;40(2):73–8.
20. Milone M, Salvatore G, Maietta P, Sosa Fernandez LM, Milone F. Recurrent varicose veins of the lower limbs after surgery. Role of surgical technique (stripping vs. CHIVA) and surgeon's experience. G Chir. 2011;32(11-12):460–3.
21. Delfrate R, Bricchi M, Franceschi C, Goldoni M. Multiple ligation of the proximal greater saphenous vein in the CHIVA treatment of primary varicose veins. Veins Lymphat. 2014;3:19–22.
22. Wang H, Chen Q, Fei Z, Zheng E, Yang Z, Huang X. Hemodynamic classification and CHIVA treatment of varicose veins in lower extremities (VVLE). Int J Clin Exp Med. 2016;9(2):2465–71.
23. Zmudzinski M, Malo P, Hall C, Hayashi A. CHIVA – a prospective study of a vein sparing technique for the management of varicose vein disease. Am J Surg. 2017;213:967–9.
24. Mendoza E, Amsler F. CHIVA with endoluminal procedures: LASER versus VNUS – treatment of the saphenofemoral junction. Phlebologie. 2017;46:5–12.

11 Perioperative Management in Saphenous Sparing Surgery

Erika Mendoza

11.1 Introduction

Saphenous sparing surgery is performed all around the world. Very different health-care systems lead to difficult diagnostic and treatment settings; in some countries, different persons perform ultrasound and surgery as a rule; in others, surgeons are educated in ultrasound and can perform their own investigation. Another problem might be the reimbursement situation, sometimes with clear differentiation between national health-care systems and private (often self-paying) medicine, sometimes with long waiting lists. So, in this chapter, the optimal settings are described, as well as the post-operative care recommendations applied in the environment of the authors. Obviously national regulations must be attended, and every unit for venous treatment will find the proper way between ideal treatment settings and local rules.

When Claude Franceschi first published his ideas about saphenous vein sparing surgery in his book *CHIVA* in 1988 [1], the idea to do venous surgery on ambulatory bases was like a revolution. Saphenous surgery (mostly stripping) was performed as in-house procedures. In most of the countries, even the diagnostics of varicose veins was performed only in specialized centres, most often attached to hospitals or big health-care centres for specialized medicine. Also in Germany, one of the only countries where specialized medicine was carried out in offices and surgery offices offered possibility to do the small surgery like crossectomy and stripping outside a hospital, varicose vein stripping was the domain of clinics and a good source of income for the house.

So, the "A" in CHIVA, which stands for "ambulatory", was sometimes more revolutionary than the theory to spare saphenous veins itself. The "A" could harm some pockets. The different country structures play a role in the acceptance or not of a new procedure. There are two examples: in Germany, the decision makers (chiefs of departments in hospitals) are paid by performance. CHIVA was not welcome in the 1990s when venous surgery was in-house based—this only changed after a reimbursement reformation in 2005. In Spain and in the context of the national health-care system, the vascular surgery is only

E. Mendoza, M.D., Ph.D.
Venenpraxis, Wunstorf, Germany
e-mail: erika.mendoza@t-online.de

P. Zamboni et al. (eds.), *Saphenous Vein-Sparing Strategies in Chronic Venous Disease*,
https://doi.org/10.1007/978-3-319-70638-2_11

performed in hospitals. Chiefs of departments in hospitals earn their money independently of the amount of procedures performed or the sales achieved. One of the best Spanish departments of vascular surgery in Barcelona learned about CHIVA between 1988 and 1992 and then decided to apply mainly CHIVA. All their residents were taught about CHIVA. They spread over Spain thereafter. Within 2005, more than 50% of all surgical venous procedures performed in Spain were CHIVA.

11.2 Preoperative Assessment

11.2.1 Preoperative Assessment of the Patient

Prior to talk about interventions, the indication to perform the treatment must be clear. The patient should be explained the therapeutic options, why a venous sparing technique is recommended, and what the advantages and disadvantages could be. He must be introduced to the risks and the things he must take care of after the surgery (see Sect. 11.5). This informed consent must be written down and signed by the surgeon and the patient.

Depending on the planned intervention and the personal risk factors of the patient, a blood sample will be taken for cell count, coagulation, and in case of a planned general anaesthesia those parameters the anaesthesiologist wishes.

Both legs might be treated at the same day or in different sessions. In case of large veins and cardiac problems, it might be recommended to treat one leg first and after at least a week the other to avoid right heart overload.

11.2.2 Contraindications for Venous Sparing Surgery

Venous sparing surgery shares most of the contraindications of general surgery.

Absolute Contraindications

- Pregnancy (because every unnecessary intervention should be avoided during pregnancy to protect the unborn child)
- Acute deep leg vein thrombosis (up to 6 moths subsequently)
- Acute infection of the leg or groin region
- All general contraindications for surgery

Relative Contraindications

- Severe arterial obstructive disease (see Sect. 11.6.4).
- If the patient does not understand the need to attend for post-operative examination and the need to possibly undergo a second intervention.
- If the patient does not understand that there may be no immediate visible improvement after the first operation or does not want to cope with the fact that the veins do not disappear immediately.
- Post-thrombotic occlusion of the deep leg veins with secondary varices acting as a bypass. Nevertheless, targeted ligations may allow some improvement to be achieved.

Indications for varicose vein surgery are discussed in Chap. 14.

11.2.3 Preoperative Assessment of Venous Reflux

Given the indication to perform the intervention, the first step is to do a cartography with a clear description of the shunt type and the recirculations involved, with exact knowledge of reflux points and drainage pathways. Then the disconnection points are marked on the skin immediately prior to the surgical intervention or sometimes—due to organizational aspects—the day prior to the surgery.

To apply CHIVA properly, the preoperative cartography of the venous system is mandatory. All steps needed to perform the duplex investigation are explained in Chap. 4 and in specialized textbooks. Usually history, physical examination, and duplex ultrasound are enough as preoperative venous examination. In case of complex disease, further explorations are needed, and the possibility to perform them or to send a patient to have these explorations done must be organized.

The marking on the skin can be performed in different ways. Permanent markers will still be visible after applying skin disinfection but will not paint on the skin when it is wet with ultrasound gel. So, some colleagues use coal eyeliners for the painting on wet surface.

The marking is performed in standing position. The course of the refluxive saphenous vein is marked on the skin, as well as relevant tributaries with their tortuosity. Then, preferably with a different colour, the places where disconnections are to be performed are marked. Different techniques of marking have been developed by different teams, so the ones presented here should only be an orientation (see Figs. 11.1, 11.2 and 11.3).

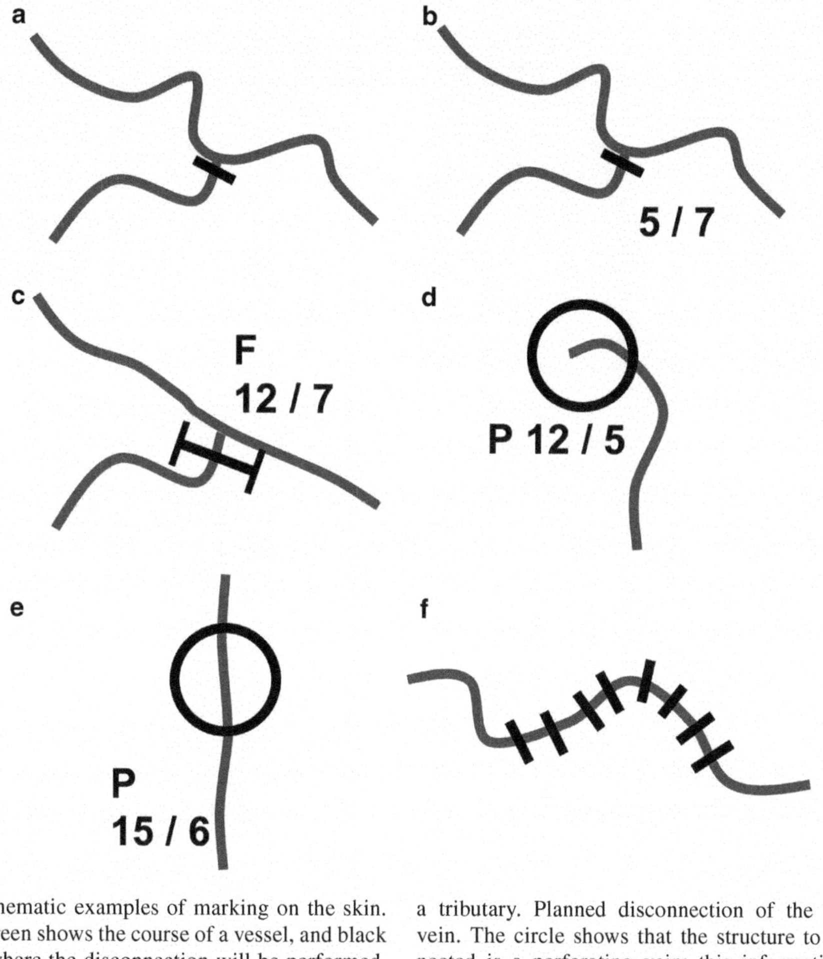

Fig. 11.1 Schematic examples of marking on the skin. In this case green shows the course of a vessel, and black is the place where the disconnection will be performed. (**a**) Marking of two connected tributaries. At the branching point, one of them will be disconnected. The black line shows the correct place. As these tributaries run immediately under the skin, no indications of the depth are necessary. (**b**) These tributaries run deeper under the skin. The black line indicates the disconnection point, the first number the depth of the vein wall, and the second number the diameter of the vein in mm. (**c**) Saphenous vein with branching tributary. The disconnection of the tributary must be performed under the saphenous fascia. To ensure this information, the F is painted on the leg, and the black line is reinforced with two crossbeams. (**d**) Incompetent perforating vein filling a tributary. Planned disconnection of the perforating vein. The circle shows that the structure to be disconnected is a perforating vein; this information is reinforced by the P written on the skin. The tributary ends in the circle. The numbers indicate the depth of the fascia from the skin and the diameter of the perforator at this level in mm. (**e**) Direct incompetent perforating vein filling a saphenous vein. The circle shows that the structure to be disconnected is the perforating vein, reinforced with the written P. As it is marked on the course of the saphenous vein, it is obvious that it is connected to the saphenous vein. The numbers indicate the depth of the fascia and the diameter of the perforating vein in mm. (**f**) Refluxive tributary. This tributary shall be treated with phlebectomy; many little interruption lines in black are the signal for this. With permission by [10]

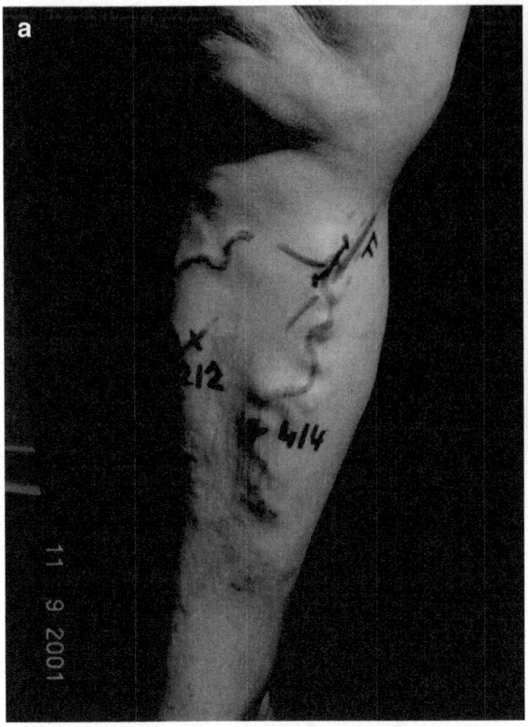

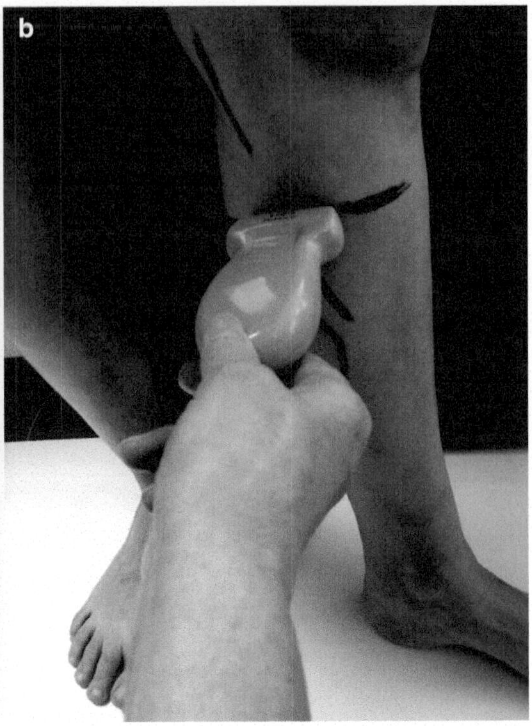

Fig. 11.2 (**a**) Image of a mapping according to Fig. 11.1. Visible veins marked in green, GSV marked with a green straight line. Shunt type 3 with incompetent GSV (competent terminal valve, incompetent preterminal valve) with reflux above and below knee, into a tributary below the knee. This "CHIVA 2 Point" is interrupted (F and Line with crossbeams), as well as two further tributary branching points with indication of depth and diameter of vein. (**b**) As the permanent markers do not paint on ultrasound gel and it is bothering to always guess, mark, double check, and correct, another way to securely mark the target on the skin is marking a crosshair, whilst the branching point or the perforator or the sapheno-popliteal junction is just below the transducer. The palpable and visible veins are marked in green, and then the longitudinal course of the saphenous vein is marked first (black line with longitudinal course), and the location of the junction between the tributary and the saphenous vein is marked afterwards crosswise. With permission by [10]

In the same way, the result of the investigation has to be written down in the records of the patient and as the base for the surgery. Also in this case, the team is free to choose one form of representation, but it should be clear to the surgeon what is expected from him, and it should be clear in case of further interventions what exactly was done in the prior occasions. Examples are shown in Fig. 11.4.

11.3 Surgical or Interventional Settings

11.3.1 Technical Aspects

In the context of CHIVA, different techniques will be applied: from sclerotherapy with or without ultrasound control, intervention on tributaries (only disconnection or phlebectomy), to surgery at the sapheno-femoral and sapheno-popliteal junctions and perforators or deep vein reconstruction. As new modalities, endoluminal heat or glue techniques are currently being introduced (see also Chap. 7 and Sect. 14.1.2).

The surgical theatre must be prepared to allow these procedures, fitted with ultrasound devices able to be used in the surgical setting, sterile material, and experienced personnel. All the locally typical regulations have to be taken into account. The physician must have a proper professional liability insurance. It must be made sure that the patient will be able to reach the surgeon or another person with knowledge of the procedures in case of possible complications after the intervention.

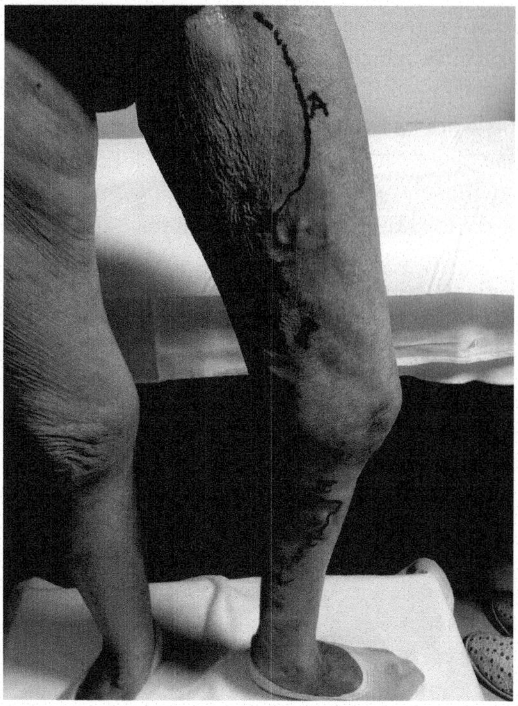

Fig. 11.3 Image of another type of mapping. Another kind of cartography, more detailed with kind permission to publish by Roberto Delfrate, Cremona, Italy (for details, see Fig. 11.4b). With permission by [10]

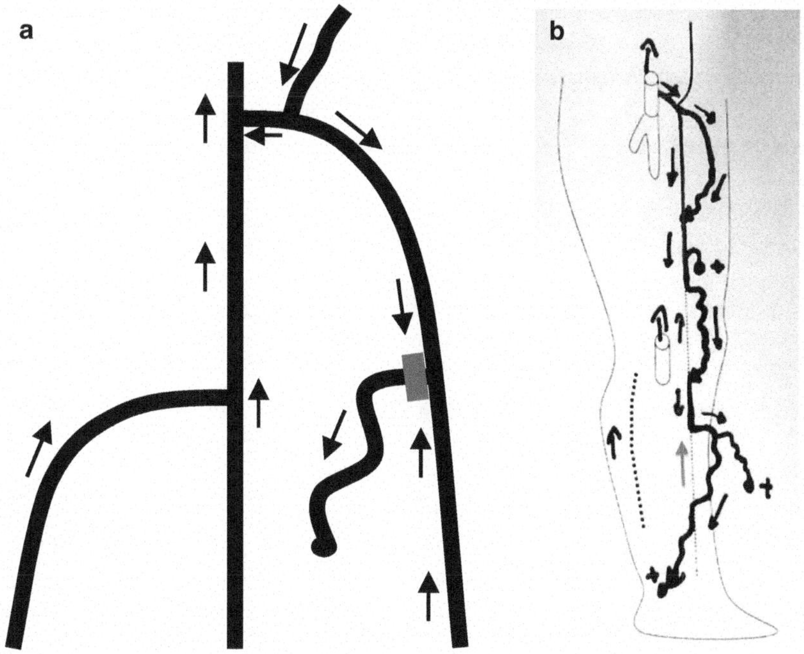

Fig. 11.4 Cartography with the result of the investigation; different types of cartography are possible; free hand painting of the reflux pathways, shunt types, and disconnection points must be marked in the scheme. (**a**) The empty scheme contains the deep and the saphenous veins as lines. During the cartography, the flow direction and relevant connections are marked. Cartography of a pelvine shunt type 5 in the great saphenous vein with drainage through a tributary and planned disconnection (CHIVA 2), corresponding to the photo in Fig. 11.2b. (**b**) Cartography with the result of the investigation corresponding to the clinical case of Fig. 11.3. The empty scheme contains the leg shape, a segment of the deep veins at knee level (popliteal vein) and at groin level, and the dotted lines for the GSV and SSV. The recirculation circuit is painted in the scheme. In this case, we find shunt types 1 and 2. With permission by [10]

If the surgeon is not the person doing the pre-operative mapping, he should know his duplex-partner perfectly and should be able to understand his markings on the skin and the different painting options he gives him. Figures 11.1, 11.2 and 11.3 display some option of marking on the skin, and Fig. 11.4 shows different options of how to draw the result of the cartography on a paper, serving as guide for the intervention.

11.3.2 Anaesthesia During the Intervention or Surgery

In regular saphenous sparing surgery, setting the intervention can be performed under local anaesthesia. Sometimes, preferences of the surgeon or the patients are to perform the intervention in sedation or general anaesthesia, this will have to be discussed with the patient.

Deep vein reconstruction (see Chap. 8) is surely best performed under general anaesthesia.

11.4 Perioperative Management

11.4.1 Anticoagulation

The normal guidelines for prophylaxis against deep vein thrombosis in leg vein operations also apply to saphenous sparing surgery. It can be performed almost always on ambulatory, usually without general anaesthesia. According to the guidelines, low-molecular-weight heparin is not required by otherwise healthy patients without a history of thrombosis. The use of this prophylactic is however still widespread in hospitals and operations under general anaesthesia, no doubt for logistic or forensic reasons.

The German CHIVA Association recommends administration of heparin in the following situations:

- After the first step of CHIVA 2 (see Sect. 6.4.1)
  Thrombosis of the saphenous trunk veins is a possible complication of CHIVA interventions. If it occurs in the proximal segment of a saphenous vein, it may ascend to the deep vein, since the junction has not been interrupted. To avoid this complication, the patient is prescribed a prophylactic dose of low-molecular heparin for 10 days.
- Shunt type 1
  If the great or small saphenous vein presents very a large calibre (greater than 8.5–10 mm diameter at mid-thigh) over long segments, post-operative superficial vein thrombosis, if it occurs, is generally painful [2]. We therefore prescribe a prophylactic dose of low-molecular heparin for 10 days.
- A prophylactic dose of low-molecular heparin is generally prescribed for 5 days in case of surgery at the sapheno-popliteal junction.

A blood count is done before the operation to count the thrombocytes, and the patient is recommended to have another check-up 5–7 days after the operation if heparin is administered for more than 5 days.

In Spain, low-molecular-weight heparin is given as a rule to every patient for 7 days after saphenous vein sparing surgery [3].

Independently of the different country customs applying anticoagulation after surgery, it is important to keep in mind that after the first step of CHIVA 2 a superficial vein thrombosis of the proximal saphenous segment could progress into the deep vein, and therefore preventive anticoagulation has to be installed after surgery, especially if the saphenous vein is dilated.

11.4.2 Compression

The indication for post-operative compression after venous sparing strategy differs from that after venous ablation. After stripping or endothermal heat ablation and phlebectomy, compression is given for oedema and haematoma reduction, thus, to reduce the pain level. After stripping, all the enlarged veins have been removed, so the compression does no longer target the veins themselves.

In case of venous sparing surgery, compression targets the treated veins: their calibre is large at first, but they carry less blood than before the intervention because the recirculation volume has been eliminated. Thus, compression takes on the role of prophylaxis against thrombosis in the superficial leg veins. The external pressure prevents the distended veins from filling when the patient is standing, reducing the flow turbulence as far as possible. This reduces the residence time of the blood in the veins. It also assists vein regeneration, since contraction of the vein wall is accelerated if distension is avoided. The period of postsurgical recovery of the vein tonus depends on the preoperative distension.

The patient is fitted with a compression stocking on the operation table. This is kept on for the first night, but thereafter it need only be worn during the day. The legs do not need to be bandaged, as there is no significant danger of secondary bleeding or haematoma formation.

The following parameters must be observed for compression:

- Compression class: Depending on the countries' and the patient's settings, compression stockings with either 15–22 or 22–32 mmHg at the ankle should be selected.
- Length of the stocking: The highest reflux source must be compressed by the stocking. It is known that compression stockings cannot apply a very high pressure on the thigh, but at the top edge of the compression stocking however, the pressure difference from stocking to no stocking is quite enough to cause a reduction in the calibre of the superficial leg veins, which can lead to thrombosis. The upper edge of the compression stocking should therefore never lie across the course of a treated vein (see Fig. 11.5). Compression tights or a long compression stocking up to the groin is recommended after treatment of great saphenous vein or perforators at the thigh region. In case of treatment of the small saphenous vein, a thigh stocking is necessary in most of the

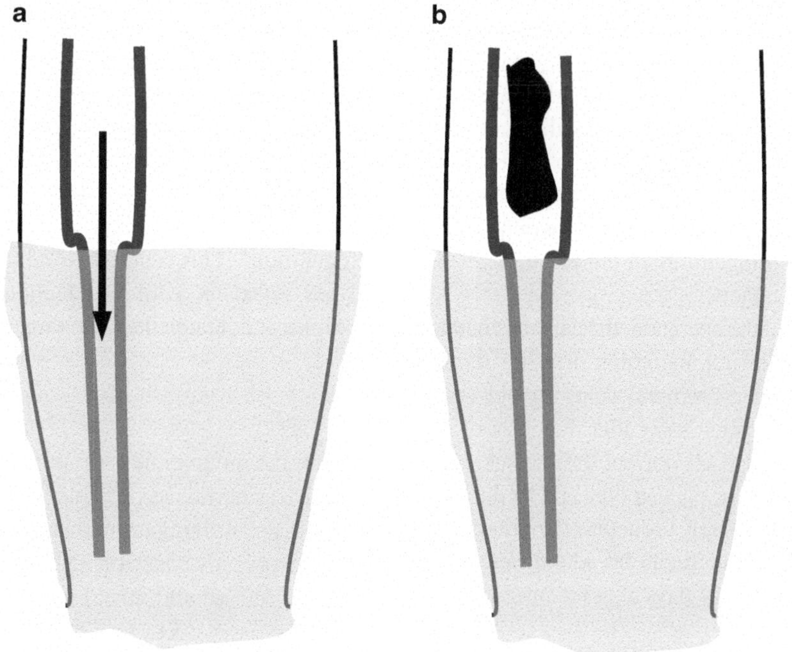

Fig. 11.5 (**a**) Diagram of a thigh with compression stocking reaching only up to mid-thigh after disconnection of the sapheno-femoral junction. The blood from thigh tributaries is draining towards the perforators at distal thigh and below knee (arrowed). The top edge of the compression stocking causes a reduction in the calibre of the treated but still distended vein. (**b**) The diameter change increases the risk of superficial vein thrombosis higher up the leg. A thrombus is shown in the vein. With Permission by [10]

cases, as the incision to treat the junction is performed in the knee fold and a knee-long stocking would not cover the region.
- Compression period: Depending on the severity of the clinics, we recommend wearing compression for 4–6 weeks after the operation. The leg should be free of compression for 1–2 weeks before the post-operative examination, to make it easier to identify any varicose connections, which may arise in duplex ultrasound. In cases of deep vein insufficiency, venous ulcer, or advanced chronic venous insufficiency, use of the compression stocking must of course be continued, even before the post-operative examination.

11.4.3 Adjunctive Prescription

As a rule, very little discomfort is caused by operation under local anaesthetic. The alternative of general anaesthesia is available for fearful patients. If pain or nervousness arise in the context of an operation under local anaesthetic, the anaesthesia can be supplemented intraoperatively with painkillers and/or an anxiolytic agent, depending on the nervousness or pain suffered by the patient.

On the day of the operation, the author gives the patient two tablets of paracetamol 500 mg, in case of immediate pain from the wounds after surgery. According to an in-house survey, only 21% need the tablets.

On the day of the operation, the patient is handed out a prescription for ibuprofen 400 mg in case thrombosis of the superficial veins should occur. Taking this medication soon after the onset of distress it will not of itself prevent thrombosis, but it can clearly reduce the pain amount and its duration. If the patient has strongly pronounced tributary convolutes, this medication can be administered as a prophylactic in the first days after the operation.

11.5 Post-operative Lifestyle Indications

Even if the patient is operated under local anaesthetic, we recommend against eating or drinking for a few hours before the operation, in case of an allergic reaction or other complications, which would make intubation necessary. The patient must also be warned that he is not allowed to drive for 24 h after the administration of local anaesthetics (under German law). He must therefore arrange to be collected or use public transport to return home.

The patient will be mobile immediately after the operation. He should walk for half an hour immediately after the operation to prevent the risk of superficial and deep vein thrombosis. The wounds may then be checked again for bleeding. The patient can then normally leave the office or hospital and can return to work the following day. Only patients whose jobs require them to lift heavy weights (including nursing staff!) should be given 1 weeks' sick leave or a medical certificate saying that they must not lift heavy weights. Lifting heavy weights may prejudice vein regeneration, especially after tributary disconnection only (CHIVA 2).

The patient is informed about the possibilities of bleeding, haematoma formation, and superficial vein thrombosis formation. In case one of these occurs, the patient is given a contact telephone number where he can request further information or is asked to return to the hospital, if the treatment was performed there.

On the day of the operation, we give every patient a sheet "What I can and cannot do after the operation". This is very helpful for the patient and has saved us a lot of telephone calls with questions. It contains the following information:

> After the intervention, it is important to behave as normal as possible. Usually there is no pain; walking around and doing usual homework are possible without restrictions. You should avoid carrying heavy weights (over 20 kg) to avoid haematoma formation in the first week. If possible, take walks of about 20–30 min twice or three times a day in the first week.
>
> If you are returning home by car over a long distance, please ask the driver to stop after every 30 min to have a little walk.

The plaster can be taken off 2 days after surgery and replaced by a new one. You can take showers 48 h after surgery; bathing is not allowed for 14 days. Seven days after surgery, the stitches have to be removed.

Compression stockings should be worn the first night and then throughout the day for 6 weeks. Please stay without compression at least 1 week before returning to the next ultrasound control.

If heparin was prescribed, please inject it every day at the same time.

In case of pain and reddening along the treated vein, a superficial vein thrombosis has to be suspected. Please start taking ibuprofen 400 mg up to three times a day after a meal immediately to reduce the pain, and contact us in case the pain did not reduce significantly after 1 day.

Please return to the scheduled visit after 2–3 months.

11.6 Surgical Management in Special Situations

Saphenous vein sparing principles are always a good option to treat a patient, because of less side effects and less recidives (see Chap. 10). But in some cases, the indication to harm less is most important, like in obese patients with comorbidities, multi-morbidity, anticoagulation, legs with infections like in the case of venous ulcers, and, above all, arterial disease that would benefit from a recovered saphenous vein to be used as a bypass later on.

11.6.1 Treatment of Obese Patients

The number of obese patients is ascending all around the world. Surgery of varicose veins in these patients is a challenge, as the veins run much deeper in the leg, they often suffer co-morbidities and are very difficult to be fitted with compression stockings.

Nevertheless, in case of reflux and obesity, the progression of skin changes at the ankle will be quicker, as the lymphatic flow reduction due to obesity plays a synergistic role.

These patients are special cases where the tissue lesion should be as little as possible to reduce infection risk and the surgery time as short as possible to reduce thrombus formation. The best choice is to close only the proximal insufficiency point, if possible with endothermal heat avoiding large incisions, and then wait for calibre reduction in the veins and decide in a second investigation some months after the first, if further steps have to be taken.

11.6.2 Treatment of Patients with High Risk of Bleeding

Atrial fibrillation and other diseases make it necessary to take anticoagulating agents. Surgery of varicose veins in these patients should be the less aggressive as possible. So, these patients are perfectly fitted with saphenous sparing surgery, as no stripping channel with haematoma formation will be produced. A simple Crossotomy can be performed under anticoagulation, as well as the endoluminal heat treatment of the sapheno-femoral or sapheno-popliteal junctions. Tributary disconnections without phlebectomies are possible under anticoagulation, too.

11.6.3 Treatment of Patients with Venous Ulceration

Chronic venous ulcers are always contaminated with bacteria. This increases the risk of infection in case of surgery with subfascial wound formation like stripping and SEPS (subfascial endoscopic perforator surgery). Venous ulcers caused by superficial venous reflux mostly depend on reflux at the junctions or large perforators. Most often the simple disconnection of these reflux sources will lead to ulcus healing without the need of stripping or ablating veins.

Zamboni et al. could demonstrate the superiority of CHIVA against compression alone in case of leg ulceration [4]; see Sect. 10.2.1.

11.6.4 Treatment of Patients with Arterial Disease

Patients with arterial obstructive disease and varicose veins always present a challenge. Clearly, they should not be caused any unnecessary wounds. Patients with severe arterial obstruction must not be treated conventionally with compression stockings. But in case of mixed ulcers, the treatment of the venous disease often improves the clinical situation significantly, sometimes allowing an arterial revascularization after reducing the risk of infection operating on a leg with a chronic wound.

Most often ulcerations occur in case of incompetent saphenous junctions. They can be treated easily with endoluminal heat occlusion without producing skin incisions. If arterial flow in the thigh is good, and only worsens in the lower leg, then a crossectomy is perfectly feasible. There is no fear of poor healing of a wound in the groin in these patients, so long as arterial flow is still good in this region. The closure of the reflux point will lead to a healing of the ulcer in most of the cases.

Post-operative compression will be applied depending on the arterial perfusion. In worst cases, no compression will do.

It is particularly important to maintain saphenous veins for bypass material in these patients, so these patients present with special indications to perform saphenous sparing surgery.

11.7 Complication Identification and Management

Duplex examination before the operation is sometimes stressful for the patient. The examination often takes quite a long time, especially in the learning phase of the doctor. Some patients may need to lie down due to orthostatic problems, requiring the examination to be interrupted. This problem is particularly common in summer.

Every surgical treatment is susceptible of provoking complications. Compared to the ablative strategy, the venous sparing strategy per definition causes less destruction of tissues, and so the risk of complications is much less than after all the other surgical therapeutic options of vein treatment.

The only complication, which is typical of the CHIVA method, is thrombosis of saphenous trunk veins, which is generally asymptomatic, except for the case of large superficial veins prior to treatment [2]. This can of course also occur after stripping—there is no longer any proximal backflow in the saphenous veins after correctly performed stripping. Thrombosis in the tributaries left in place, which is known from stripping operations, is likewise observed with CHIVA.

11.7.1 General Complications

General surgical complications, like bleeding, haematoma, lymph cyst, and thrombosis, may occur after any type of surgery but are less often after CHIVA as demonstrated in the Cochrane review [5]. The patient must be able to contact someone of the team of the surgeon in case of questions or pain, bleeding, or haematoma. If necessary, a physical investigation is performed, and a duplex investigation might enlighten the problem. The treating team has to be able to cope with complications by themselves or cooperate with a centre able to do so.

11.7.2 Superficial Vein Thrombosis

Superficial vein thrombosis is the most frequent post-operative complication, occurring in around 10% of patients [2]—in saphenous veins and/or tributaries. It is caused by alterations in their haemodynamics: after the interruption of the reflux source, a large-calibre vessel is left with a clearly reduced blood flow. Compression and movement are the best prophylactic measures to keep the veins well drained and to enhance the retonification of the vein wall, as well as heparin in prophylactic doses. Sometimes an ill-fitting compression stocking can cause superficial vein thrombosis, if differences in pressure occur along the course of the vein (Sect. 11.4.2).

In some patients, thrombosis occurs in subcutaneous tributaries above the knee joint. In these cases, it is necessary to check whether the stocking forms fold at the knee, as these folds may constrict the vein if the patient sits or crouches for a long time. In these cases, the best treatment for thrombosis in the great saphenous vein or the tributary is to remove the ill-fitting compression.

Thrombus of the saphenous vein occurs in up to 10–15% of the cases [2, 3], but interestingly most patients present no symptoms of superficial vein thrombosis—it is only noticed in the post-operative examination. The most frequent setting is after closure of the junction and simultaneously distal tributaries, if the saphenous vein is left with too little flow volume in relation to its diameter. After CHIVA 2 with interruption of the tributary flush at the saphenous vein, a thrombus in the saphenous vein might occur if the distal saphenous vein is very small calibre. In this case, a thrombus progression to the deep vein is possible.

If the superficial thrombosis causes distress, it generally disappears after 1 or 2 days under administration of an anti-inflammatory drug as soon as pain is noticed—e.g. give ibuprofen, 3 × 400 mg/day. Local measures such as chilling and the application of anti-inflammatory creams can help. Prescription of heparin may be considered for patients with severe pain during thrombosis of the tributaries, which does not become asymptomatic within a few days under anti-inflammatory drugs and for those with symptomatic thrombi in the saphenous vein after closure of the junction. In case of patent junctions, heparin is mandatory to prevent ascension.

11.8 Follow-Up Timeline

The operation can be carried out at any time of year, although it is more uncomfortable for the patient to wear a compression stocking after the operation in summer.

Vein regeneration is assessed approximately 8 weeks to 6 months after the operation, as it is not complete until then. After this period, it is possible to decide whether a further operation is necessary or if the patient only needs to come in again for check-ups.

The follow-up timeline depends on the healthcare system. It is mandatory to have the patient checked until the treatment is ready that means sometimes after a second intervention in case of CHIVA in two steps. Afterwards, often the surgery team has no possibilities to see the patient, until a recidivant vein appears and the follow-up is performed by other centres for diagnostics or of ambulatory assistance.

The patient should be seen after 1 year and then depending on the evolution after 5 and 10 years.

11.9 Outcome Measures

The first outcome measures applied in studies were those described by Hobbs, to make CHIVA results comparable to stripping series (see Chap. 10). Hobbs [6] divided the subjective result of the patient and the objective findings after surgery into:

- Cured
- Improvement
- No changes
- Worse

Other measures applied in further studies are duplex investigation of reflux in visible veins and cartography of reflux point as in the preoperative investigation.

Diameter at proximal thigh preoperatively and in the evolution after surgery will first show a clear reduction [7–9] and then could possibly be used as a marker of recurrence, if again increasing. The diameter decrease of the common femoral vein after CHIVA has also shown that the deep vein diameter reduction follows the varicose vein treatment. Thus, the measurement of the diameter of the common femoral vein could orientate to a recurrence when increasing in the follow-up timeline.

Some authors apply plethysmography as a global measurement in study situations, which has shown to improve significantly after CHIVA [7–9].

Literature

1. Franceschi C. Théorie et Pratique de la Cure Conservatrice et Hémodynamique de l'Insuffisance Veineuse en Ambulatoire. Armançon: Précy-sous-Thil; 1988
2. Pintos T, Senin E, Ramos R, Rodríguez E, Martínez-Pérez M. Trombosis de safena interna post- CHIVA. Incidencia, factores condicionantes y repercusiones clínicas. Presented at the XLVII National Congress of the Spanish Society of Angiology and Vascular Surgery, Valladolid; 2001.
3. Juan J, Escribano JM, Criado E, Fontcuberta J. Haemodynamic surgery for varicose veins: surgical strategy. Phlebology. 2005;20(1):2–13.
4. Zamboni P, Cisno C, Marchetti F, Mazza P, Fogato L, Carandina S, De Palma M, Liboni A. Minimally invasive surgical treatment of primary venous ulcers vs compression treatment: a randomized trial. Eur J Endovasc Surg. 2003;25(4):313–8.
5. Bellmunt-Montoya S, Escribano JM, Dilme J, Martinez-Zapata MJ. CHIVA method for the treatment of chronic venous insufficiency. Cochrane Database Syst Rev. 2013,(2):CD009648. https://doi.org/10.1002/14651858.CD009648.
6. Hobbs JT. Surgery and sclerotherapy in the treatment of varicose veins. A random trial. Arch Surg. 1974;109:793–6.
7. Mendoza E, Berger V, Zollmann C, Bomhoff M, Amsler F. Kaliberreduktion der V. saphena magna und der V. femoralis communis nach CHIVA. Phlebologie. 2011;40(2):73–8.
8. Mendoza E. Diameter reduction of the great saphenous vein and the common femoral vein after CHIVA long-term results. Phlebologie. 2013;42:65–9.
9. Mendoza E, Amsler F. CHIVA with endoluminal procedures: LASER versus VNUS—treatment of the saphenofemoral junction. Phlebologie. 2017;46:5–12.
10. Mendoza E. Handbuch CHIVA. Arrien GmbH; 2002.

Part III

Other Venous Sparing Techniques

Ambulatory Selective Varices Ablation Under Local Anaesthesia (ASVAL)

12

Paul Pittaluga and Sylvain Chastanet

12.1 History

For many decades, the so-called "radical" therapeutic approach to varicose disease has aimed to eliminate saphenous reflux using surgical treatment combining crossectomy and stripping of the saphenous vein as a reference [1, 2]. This first treatment fits in with the traditional physiopathological description of varicose disease, which is considered to develop from the junctions between the deep venous system and the saphenous veins. According to this theory, the appearance of reflux at the terminal valve of the saphenous vein is the key point in the progression of saphenous insufficiency, leading to the appearance of varicose veins in the collaterals throughout the saphenous veins from the top to the bottom [3, 4].

The description of a new haemodynamic theory of varicose disease treatment by Franceschi at the end of the 1980s [5] has been an exception among the mainstream concept for pathophysiology.

It was research into a less invasive approach to surgical treatment in the late twentieth century that led to the appearance of new methods and techniques, with the option of the endovascular route just as with arterial surgery, using thermal laser energy or radiofrequency [6, 7]. At the same time, sclerotherapy was revolutionized by the use of foam sclerosants which are considerably more effective in larger veins [8–10] and which therefore provided a serious competitor to traditional surgical and endovenous techniques.

These technique developments took place without calling into question the principle behind surgical treatment, namely, the systematic ablation of the refluxing saphenous vein, which is supposed to be responsible for the appearance of varices in its collaterals. However, to make procedures less invasive, crossectomy no longer accompanied thermal ablation or sclerotherapy of the saphenous vein. This technique-related "detail" caused the utility of crossectomy—which was indissociable from traditional surgical treatment—to be called into question. The absence of direct elimination of ostial reflux led to the relevance of the descending haemodynamic theory of varicose disease with progression from the saphenous vein being called into question [11]. This was supported by a work based on increased haemodynamic understanding, thanks to developments in ultrasound technology [12–17]. Some observations support the idea that varicose disease develops from the distal superficial venous network in an ascending or a multifocal way [11–17] and that the elimination of varicose tributaries can lead to the reduction of the diameter of the saphenous vein or the disappearance of the saphenous vein reflux [18–20]. A mini-invasive surgical approach has therefore

P. Pittaluga, M.D. (✉) • S. Chastanet, M.D.
Riviera Veine Institut, Monaco, France

P. Zamboni et al. (eds.), *Saphenous Vein-Sparing Strategies in Chronic Venous Disease*,
https://doi.org/10.1007/978-3-319-70638-2_12

appeared, based on treatment of the superficial varicose reservoir by means of phlebectomy and conservation of the saphenous vein, even if the saphenous vein presents reflux [11, 21, 22]. Supporters of this conservative approach cite the physiological role played by the saphenous vein, as well as the haemodynamic and clinical efficacy in the midterm of a rigorous isolated resection of the superficial varicose reservoir, in addition to the benefit to preserve the saphenous vein as a potential material for a coronary or a distal arterial bypass in the patient's future.

12.2 Theoretical Foundations: Principles of Treatment

12.2.1 Theoretical Foundations of ASVAL

The "haemodynamic hypothesis" is based on the idea of upstream saphenous vein insufficiency being caused by insufficiency of the terminal valves of the saphenous vein or the valves in the perforating femoral veins. This theory has been widely accepted for a long time, but it is now being called into question by the well-substantiated arguments put forwards by supporters of the "parietal hypothesis". These arguments essentially concern an initial alteration to the venous wall leading to venous dilation, which in turn causes incontinence of the valves as their leaflets no longer meet properly [23–26]. A new physiopathological concept has been mentioned recently: varicose disease could come about at the level of the epifascial tributaries, which are the most superficial and the most exposed and whose walls are the thinnest [27]. The epifascial veins could be the first to dilate through decompensation of their parietal weakness. Progression could initially remain epifascial, creating a dilated and refluxing venous network. When this refluxing network becomes large enough, it could create a "filling" effect in the subfascial saphenous vein, leading to the decompensation of the saphenous vein wall, moving forwards to reach the saphenofemoral or saphenopopliteal junction (see Fig. 12.1).

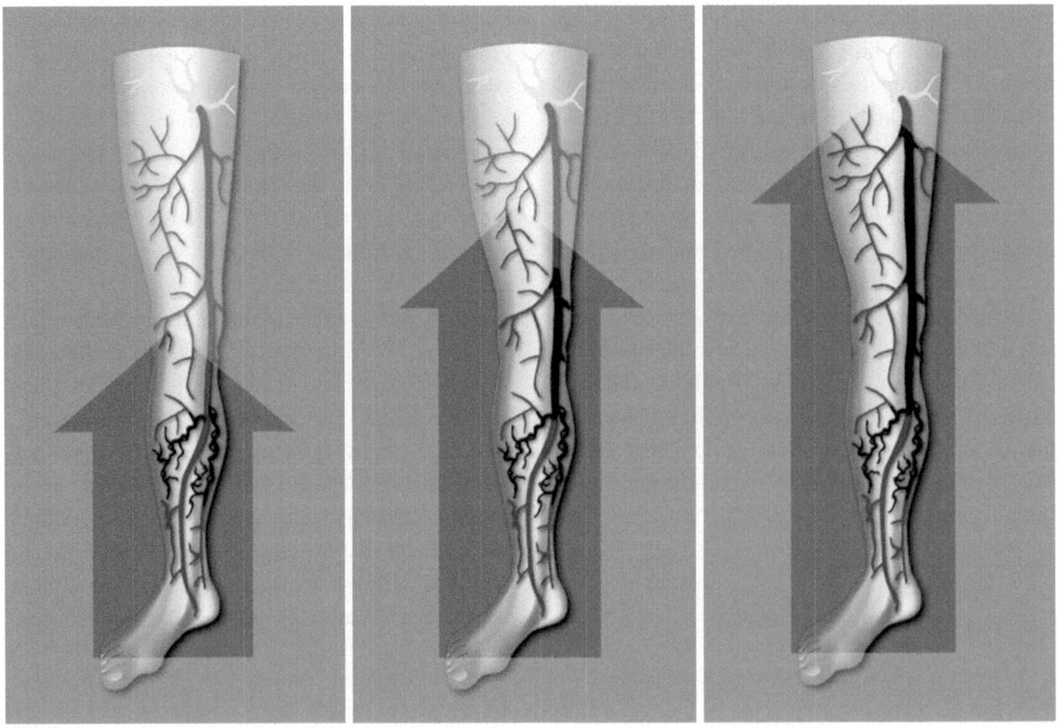

Fig. 12.1 Concept of ascending evolution of the varicose disease. With permission In Bergan JJ ed. Foam sclerotherapy London: The Royal Society of Medicine Press, 2008, pp. 163–176

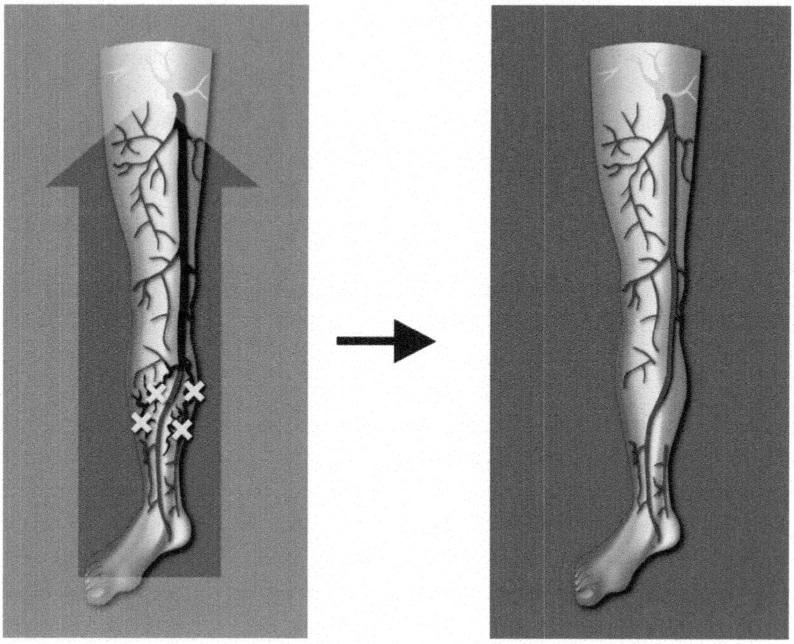

Fig. 12.2 Haemodynamic effect on the great saphenous vein of the treatment by ASVAL technique. The yellow "x" on the left image refers to the veins that are ablated. With permission: In Bergan JJ ed. Foam sclerotherapy. London: The Royal Society of Medicine Press, 2008, pp. 163–176

The saphenous vein is the superficial vein with the thickest and most muscular wall. Furthermore, the saphenous vein is protected by the splitting of the subcutaneous fascia in which it flows. It would therefore be the last vein to experience decompensation as varicose disease progressed. The fact that the ostial valve is frequently continent (>50%) when there is trunk reflux has been clearly proven [28]. Numerous publications challenge the theory of descending progression, citing the possibility of local or multifocal early distal evolution, sometimes ascending or anterograde, based on precise and detailed echo-Doppler explorations.

12.2.2 Therapeutic Principle of ASVAL

This physiopathological theory has two consequences:

1. If there is no saphenous vein reflux, early treatment of all varicose tributaries that define the varicose reservoir would be useful in order to prevent the reflux to spread to the saphenous vein.
2. If there is saphenous vein reflux, and up until a certain stage of the disease, first-line therapy should include ablation of the varicose reservoir and not elimination of the saphenous reflux which is potentially reversible (see Fig. 12.2).

Saphenous stripping or ablation would only be indicated in cases for which saphenous reflux seems to be irreversible. This approach therefore involves selective management of superficial venous reflux, depending on the clinical and haemodynamic context found in each case.

The main argument in favour of this saphenous-sparing approach is the physiological **role that the saphenous vein could play in superficial drainage and, to a lesser extent, its availability as revascularization material. In the literature, there are reports of the harmful effect that resection of the saphenous vein has on the long-term progression of saphenous vein insufficiency** [18].

12.3 Evaluation of the Patient

12.3.1 Technique of Evaluation

The evaluation of the patient is performed by a clinical examination and by a duplex ultrasound assessment both performed with the patient standing upright.

For the clinical examination technique, each lower limb is divided into four surface areas (anterior, posterior, lateral, and medial), and then each surface area was divided in eight zones: the thigh into three zones (the upper third, middle third, and lower third), the calf into three zones (the upper third, middle third, and lower third), plus one zone for the knee and one zone for the foot. Therefore, each limb is divided into 32 zones in the preoperative clinical mapping (Fig. 12.3). On the virgin figure, the varicose veins are drawn that are visible or palpable during the examination of each side, and the number of zones in which varicose veins are present is counted. The total number of zones is called the number of zones to be treated (NZT) by phlebectomy. In the example in Fig. 12.4, the NZT is seven, which means that there are seven zones occupied by varicose veins. The extent of the varicose reservoir is evaluated according to this NZT.

The duplex ultrasound scanning uses the manual venous flushing manoeuvre in the calf region, and venous haemodynamics are recorded at the moment of the sudden release of manual compression of the calf. Under these conditions, a reflux is considered to be pathological if the reflux duration (RD) exceeds 0.5 s for the superficial veins and 1 s for the deep veins.

12.3.2 Selection of Patients Eligible for ASVAL

According to more than 10 years of experience, and according to the results published in literature, we can bring out some simple tools in order to determine the patients that will profit from ASVAL:

1. Haemodynamic/anatomical criteria
   (a) Saphenous vein reflux patterns: The presence of a competent junction or of a segmental saphenous vein reflux [17, 21, 27, 31], a saphenous vein reflux limited at the thigh [21, 22, 31], and a limited dilatation of the saphenous vein [21, 27]
   (b) The reflux elimination test (RET) is considered as positive if the reflux of the saphenous vein is completely abolished by the compression of the varicose tributary at the moment of the sudden release of manual compression on the calf, during a duplex ultrasound examination performed with the patient standing upright. The positive predictive value of the RET for the abolition of reflux of the great saphenous vein has been reported as 95.7% and 94.7% at 1 and 2 years of follow-up [29, 30].
2. Clinical and demographic data
   (a) The extent of the varicose reservoir is a determinant factor for the haemodynamic and clinical efficiency of ASVAL [27]. A significant linear trend between the outcomes after ASVAL and the NZT has been shown [1].
   (b) The presence of a unique or limited number of varicose tributaries, especially at the thigh, increases the likelihood for the freedom of varicose vein recurrence at midterm [21]
   (c) The nulliparity is a criterion that should be taken in account for the preservation of the saphenous vein in young women. The benefit of the ASVAL treatment for nullipara patients has been reported for the reduction of complexity, signs, and symptoms in the event of varicose vein recurrence after pregnancy [29].
   (d) The young age [27] and the absence of symptoms with a cosmetic concern [27, 31] are also criteria that plead in favour of the preservation of the saphenous vein.
3. Predictive Score
   Biemans et al. [21] have reported a PREST prediction model including CEAP classification, number of refluxing segments, great saphenous vein diameter (above the tributary), and RET result, in order to give a preoperative score that correlates with a probability of restoring great saphenous vein competence. For example, for patients with great saphenous vein reflux in one segment (3 points), C2 (3 points), positive reflux

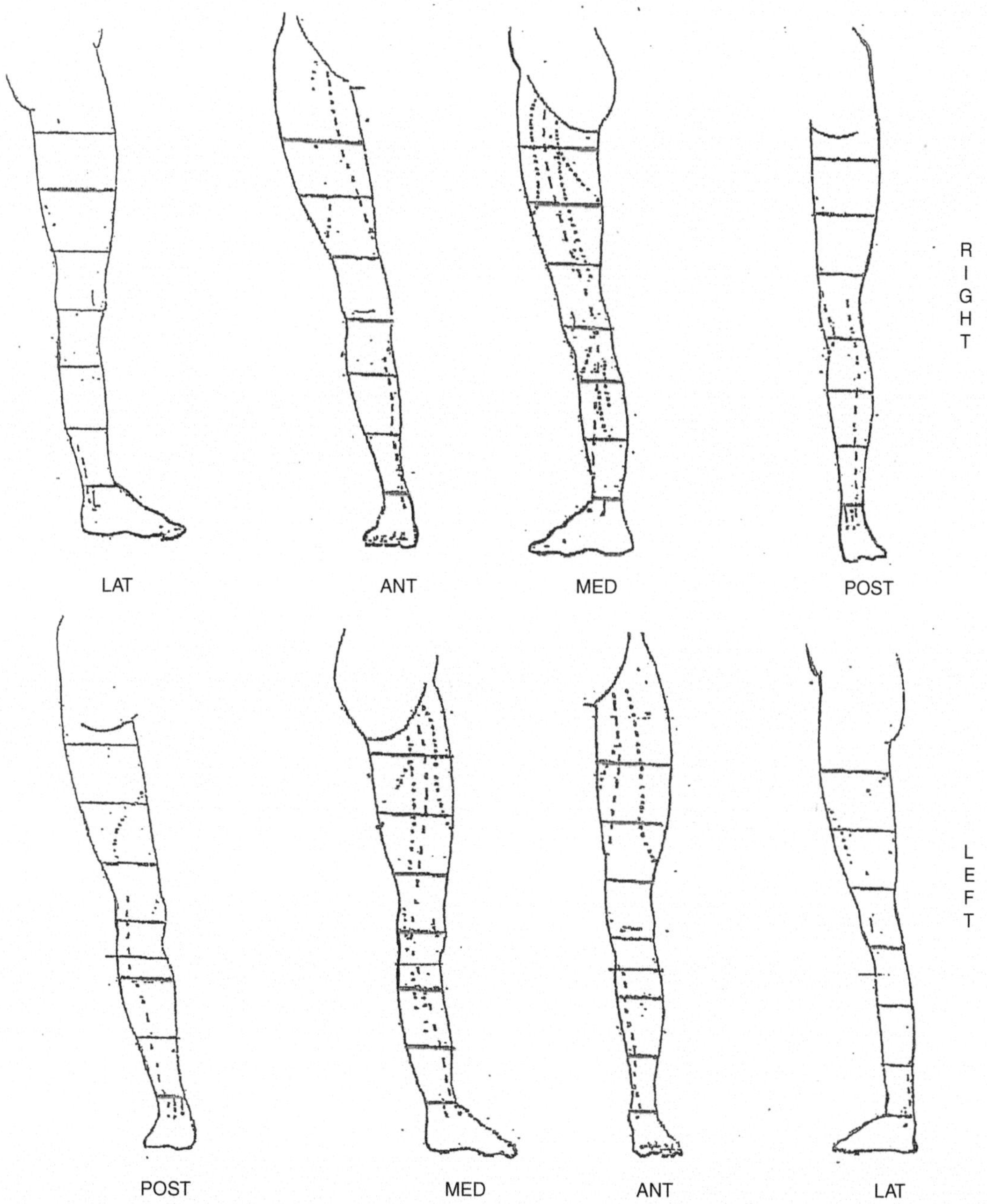

Fig. 12.3 Diagram used for the preoperative mapping during the clinical examination. Copyright: [Paul Pittaluga]

elimination test result (2 points), and great saphenous vein diameter of 5 mm at proximal thigh (approx. 15 cm away from the sapheno-femoral junction) (6 points), the model can predict that phlebectomy will be effective in 90% (total of 14 points).

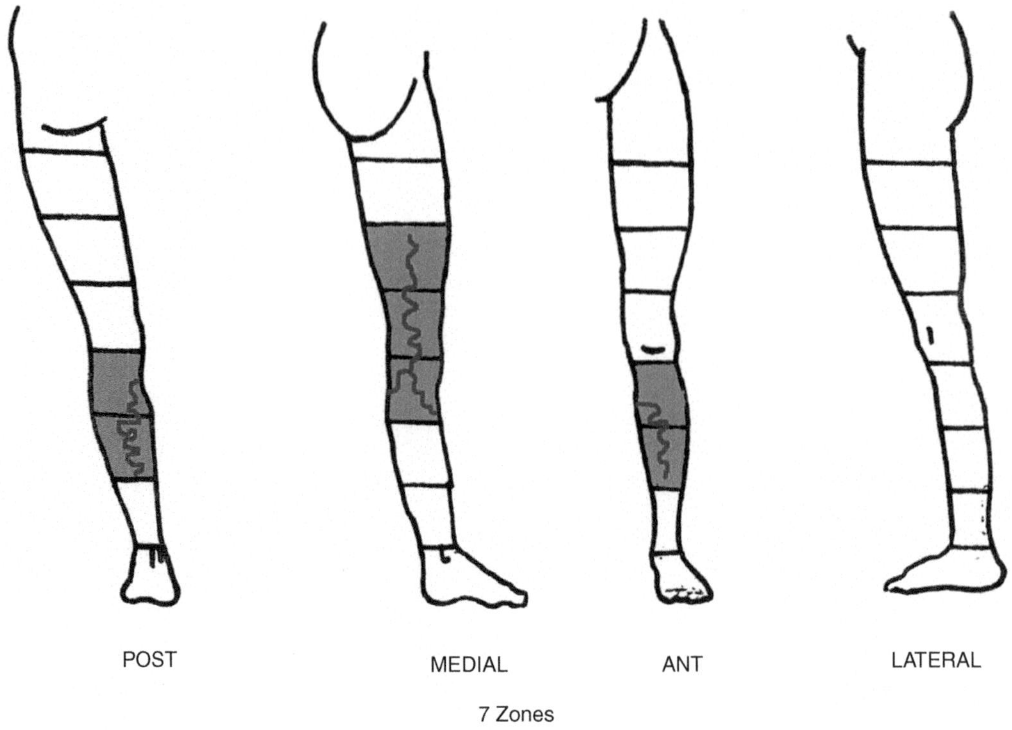

Fig. 12.4 Example of varicose veins with seven number of zones to be treated (NZT). With kind permission by Elsevier from: Pittaluga P, Chastanet S, Rea B, Barbe R "Midterm results of the surgical treatment of varices by phlebectomy with conservation of a refluxing saphenous vein". J Vasc Surg 2009;50: 107–118

12.4 Surgical Technique

12.4.1 Preoperative Skin Marking

Skin marking before the surgery is mandatory to perform a thorough ablation of the varicose reservoir, which is essential since we have reported that the removal of a large varicose reservoir is one of the keys to get good clinical and haemodynamic result after ASVAL [27]. A precise skin marking enables a more precise and less aggressive surgical gesture, enabling to reduce the risk of lymphatic complication after varicose vein surgery [32]. Ideally this skin marking should be done by the surgeon treating the patient. The first step of the skin marking procedure has to be done by clinical examination with the marking of visible and palpable varicose veins, followed by the ultrasound location of deeper veins (subfascial veins or epifascial veins in obese patients) as complement of the clinical marking (Fig. 12.5). It is advised to store the picture of the skin marking before the surgery.

12.4.2 Tumescent Local Anaesthesia

Tumescent local anaesthesia is essential for the performance of the surgical procedure for ASVAL. It is very efficient for the pain abolition, and it reduces dramatically the bleeding by the subcutaneous high pressure, thanks to a large infiltration of liquid. It gives to the surgeon an excellent comfort for removing the varicose veins. It has been reported that the use of isotonic bicarbonate improves furthermore the efficiency of the lidocaine and allows to reduce the total amount of lidocaine, enabling to inject large

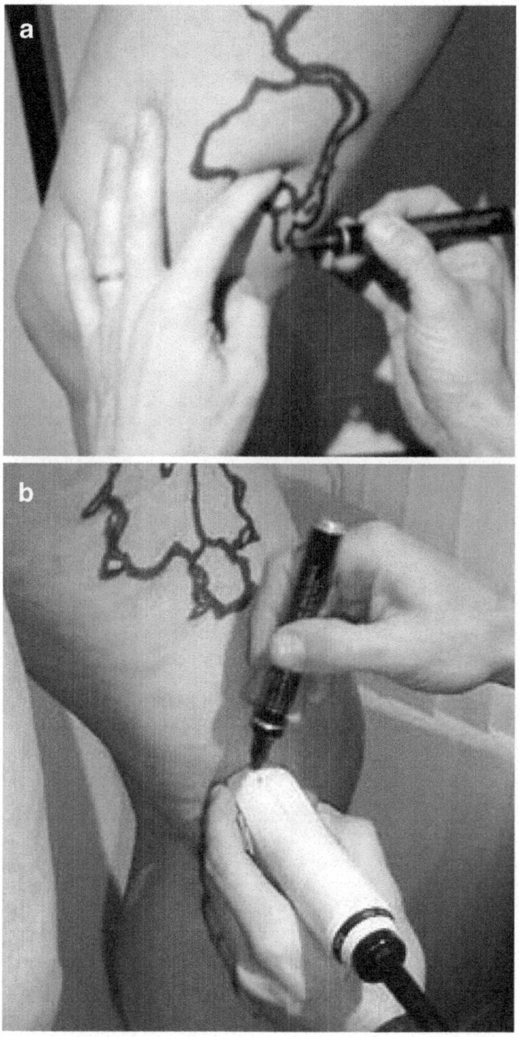

Fig. 12.5 The two consecutive steps of the preoperative skin marking: (**a**) (left) 1st clinical marking. (**b**) (right) 2nd ultrasound marking. Copyright: [Paul Pittaluga]

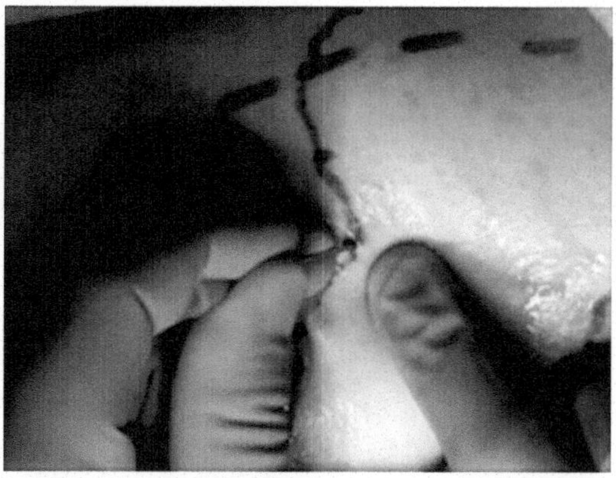

Fig. 12.6 Technique applying ASVAL: After exact skin marking and application of tumescent anaesthesia, little incisions are performed with an 18-gauge needle making a skin flap. Copyright: [Paul Pittaluga]

volume of tumescence and therefore to treat a large surface on the lower limb [33].

12.4.3 Microsurgical Technique

The varicose veins are extracted by micro-phlebectomy. The use of magnificent glasses is mandatory to perform the micro-phlebectomy properly. The incisions are done with an 18-gauge needle (see Fig. 12.6). The bevel of the needle makes a flap on the skin that facilitates the penetration of the hook through the skin and gives an excellent cosmetic result (Fig. 12.7). As it is a tangential flap, the skin healing will be invisible. In the authors' experience, the best tool is the Muller hook n°0. The phlebectomy should be atraumatic, thanks to a precise skin marking that enables to make the micro-incision directly above the vein, avoiding the scraping of the subcutaneous tissues with the hook to get the veins. In order to get the best cosmetic result, it is recommended to avoid leaving a piece of varicose, since it limits the risk of staining. The force of pulling should be gently exerted in the axis of the vein (and not perpendicularly) so to pull out the entire segment of the vein without rupture between two incisions (Fig. 12.8).

12.4.4 Postoperative Management

The use of stiches is not necessary, thanks to the limited size of the micro-incisions performed with the 18-gauge needle. Stretch sterile strips are recommended in order to avoid blisters. The patient is invited to walk immediately at the end of the procedure and can usually leave the hospital or office 1 h after the end of the procedure.

In the authors' experience, wearing of compression stockings is not necessary after the first 24 h following a mini-invasive procedure [34].

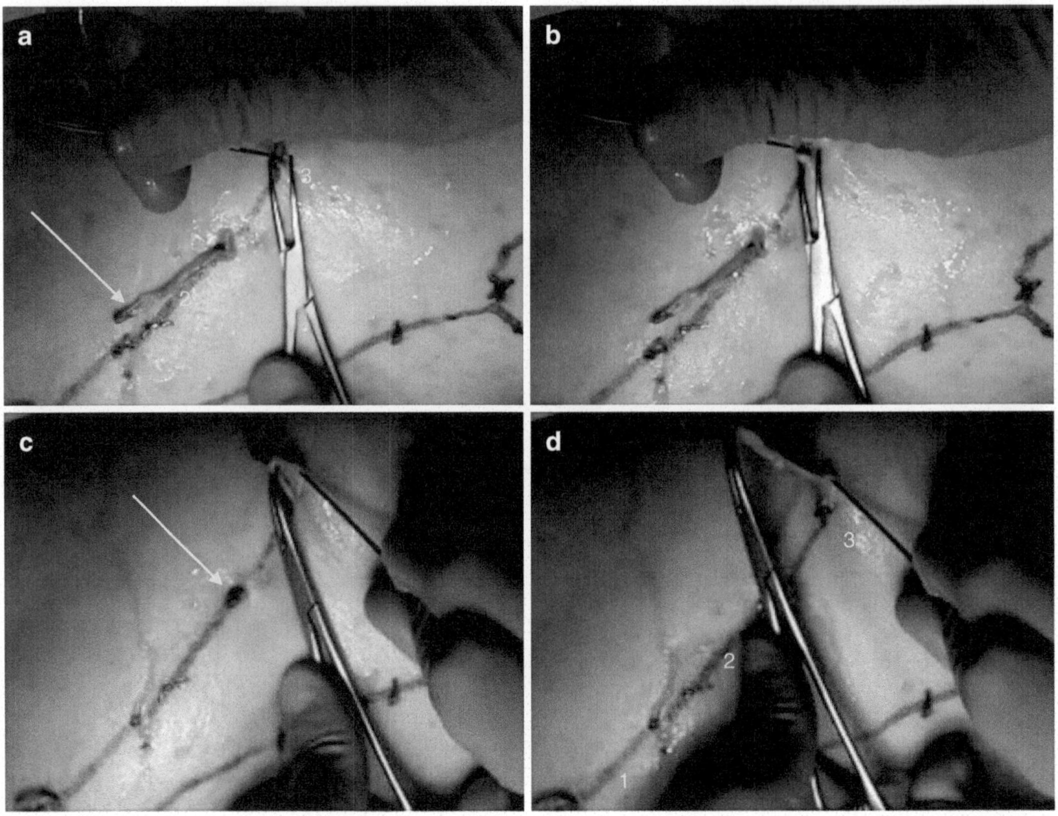

Fig. 12.7 Technique for vein extraction. Between incisions 1 and 2, the vein segment has already been extracted (arrow); now the hook is inserted in incision number 3. (**a**) The first segment of the vein is already extracted (arrow). Introduction of the hook in the next incision place. (**b**) The vein is emerging through the skin flap at position 3 (see **a**); the mosquito clamp is used to fix the skin down and gently pull the vein outside the little skin lesion. (**c**) The mosquito clamp is used to pull the vein out after a loop of the vein is visible on the surface; note that the visible vein in image a has disappeared through incision 2 (arrow), because the vein is being pulled out through to the next incision. (**d**) The vein is now completely extracted through incision number 3. Copyright: [Paul Pittaluga]

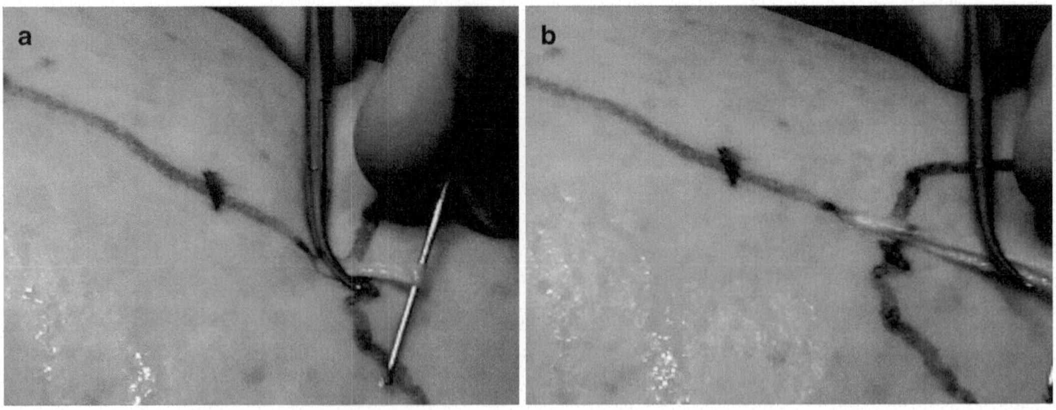

Fig. 12.8 (**a**) Extraction of the varicose tributary at the last incision by a gentle force of pulling exerted in the axis of the vein in order to take out the entire segment of the vein without rupture between two incisions. (**b**) A vein loop can be seen emerging from the skin incision. (**c**) The vein is extracted completely. (**d**) Checking that the full length of the vein has been extracted. Copyright: Paul Pittaluga, with kind permission from Tips & tricks in angiology. Eds: C. Allegra, P.L. Antignani, E. Kalodiki. Edizioni Minerva Medic, Torino, 2016, 161–165

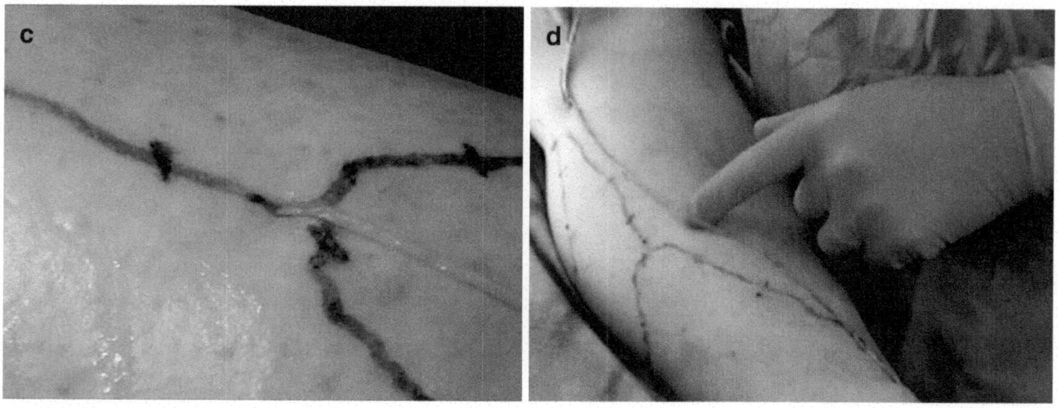

Fig. 12.8 (continued)

12.5 Results Published in Literature

Since the publication of the preliminary results of the ASVAL method (303 lower limbs with a mean follow-up period of 7 months) [11], with a disappearance of the saphenous vein reflux in 69.1%, a relief of symptoms in 91.8%, and a cosmetic benefit in 90.4%, this initial cohort has been followed up regularly, and the medium-term results were published [27] and are shown in Table 12.1. The abolition of the saphenous vein reflux at 4 years was observed in 66.3% of the limbs, and the diameter of the saphenofemoral junction significantly decreased, as measured at the saphenous confluence, in 243 lower limbs after 6 months (5.87 vs. 7.87 mm preoperatively, $P < 0.0001$). Symptom relief after 4 years was still present in 78.0%. Mean venous disability score was significantly lower at 6 months postoperatively for the symptomatic limbs (0.64 vs 1.30 preoperatively, $P < 0.001$) and remained until the 4th year of follow-up. At last, the freedom of varicose vein recurrence in the treated lower limbs was 88.5% after 4 years. In this study, we found a significant link between the NZT and the postoperative evolution of saphenous reflux and existence of symptom relief: when the NZT was above seven, an abolition of the saphenous reflux was 6.81 times more likely obtained ($P = 0.037$) and a symptom relief 2.91 times more likely achieved ($P = 0.004$).

Biemans et al. showed a lower frequency of abolition of the great saphenous vein reflux after single phlebectomy at 1 year (50%), with an abolition of symptoms in 66%, but this study included unselected patients [21]. However, he found that after the ASVAL procedure, the diameter of the great saphenous vein was significantly reduced, the CEAP classification decreased and the VCCS and VCSS scores were improved for all patients, independent of the haemodynamic evolution. The authors stated in this paper that "phlebectomies probably reduce the total refluxing volume, explaining the clinical and haemodynamic improvements, even if saphenous reflux persists". We found the same evolution in a study in which we followed 1010 limbs treated by ASVAL until the 5th year [31]: at 5 years, the freedom of presence of a persistent or recurrent great saphenous vein reflux >0.5 s in the treated limb was at 66.2% and the freedom of clinical varicose veins recurrence at 87% and the absence of need of a secondary surgical procedure at 95.5%. It was obvious that a significant proportion of patients had a persisting reflux without clinical consequence (Fig. 12.9). As Biemans stated this quasi-systematic clinical improvement after ablation of the varicose reservoir is probably explained by the dramatic reduction of the refluxing volume in the saphenous vein which has been spared during the ASVAL procedure. It has been already reported that single phlebectomy has a haemodynamic effect on a saphenous vein [17–19]. We have been also able to determine groups of patients with lower risk of recurrence after ASVAL in this 5 years of follow-up study: the patients with a great saphenous vein reflux

Table 12.1 Outcomes at midterm after ASVAL [27]

	6 months	1 year	2 years	3 years	4 years
Abolition of saphenous reflux	69.6%	69.2%	68.7%	68%	66.3%
Symptom relief	84.2%	84.2%	83.4%	81.4%	78%
Freedom of varicose vein recurrence	98.9%	95.5%	94.6%	91.5%	88.5%

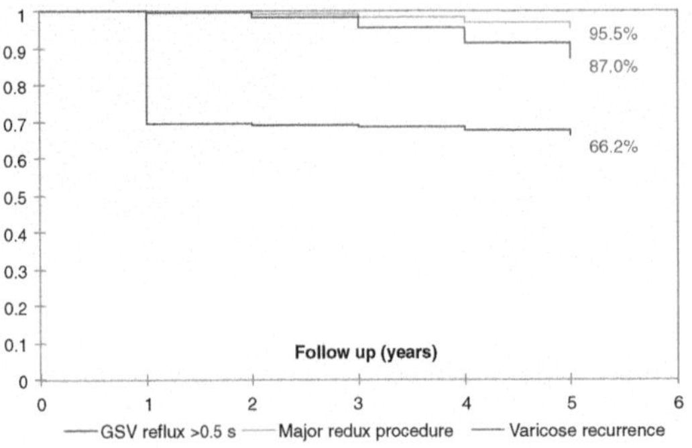

Fig. 12.9 Freedom of saphenous reflux, clinical varicose vein recurrence, and need of a secondary surgical procedure till 5 years of follow-up (With permission from Pittaluga and Chastanet, Phlebology 2015; 30: 98–106)

Table 12.2 Outcomes at long term after ASVAL [35]

	2 years	5 years	7 years	10 years
Abolition of saphenous reflux	71%	69.7%	68.5%	64.4%
Absence of clinical varicose vein recurrence	93.1%	84.7%	75.5%	68.8%
Functional improvement	86.7%	83.8%	78%	69.9%
Aesthetic improvement	92.2%	86%	77.2%	65.7%
Absence of surgical re-intervention	96.9%	90%	83.6%	76.7%

limited to the thigh had a significant lower risk of clinical varicose vein recurrence at 5 years than with a reflux extended below the knee; that was also the case when the emergence of varicose veins was limited at the thigh in comparison with multiple emergences of varicose veins below the knee [31]. Biemans defined preoperative predictors for haemodynamic success after ASVAL: a lower frequency of C3 or C4, a lower VCSS and quality of life score (AVVQ), a limited length of refluxing saphenous vein (<10 cm), a limited dilatation of the saphenous vein, and the positivity of the RET were associated with a higher frequency of disappearance of the saphenous vein reflux at 1 year of follow-up.

Zolotukhin has also recently published his experience of ASVAL at short term [22]. He reported an abolition of the great saphenous vein reflux in 66% of the cases at 1 year of follow-up after an ASVAL procedure performed in an unselected population. The diameter of all the veins decreased significantly no matter if reflux disappeared or not. The overall frequency of clinical varicose vein recurrence was at 13.5%. He observed that the reflux disappearance during the reflux elimination test (RET), a great saphenous vein diameter below 8 at the proximal thigh approximately 15 cm below the inguinal fold and a great saphenous vein reflux limited above the knee were associated with a lower frequency of clinical varicose veins recurrence.

At last the authors have recently published the long-term results of a cohort of patients treated by ASVAL [35]: survival curve analysis showed an absence of saphenous reflux in 64.4% of the cases, an absence of clinical varicose veins recurrence in 68.8% of the cases, an absence of surgical re-intervention in 76.7% of the cases, a functional improvement in 69.9% of the cases, and aesthetic improvement in 65.7% of the cases at 10 years (see Table 12.2).

These results showed a stable evolution of the saphenous vein reflux, while the clinical evolution was slightly but continuously worsened throughout the follow-up until year 10 (Fig. 12.10). Therefore, it seems that the evolution of the venous insufficiency follows the natural evolution of the disease, mostly independent of the reflux.

In so much as the recurrence rate for the ASVAL method in the short, medium, and long

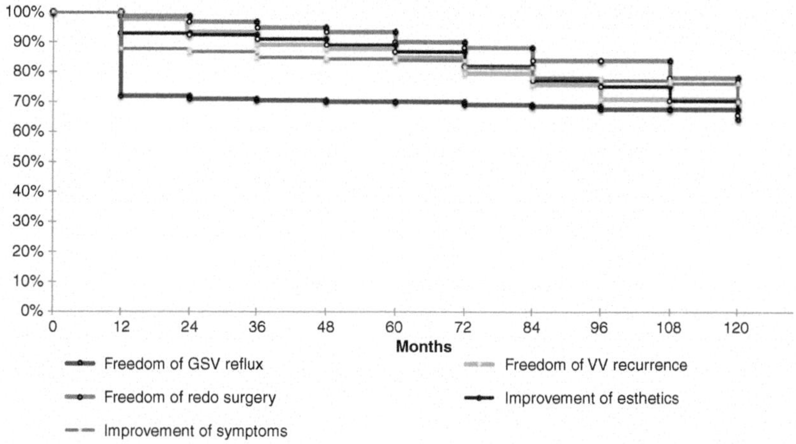

Fig. 12.10 Freedom of saphenous reflux, presence of symptoms, cosmetic concern, clinical varicose vein recurrence, and need of a secondary surgical procedure till 10 years of follow-up [35]. With kind permission by Elsevier from: Pittaluga P, Chastanet S "Treatment of varicose veins by ASVAL: 1 results at 10 years". Ann Vasc Surg. 2017 Jan;38:e10. doi: https://doi.org/10.1016/j.avsg.2016.07.021. Epub 2016 Oct 11

term is not higher than for techniques that involve removal or ablation of the saphenous vein, it is worth to ask ourselves whether a saphenous vein-sparing approach is not therefore justified as a first-line therapy when there is only partial saphenous vein reflux and when the saphenous vein is only moderately dilated. The main argument in favour of this conservative approach is the physiological role that the saphenous vein could play in superficial drainage and, to a lesser extent, its availability as revascularization material.

As a consequence there is no longer any place for systematic elimination of the saphenous vein: numerous studies show that extensive axial reflux is involved in only a minority of cases. Regardless of the technique chosen, the procedure should be adapted to each individual case and should involve the less aggressive option.

Therefore, it seems that first-line therapy should always consider the option of sparing the saphenous vein, depending on the clinical examination, the duplex ultrasound assessment, and the patient's concern for consulting. Isolated treatment of the varicose reservoir by ASVAL procedure at stage C2 of the CEAP classification will probably therefore often be the most appropriate course of action. Ablation of the saphenous vein using traditional surgery, endothermal ablation by laser, or radiofrequency and chemical ablation by foam sclerotherapy should then only be indicated at the advanced stages of the varicose disease.

In terms of isolated treatment of the varicose reservoir, micro-phlebectomy seems to be the most appropriate technique, but ultrasound-guided foam sclerotherapy of the tributaries is possible [10], provided that it blocks the sclerosant from entering the saphenous vein, which is, however, not an easy thing to do.

Literature

1. Mayo CH. Treatment of varicose vein. Surg Gyn Obst Br J Surg. 1906;2:385–8.
2. Babcock WW. A new operation for the extirpation of varicose veins of the leg. N Y Med J. 1907;86:153–6.
3. Trendelenburg F. Ueber die Unterbindung der Vena Saphena magna bei Unterschenkel Varicen. Beitr Klin Chir. 1890–1891;7:195–210.
4. Ludbrook J, Beale G. Femoral venous valves in relation to varicose veins. Lancet. 1962;1:79–81.
5. Franceschi C. Théorie et Pratique de la Cure Conservatrice Hémodynamique de l'Insuffisance Veineuse en Ambulatoire, Percy sous thil, Editions de l'Armaçon, 1988.
6. Navarro L, Min RJ, Bone C. Endovenous laser: a new minimally invasive method of treatment for varicose veins--preliminary observations using an 810 nm diode laser. Dermatol Surg. 2001;27(2):117–22.

7. Chandler JG, Pichot O, Sessa C, Schuller-Petrovic S, Kabnick LS, Bergan JJ. Treatment of primary insufficiency by endovenous saphenous vein obliteration. Vasc Surg. 2000;38:201–14.
8. Cabrera Garrido JR, Cabrera Garcia Olmedo JR, Garcia Olmedo D. Nuevo metodode esclerois en las varices trunculares. Pathol Vasc. 1993;1:55–72.
9. Hamel-Desnos C, Desnos P, Wollman JC, Ouvry P, Mako S, Allaert FA. Evaluation of the efficacy of polidocanol in the form of foam compared with liquid form in sclerotherapy of the greater saphenous vein: initial results. Dermatol Surg. 2003;29:1170–5.
10. Guex JJ. Foam sclerotherapy: an overview of use for primary venous insufficiency. Semin Vasc Surg. 2005;18:25–9.
11. Pittaluga P, Réa B, Barbe R, Guex JJ. Méthode ASVAL (Ablation Sélective des Varices sous Anesthésie Locale): principes et résultats préliminaires. Phlebologie. 2005;58:175–81.
12. Labropoulos N, Leon L, Kwon S, Tassiopoulos A, Gonzalez-Fajardo JA, Kang SS, Mansour MA, Littooy FN. Study of the venous reflux progression. J Vasc Surg. 2005;41(2):291–5.
13. Cooper DG, Hillman-Cooper CS, Barker SG, Hollingsworth SJ. Primary varicose veins: the sapheno-femoral junction, distribution of varicosities and patterns of incompetence. Eur J Vasc Endovasc Surg. 2003;25(1):53–9.
14. Engelhorn CA, Engelhorn AL, Cassou MF, Salles-Cunha SX. Patterns of saphenous reflux in women with primary varicose veins. J Vasc Surg. 2005;41(4):645–51.
15. Pittaluga P, Chastanet S. Classification of saphenous refluxes: implications for treatment. Phlebology. 2008; 23:2–9.
16. Pittaluga P, Chastanet S, Réa B, Barbe R, Guex JJ. Saphenous vein preservation: is it the new gold standard? Torino: Minerva Med; 2007. p. 391–9.
17. Labropoulos N, Kokkosis AA, Spentzouris G, Gasparis AP, Tassiopoulos AK. The distribution and significance of varicosities in the saphenous trunks. J Vasc Surg. 2010;51:96–103.
18. Creton D. Diamater reduction of the proximal long saphenous vein after ablation of a distal incompetent tributary. Dermatol Surg. 1999;25:394–7.
19. Zamboni P, Cisno C, Marchetti F, Quaglio D, Mazza P, Liboni A. Reflux elimination without any ablation or disconnection of the saphenous vein. A haemodynamic model for venous surgery. Eur J Vasc Endovasc Surg. 2001;21:361–9.
20. Pittaluga P, Chastanet S, Locret T, Barbe R. The effect of isolated phlebectomy on reflux and diameter of the great saphenous vein: a prospective study. Eur J Vasc Endovasc Surg. 2010;40:122–8.
21. Biemans A, Van den Bos R, Hollestein LM, et al. The effect of single phlebectomies of a large varicose tributary on great saphenous vein reflux. J Vasc Surg Venous Lymphat Disord. 2014;2:179–87.
22. Zolotukhin IA, Seliverstov EI, Zakharova EA, Kirienko AI. Short-term results of isolated phlebectomy with preservation of incompetent great saphenous vein (ASVAL procedure) in primary varicose veins disease. Phlebology. 2016. https://doi.org/10.1177/0268355516674415.
23. Rose SA, Ahmed A. Some thoughts on the etiology of varicose vein. J Cardiovasc Surg. 1986;27:534–43.
24. Clarke GH, Vasdekis SN, Hobbs JT, Nicolaides AN. Venous wall function in the pathogenesis of varicose veins. Surgery. 1992;111:402–8.
25. Travers JP, Brookes CE, Evans J, Baker DM, Kent C, Makin GS, Mayhew TM. Assessment of wall structure and composition of varicose veins with reference to collagen, elastin and smooth muscle content. Eur J Vasc Endovasc Surg. 1996;11:230–7.
26. Labropoulos N, Giannoukas AD, Delis K, Mansour MA, Kang SS, Nicolaides AN, Lumley J, Baker WH. Where does venous reflux start? J Vasc Surg. 1997;26:736–42.
27. Pittaluga P, Chastanet S, Réa B, Barbe R. Midterm results of the surgical treatment of varices by phlebectomy with conservation of a refluxing saphenous vein. J Vasc Surg. 2009;50:107–18.
28. Abu-Own A, Scurr JH, Coleridge Smith PD. Saphenous vein reflux without incompetence at the saphenofemoral junction. Br J Surg. 1994;81:1452–4.
29. Pittaluga P, Chastanet S. Predictive value of a preoperative test for the reversibility of the reflux after phlebectomy with preservation of the great saphenous vein. J Vasc Surg Venous Lymphat Disord. 2014a;2:105.
30. Pittaluga P, Chastanet S. Varicose vein recurrence after pregnancy: influence of the preservation of the saphenous vein in nullipara patients. Blucher Med Proc. 2014b;1:81–2.
31. Pittaluga P, Chastanet S. Persistent incompetent truncal veins should not be treated immediately. Phlebology. 2015;30:98–106.
32. Pittaluga P, Chastanet S. Lymphatic complications after varicose veins surgery: risk factors and how to avoid them. Phlebology. 2012;27(Suppl 1):139–42.
33. Creton D, Rea B, Pittaluga P, Chastanet S, Allaert FA. Evaluation of the pain in varicose vein surgery under tumescent local anaesthesia using sodium bicarbonate as excipient without any intravenous sedation. Phlebology. 2012;27:368–73.
34. Pittaluga P, Chastanet S. Value of postoperative compression after mini invasive surgical treatment of varicose veins. J Vasc Surg Venous Lymphat Disord. 2013;1:385–91.
35. Pittaluga P, Chastanet S. Treatment of varicose veins by ASVAL: results at 10 years. Ann Vasc Surg. 2017;38:e10. https://doi.org/10.1016/j.avsg.2016.07.021. Epub 2016 Oct 11

External Valvuloplasty of the Sapheno-Femoral Junction

13

Paolo Zamboni and Sergio Gianesini

13.1 Surgical Rationale

In 1940 two Boston researchers, Edwards and Edwards [1], published an article in the *American Heart Journal* to demonstrate the possibility of studying varicosity based on an autopsy examination of varicose patients. They stratified the possible findings in four different stages (see Fig. 13.1) according to the image of the valves at the level of the ostium (sapheno-femoral junction).

It is visible that no direct lesions of the valvular structure are detectable in the first two stages. The postulated explanation was that in early stages, valvular insufficiency is secondary to wall dilation, which by separating the valvular cusps from one another makes them incompetent. In later stages, atrophy, retraction and other damage are found, directly affecting the tiny valvular leaflets, due either to the turbulence created by reflux or to the progression of the disease. These histological observations have also been confirmed by other authors [2, 3].

P. Zamboni, M.D. (✉)
School of Vascular Surgery and Vascular Diseases Center, University of Ferrara, Ferrara, Italy

Unit of Translational Surgery, AOU Ferrara, Ferrara, Italy
e-mail: zmp@unife.it

S. Gianesini, M.D., Ph.D.
Vascular Diseases Center, University of Ferrara, Ferrara, Italy

USUHS University, Bethesda, MD, USA

Figure 13.2 provides an example of histologically intact valves of the great saphenous vein following stripping procedure. Quite recently, several authors demonstrated that about 50% of the terminal valves when investigated by duplex are competent, challenging the vision of the obliging treatment with high tie of the sapheno femoral junction [4–6].

From the cases A and B showed in Fig. 13.1, it seems that a saphenous vein with healthy valvular cusps and a wall with early dilation might be restored to normal hemodynamic function by rectifying the dilated wall alone. This is the aim of the external valvuloplasty: to correct the wall defect and to permit a normal functioning of healthy valvular cusps.

This simple surgical idea was first tested, paradoxically, on the most difficult deepest vein system [7, 8].

Subsequently other authors demonstrated the efficacy of external valvular banding in the treatment of primary valvular insufficiency of the sapheno-femoral junction, with various techniques of external banding [9–17].

13.2 Patient Selection

The biggest problem associated with testing intuitions about possible new beneficial surgical techniques involves the definition of indications and creation of a patient selection protocol. This

P. Zamboni et al. (eds.), *Saphenous Vein-Sparing Strategies in Chronic Venous Disease*,
https://doi.org/10.1007/978-3-319-70638-2_13

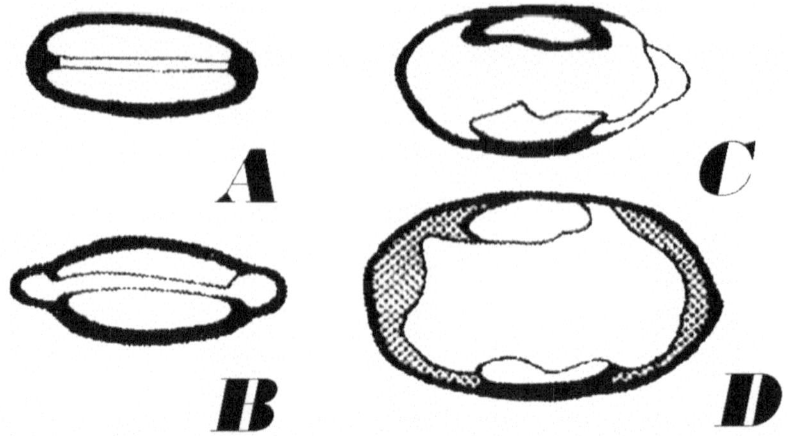

Fig. 13.1 Progression of saphenous ostial valve insufficiency. In the first two stages, A and B, wall dilation is causing separation of the valvular cusps. In stages C and D vein wall degeneration has occurred, as well as valve alterations. Modified from Am. Heart J. 19:338–351, 1940. © P. Zamboni

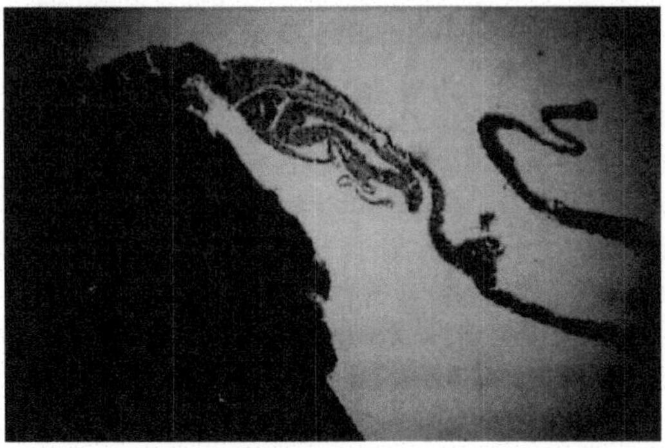

Fig. 13.2 Histological examination of integral valve leaflets inserted on a dilated vein wall. © P. Zamboni

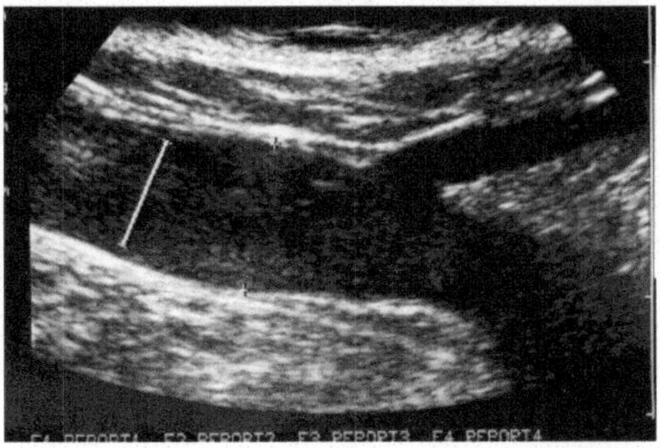

Fig. 13.3 Duplex scanning of the sapheno-femoral junction with measurement of the diameter of the valvular site for repair. © P. Zamboni

procedure has been successfully used with patients who have the following characteristics:

13.2.1 Clinical Criteria

These criteria have been chosen to apply extraluminal valvuloplasty:

- Patients with moderate varices of recent onset Clinical Class C2
- Patients without previous surgical intervention or sclerotherapy
- Patients without previous thrombosis of the saphenous veins

The last two clinical exclusion criteria are important to prevent postoperative saphenous thrombosis, which is more easily induced by previous endothelial damage. Corcos excluded also patients for whom ablation of varicose veins is considered as an important prophylactic preparation for major abdominal or orthopaedic surgery [10].

13.2.2 Ultrasound Criteria

Apart from a sapheno-femoral reflux in ultrasound, mobile valvular leaflets in the terminal and subterminal valves of the great saphenous vein should be visible. The dilation of the valvular site should also be measured relative to the segments above and below it (Fig. 13.3).

The number of millimetres that the valvular commissure is dilated beyond the adjacent saphenous trunk needs to be calculated. To establish this, it is important to perform scans that provide visualization of the valve in relation to the lumen. Finally, sapheno-femoral reflux and the competence of the deep venous circulation must be confirmed.

13.3 Anaesthesia and Preparation of the Patient

13.3.1 Type of Anaesthesia

The procedure can be performed under local or general anaesthesia. The authors have always used loco-regional anaesthesia when performing external banding of the sapheno-femoral valves. Such anaesthesia permits outpatient surgery and rapid mobilization of the patient and at the same time total control of intra- and postoperative pain. In fact, no patient asked for postoperative pain medication.

The patient is monitored on ECG, and a sphygmomanometer is placed on the arm contralateral to venous access. Resuscitative equipment and skilled emergency personnel are available during the procedure; the intervention is performed without an anaesthesiologist.

For local anaesthesia, 15 cc. of lidocaine 1% are injected. Lidocaine is preferred, because of its very rapid action and because its half-life is sufficiently protracted to guarantee coverage of this type of surgery.

The injection is performed along the preferred line of incision, from the femoral pulse medially for 5 cm along the inguinal crease, using an insulin needle and infiltrating the hypoderm somewhat superficially, about 1 cm deep. Besides injecting the line of incision, it is necessary to infiltrate the superior and surrounding tissue in a half circle and at the same depth, with provision for aspiration to prevent accidental systemic injection of the anaesthetic into a dilated varix, or it may be administered using the "mesotherapeutic" technique (consult Chap. 7).

After a usually brief interval, 3 min on average, disappearance of pain sensation is tested by pricking the skin with the point of the scalpel. In case of missing anaesthesia, the site can be sprayed with an additional 5–10 cc of lidocaine 1%. After at least 30–60 s, the field can be dried and the procedure continued.

We used this diluted anaesthetic because of its more prolonged anaesthetic action. If the indications we have listed are followed, the mean amount of anaesthetic needed is never greater than 20 cc of mepivacaine 1%.

Valvuloplasty under angioscopic monitoring is very well tolerated under local anaesthesia and does not require any additional use of drugs or devices.

13.3.2 Premedication

The patient is placed supine on the operating table. A peripheral vein is cannulated through which a 5% glucose solution is administered. If a patient is particularly anxious despite the prior requisite informational session, it may be advisable to administer a slow-drip benzodiazepine by the open intravenous route. In the case of patients with a history of peptic or gastroduodenal ulcer disease, a bolus of two vials of ranitidine (100 mg) can be given. All patients receive intravenous 1 g of ceftriaxone for ultra-short-term antibiotic prophylaxis. Administration of antibiotics is indicated if a heterologous prosthesis is used, regardless of small size or even if implanted extravascularly as in this case.

13.3.3 Heparin Prophylaxis

Although delicate in execution, extensive manipulation takes place on the junction, the valvular structures and the femoral vein. In addition, this is the only surgical procedure that manipulates at the sapheno-femoral junction and maintains the sapheno-femoral ostium patent and in continuity with deep vein circulation. Therefore, the possibility of a thrombosis has a very different clinical significance.

Thus, a heparin prophylaxis is indicated with low-molecular heparin at the day of the intervention, in case of high-risk patients for 1 week.

13.4 Manual Valvuloplasty

13.4.1 General Principles of Manual Valvuloplasty

During the initial attempts, the procedure has been performed in a number of different ways. By increasing experience, the parachute technique demonstrated to be the more rapid and effective (Fig. 13.4). Whatever technique of external banding the surgeon should prefer, he/she has to be compliant with the following principles:

1. The valvular repair location must be enclosed externally in a prosthetic material of similar circumference to match the orthostatic circumference of the zone inferior to the valvular site (rectification of the saphenous diameter). To do this, the required circumference may be extrapolated on the basis of diameters obtainable from vascular sonography.
2. Should any intraoperative monitoring system for restoration of valvular competence (strip test, Doppler, angioscopy) detect failure of the finished repair, a revision procedure should be performed or the repair should be converted to a standard high ligation of the saphenofemoral junction.
3. The intervention should be very "clean" and careful in its approach to haemostasis and exposure of the structures. Indeed, if dead space is left between the prosthetic material and the external surface of the saphenous vein, the result may well be crushing of the vein (because of the low internal venous pressure) leading to thrombus formation or it may promote onset of infection.
4. Surgical asepsis rules must be rigorously followed, even with outpatient surgery, since heterologous material is being implanted. It is absolutely critical to avoid all contact between the prosthetic material and the patient's skin.

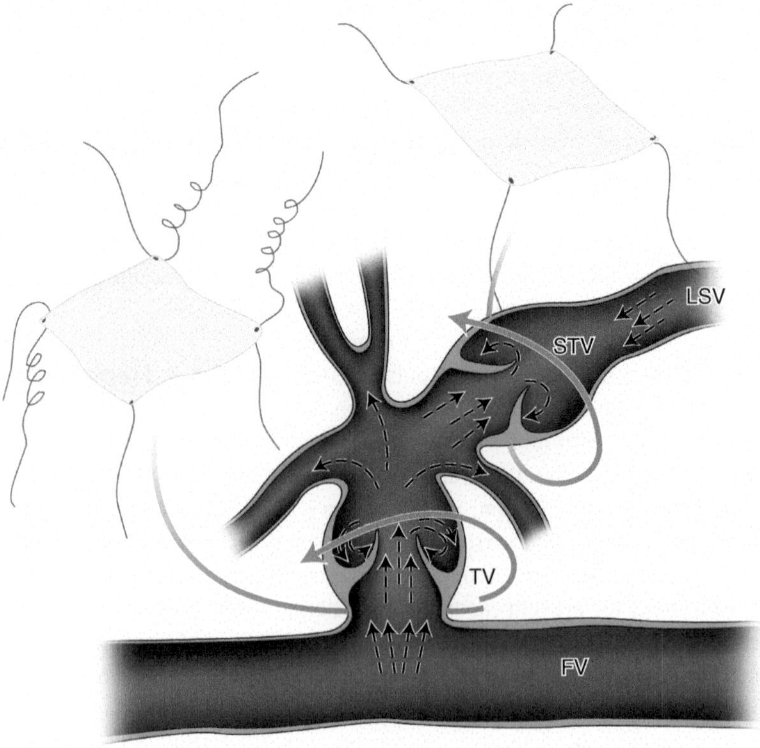

Fig. 13.4 Parachute method of placing ultrafine PTFE around respectively the terminal (TV) and subterminal (STV) valves of the saphenofemoral junction. *FV* femoral vein. © P. Zamboni

5. In the author's opinion, all collaterals should be saved, if at all possible. In a procedure that is intended to be conservative, preservation of competent tributaries at the sapheno-femoral junction potentiates drainage of the superficial and pelvic venous circulation and increases inflow into the saphenous, which in turn will preserve long-term patency of the saphenous trunk.

13.4.2 Surgical Technique

The authors prefer a transverse incision at the inguinal crease and extending 4–5 cm medially from the femoral pulse mark. The incision is deepened to the subcutaneous fascia; this is dissected with the scissors and retracted with three Farabeuf forceps. Generally, this procedure is used to expose the proximal segment of the great saphenous proceeding approximately 4–5 cm from the confluence with the femoral vein.

Skeletisation of the saphenous trunk proceeds cephalad, including skeletisation of all the tributaries of the sapheno-femoral junction. Both the proximal saphenous and tributaries must be secured with an elastic sling (Fig. 13.5).

Particular care must be taken while dissecting the cribriform fascia against penetration of the oval fossa. This segment of the saphenous vein

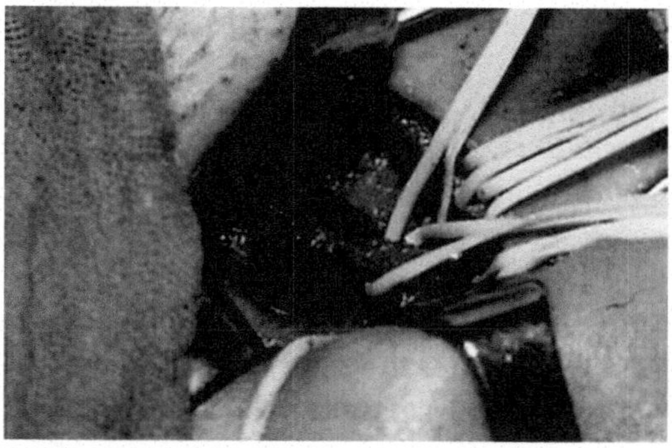

Fig. 13.5 Intraoperative view of the dilated wall from the sapheno-femoral junction, with the ostial valve well apparent. All the tributaries are preserved and encircled by elastic slings. © P. Zamboni

that courses from the origin of the final tributaries to the femoral vein should be carefully prepared by removal of excess adventitia and elevated likewise on an elastic sling.

Using blunt dissection, it is necessary also to expose the superior surface of the femoral vein, retracting it more cephalad with a Farabeuf forceps in order to leave the sapheno-femoral junction with its ostial valve clear and visible (Fig. 13.5).

During this stage of the procedure, an arteriole may be encountered with origin in the common femoral artery. If there is a tight adhesion between the arteriole and the posterior surface of the terminal saphenous vein, it should be ligated and divided between the two ligatures.

Sometimes, however, this arteriole crosses the sapheno-femoral junction superiorly — or passes beneath it — but does not adhere tightly. In many cases, it is sufficient simply to run a sling or tie underneath and apply traction on it to obtain space without sacrificing the vessel.

Other possible encounters are outlets of tiny tributaries of less than 1.5 mm at the sapheno-femoral junction or perforating veins usually originating from the deep femoral vein. Since these have a tiny diameter, they should be ligated and divided, flush with the wall using a 4/0 absorbable tie (see Sect. 13.4.4).

But whenever a collateral vein with diameter greater than 1.5 mm is encountered at the level of the valve to be repaired (and this is very rare), it should be ligated and divided, first taking care to leave a long stump. This will help to facilitate the protrusion of the stump itself through the prosthesis. The stump will then protrude either through a perforation created in the prosthesis with the scissors or a punch-type instrument or even through a suture hole (see Sect. 13.4.4). As will be explained, as soon as the valvular repair is completed, the stump should be ligated as closely as possible to the saphenous wall.

Once the terminal saphenous has been prepared, a Valsalva manoeuvre is performed on the patient; this manoeuvre reveals very well any excessive dilation of the valvular wall, which

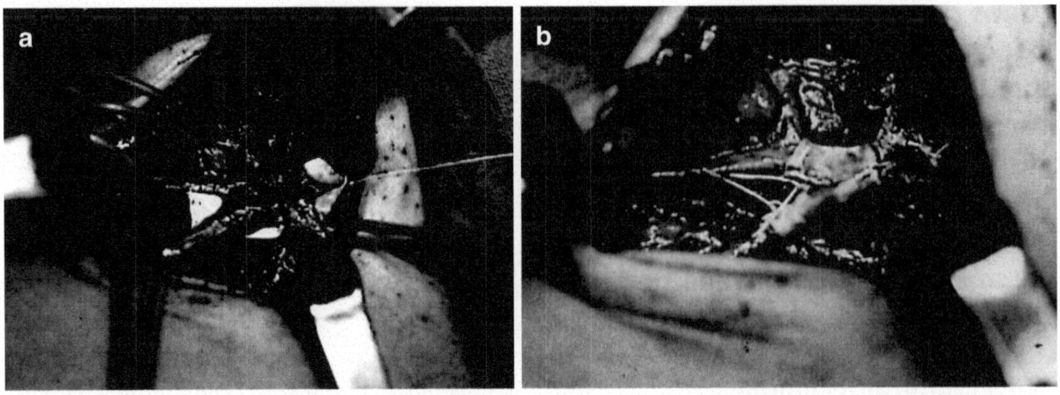

Fig. 13.6 (**a**) Example of a method for configuring a PTFE prosthesis in such a way that the tributaries may be preserved. (**b**) In this particular case—insertion of a single prosthesis over a lambdoid saphenous vein—the terminal valve and two subterminal valves are each banded at the location of the outlet of the confluence of the anterior accessory with the great saphenous vein. © P. Zamboni

sometimes also involves the superior surface of the femoral vein whenever one of the two valvular cusps is inserted at this location.

13.4.3 Measurement and Preparation of the Prosthesis

The authors have always used 0.4 mm single-velour Dacron patches and e-PTFE cardiovascular patches as prosthetic materials. The latter material has proved to be the most adaptable and suitable for this type of intervention. Other investigators have tried to use biological and absorbable materials.

A very fine stamp-size segment is cut from the e-PTFE patch, equivalent in circumference to that of the saphenous vein in the segment below the terminal valve. This dimension should be increased by at least 2–3 mm, to compensate for the space “stolen” by the suture. The length is approximately 12–15 mm (see Fig. 13.4). The authors have found that this tiny external prosthesis is adequate to correct dilation of the valve site and restore valvular competence.

Banding the valvular site with the prosthesis is not always easy; to facilitate the procedure, therefore, we advise anchoring two or even all four corners of the prosthesis with 7/0 PTFE ties. The terminal saphenous vein can be elevated by working it up and down and applying traction to the slings that were passed under the saphenous vein and tributaries.

The PTFE ties anchoring the corners of the prosthesis may be passed easily beneath the terminal valve (see Figs. 13.4 and 13.6); by crossing them on the superior surface of the great saphenous vein, the terminal valve is banded, and the prosthetic edges are approximated.

The prosthesis is attached around the valve using 4–5 interrupted sutures of 7/0 PTFE; be sure to barely bite the prosthesis edge so as not to reduce the diameter of the prosthesis. If, as mentioned, the ostial valve presents a cusp with femoral vein insertion, the authors bite the adventitia of the superior surface of the femoral vein with the needle. In this way, besides positioning and attaching the prosthesis, PTFE is also stitched on the insertion point of the valvular cusp and reinforce the wall at this delicate point (see Fig. 13.7).

13.4.4 Intraoperative Testing of Valvular Function

As soon as the terminal valve repair has been completed, it is imperative to evaluate the closure of the valves intraoperatively. Because of this, intraoperative Doppler testing has been performed in all the surgical cases. The authors have used an 8 MHz continuous wave sterile probe or a probe introduced in the finger of a sterile glove filled with gel

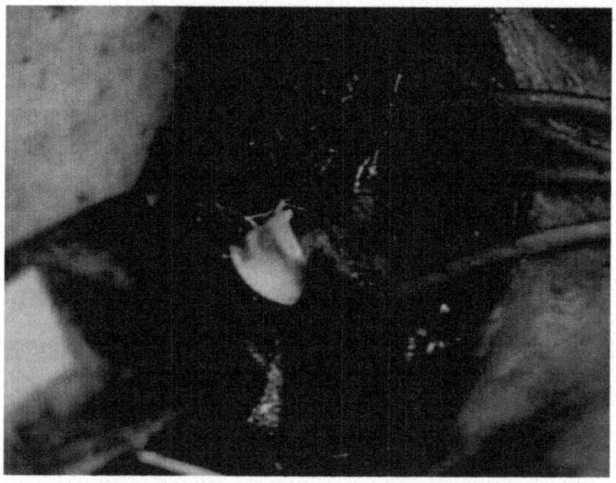

Fig. 13.7 External banding of the terminal valve by using parachute technique and a 0.4 mm thick ePTFE. The light of the angioscopy controlling the valve repair is visible in the great saphenous vein. © P. Zamboni

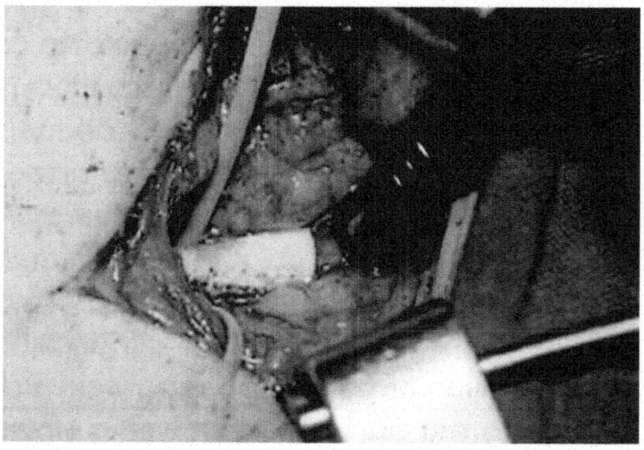

Fig. 13.8 Intraoperative Doppler test of the valvular function respectively under Valsalva and deep breathing. © P. Zamboni

(Fig. 13.8). This instrument is supported lightly (so as not to crush it) on the great saphenous vein immediately downstream from the valvuloplasty.

The test is performed with the use either of the Valsalva manoeuvre or the compression/release test. Activation of the thoracic pump can be achieved also through deep inspiration to test the saphenous vein patency.

The authors performed 21 cases under video angioscopic monitoring of valvular competence (Figs. 13.7 and 13.9).

The angioscope is introduced into the saphenous vein through one of the leg collaterals with an outlet close to the saphenous vein, located during preoperative mapping with the duplex scanner. Under local anaesthesia, the collateral is exposed through a micro-incision of the skin. The angioscope is introduced into the saphenous vein through this collateral and continued upwards as far as the inguinal cleft. Cross illumination of the vessel facilitates placement immediately downstream from the terminal valve.

Continuous flushing and traction on the sling passed around the saphenous vein and its tributaries permit flow reduction in the saphenous vein and visualization of the valvular cusps from below. The primary data coming from the test should confirm the preoperative diagnosis of macroscopically healthy valvular cusps inserted on a dilated wall.

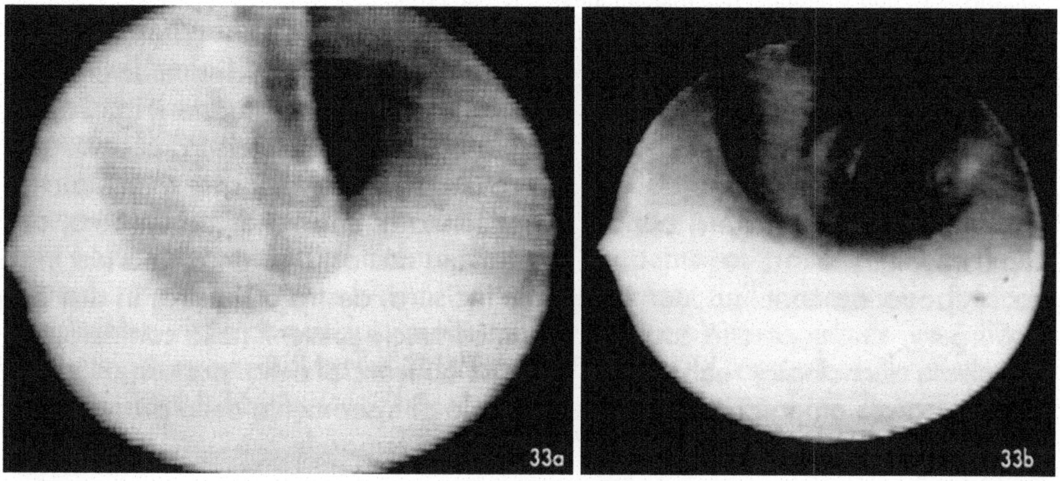

Fig. 13.9 Left: Preoperative angioscopy showing the terminal valve of the sapheno-femoral junction with lack of contact of the two cusps. Right: Postoperative control after banding demonstrating an effective valve closure. © P. Zamboni

The angioscopic view (Fig. 13.9a) demonstrates two valvular leaflets more or less distanced from each other, free of perforations, fissures, atrophic changes, collapse, or other abnormalities specific to pathological valvular cusps. Postoperative check can demonstrate the effectiveness of the procedure (Fig. 13.9b).

Although the angioscopic procedure is well tolerated under local anaesthesia, it does not increase the intervention time by more than 20–30 min and requires no more than 1000 cc of flushing solution; still, it is obvious that it cannot be routinely used for interventions on a day-surgery basis.

Another intraoperative test of valvular competence that has long been used in valvular surgery of the deep venous system is the so-called strip test, which is a type of manual squeezing at the level of the repaired valve. The authors have never used it because the method involves venous clamping and any kind of unnecessary injury to the vein should be avoided.

13.4.5 Tributary Management

During preparation of the sapheno-femoral junction, therefore, the tributaries should be skeletonized over the first few centimetres that separate them from the saphenous lumen and elevated on elastic slings (see Fig. 13.5).

In this way, applying moderate traction alternately up and down, it is possible to position the prosthesis around the valve without allowing the outlet of a tributary to fall within the range of contact of the prosthesis.

In cases of very severe anatomical anomaly, such as the emergence of tributaries barely 1–1.5 cm from the femoral vein, it becomes necessary to sacrifice the tributary by ligating and dividing it. Should the lumen of this tributary measure less than 1.5 mm, ligation should be performed flush with the saphenous vein using a 4/0 thread.

A small stump of this size, even if crushed between the prosthesis and the saphenous wall, will not cause significant modification or deformation of the venous lumen. But if the tributary diameter is greater than 1.5 mm at the time it is ligated and divided, it is better to allow the stump to emerge from the saphenous for a few millimetres rather than to perform a flush ligation.

Once the valvuloplasty is completed, a perforation at the level of the ligated tributary can be created in the prosthesis with a stab of the scissors. Grasping the loops of the previous ligation with forceps, the tributary can be retracted and retied flush with the perforation. The benefit of perforation is that it prevents crushing of the small stump of the collateral vein in the dead space between the prosthesis and the saphenous wall. Crushing may lead to lumen deformation, turbulence with associated thrombosis risk, or interference with the operation of the valve resulting from the protrusion of the stump.

13.5 Stapler Valvuloplasty

In 1988 Jessup and Lane described a device that had been used initially on experimental animals and later successfully marketed under the name Venocuff. It was capable of installing a silicone-reinforced Dacron external sleeve around the valve designated for repair.

The system proposed by Lane, supported as it was by appropriate technology, obviously drew more attention and led to the marketing of the Venocuff device which is illustrated in Figs. 13.10 left and right [11].

The device is equipped with a gage that permits the desired degree of tightening of the prosthesis around the valve; it displays the attained diameter of the dilated vein in millimetres. When the desired diameter is reached, the suture is inserted by activating the two release tabs; at the same time, the excess prosthesis material projecting over the suture staple is trimmed (Fig. 13.10).

When external repair of the sapheno-femoral junction is contemplated, the approach and preparation of the junction follows the principles already enunciated in the previous section.

The stapler is certainly more awkward to use than the tiny PTFE "parachute" used in the manual method. To simplify, therefore, the positioning of the cartridge-mounted prosthesis around

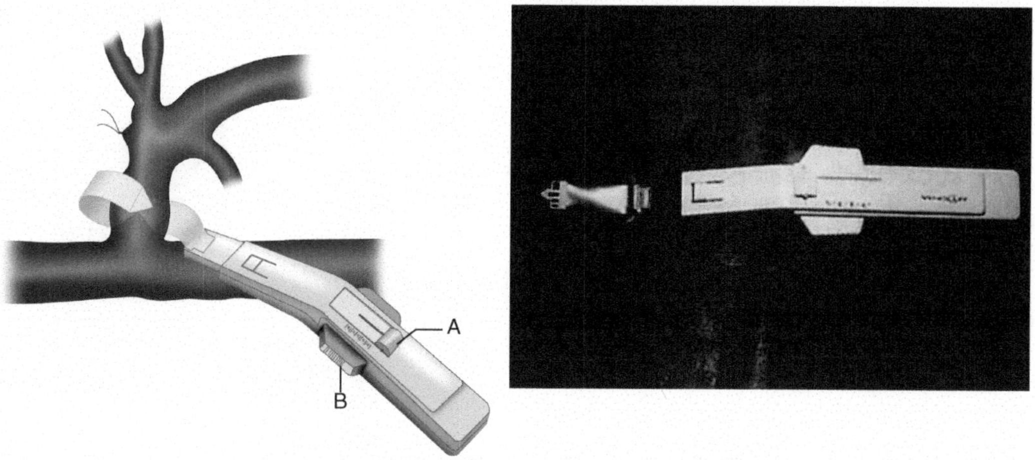

Fig. 13.10 Left: Stapler valvuloplasty of the terminal valve. A Indicates the Venocuff gage and B a release tabs. Right: The original venocuff device. © P. Zamboni

the ostial valve, it is advisable to sacrifice one or two tributaries immediately adjacent to the outlet of the femoral vein.

The sling that passes under the vein should be manipulated to elevate the terminal saphenous vein. The cartridge-mounted prosthesis is passed beneath the valvular site and an attempt is made to push the notch on the prosthesis into the angle of contact of the saphenous vein at the femoral vein.

When a diameter is reached that matches the straight vein segment underneath (determined by B mode imaging, with the patient standing) and excessive dilation is corrected, the release tabs on the side of the device are pressed; the excess prosthetic material is trimmed, and simultaneously the stapler automatically fires a single metallic staple which will fasten the prosthesis at the selected diameter.

Theoretically, a valve competence test could be performed with intraoperative Doppler imaging before the staple is released, through selection of a diameter equal to the diameter that causes the reflux signal to disappear on ultrasound.

In practice, however, although there is an undeniable advantage in adjusting the prosthesis diameter before trimming and suturing begin, this test is not easy to perform. The stapler shuts out a lot of the surgical lighting and makes it difficult to position the Doppler probe beneath the valve during the repair, at least when the surgical approach described is being used. There is no difficulty, however, in choosing the appropriate diameter when the more complicated but also more accurate angioscopic monitoring is used.

Visualization of the correctly approximated cusps is a sufficient criterion for safely proceeding with firing the cartridge.

13.6 Results

The authors have used this surgical technique in 72 cases: 42 manual and 30 with Venocuff; follow-up is 72 months; the indications listed above were observed.

The results obtained in this carefully selected patient group were a surprise to anyone who, like the authors, supports a true challenge to the progression of varicose disease rather than just performing another clinical experiment.

This very carefully selected group of patients was for obvious reasons followed with extreme care by members of the author's medical group. The results have been analysed from different perspectives: clinical, sonographic, radiological and hemodynamic; the postoperative changes in superficial blood pressure and the filling time for the limb using photoplethysmography have been measured.

13.6.1 Clinical Results

All procedures were performed under local anaesthesia under an outpatient surgery regimen without ever having to use analgesics. The patients were discharged with an 18–20 mmHg prophylactic elastic stocking and quickly resumed their normal daily schedules.

Two cases of superficial postoperative thrombosis were recorded which required an immediate re-intervention involving short stripping of the proximal saphenous vein.

After a learning curve, there was no longer any type of problem, so that the procedure can be proposed as safe.

During the follow-up, in 91% of cases the disappearance or fusion of moderate peripheral varices involved in sapheno-femoral reflux were observed [16]. Varicosity recurrence occurred in 6% of cases due to perforating veins not refluxing at the time of intervention.

This percentage is indeed very low and does not represent a failure of the technique in question, although it does represent one aspect of the natural progression of the varicose disease.

13.6.2 Results on Ultrasonography

Although the initial application of external valvuloplasty was performed on a very carefully selected group of patients, which has no comparison in the literature, the procedure provided surprising results.

Recurrence of sapheno-femoral reflux was observed only in 6% of the group (Fig. 13.11). Another important feature is the low number of saphenous veins lost after the procedure.

Duplex scanning data shows us a 94% saphenous patency rate with a mean diameter of 4 mm at the thigh, ideal therefore for an autologous arterial graft and in the ranges of normal population [18].

An investigation by Rutherford demonstrated a 21% rate of saphenous occlusion after high ligation of the sapheno-femoral junction, and therefore these were unusable as arterial grafts [19]. Fligelstone obtained only a 64% total patency rate for the saphenous vein despite excellent results in controlling the varicosity syndrome with high ligation of the sapheno-femoral junction and peripheral phlebectomy [20].

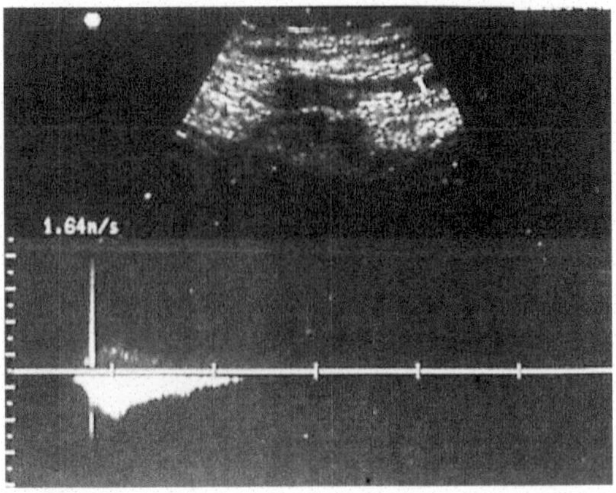

Fig. 13.11 Manual squeezing of the calf demonstrated an upward flow and reflux disappearance in 94% of patients operated on by external valvuloplasty. © P. Zamboni

Such evidence confirms the importance of maintaining saphenous drainage to stabilize the superficial venous system.

With regard to Doppler ultrasound evaluation of sapheno-femoral valvuloplasty, no vascular ultrasound probe has the resolution power capable of visualizing the fine valvular leaflets after they have been banded by the external prosthesis.

On vascular ultrasonography, the ultrafine PTFE we have suggested, 0.4 mm thick, and the silicone-reinforced Dacron mesh mounted on a Venocuff create the appearance of a hyperechoic line around the saphenous lumen. By placing the sample volume of the pulsed Doppler beneath the repaired segment, it is easy to test for valvular competence. Duplex scanning also enables determination of continued stability of the saphenous diameter at the level of the valvular site.

But the most reassuring result from ultrasonography is the evidence of saphenous anterograde drainage, which restores physiologic emptying of the superficial system at systole (Fig. 13.11).

13.6.3 Radiographic Results

The authors had been using prostheses derived from arterial vascular surgery during the first pioneering years of performing this intervention and, as mentioned previously, found that they are not suitable for postoperative imaging.

In the initial years, the patients had to undergo descending venographic testing in order to document the restoration of valvular function. In Fig. 13.12, descending venography clearly depicts the restored terminal valve function.

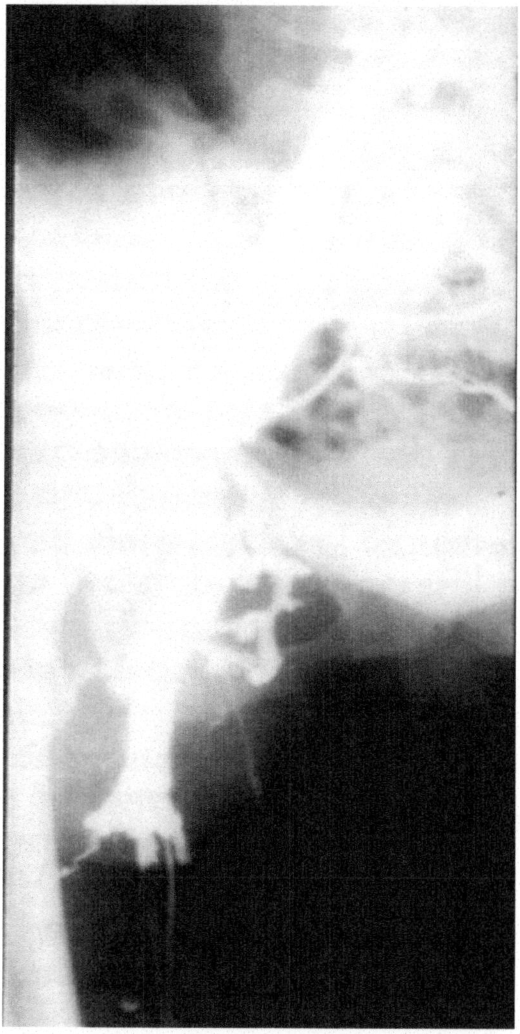

Fig. 13.12 Kistner descending venography showing disappearance of the sapheno-femoral reflux following external valvuloplasty of the sapheno-femoral junction. © P. Zamboni

13.6.4 Haemodynamic Results

Saphenous anterograde emptying with elimination of primary and secondary reflux is the basic factor behind the highly significant (statistically speaking) reduction in ambulatory venous pressure (AVP) and protraction of refilling time (RT) recorded in this group of patients. The authors believe that this evidence lends even greater support to the proposed procedure [13].

Conclusion

On the basis of their experience, the authors consider external valvuloplasty of the sapheno-femoral junction to be the procedure of choice in cases of sapheno-femoral reflux in the presence of valvular cusps that are shown to be mobile and intact on sonogram at the level of the proximal saphenous vein, if concomitant presence of other reflux sites on incompetent perforating veins are regarded as an exclusion criterion for the procedure.

The intervention is always possible under local anaesthesia with ligation of incompetent tributaries and adjunctive vein avulsion with multiple stab incisions. Experience reported in the literature indicates that this approach enables slowing of the progression of varicosity while “saving the saphenous” in its function of anterograde emptying.

Intraoperative testing of valvular competence is more than adequate using Doppler; there is no need to have recourse to strip tests or angioscopy.

There is room for improvement in the area of banding materials, and so the authors still have research in progress on a material that is more compliant and generates very little fibrotic reaction in the wall, so that removal should be made easier.

Literature

1. Edwards JE, Edwards EA. The saphenous valves in varicose veins. Am Heart J. 1940;19:338–51.
2. Bassi GL. Le varici degli arti inferiori. Turin: Minerva Medica; 1962.

3. Rose SS, Ahmed A. Some thoughts on the etiology of varicose veins. J Cardiovasc Surg. 1986;27:534–43.
4. Somjen GM, Donlan J, Hurse J, Bartholomew J, Johnston AH, Royle P. Venous reflux at the sapheno-femoral junction. Phlebology. 1995;(4):132–5.
5. Van Bemmelen PS, Summer DS. Laboratory evaluation of varicose veins. In: Bergan JJ, Goldman MP, editors. Varicose veins duplex examination of the sapheno-femoral junction and telangiectasias, diagnosis and treatment. St. Louis, MO: Quality Medical Publishing; 1993. p. 73–84.
6. Zamboni P, Gianesini S, Menegatti E, Tacconi G, Palazzo A, Liboni A. Great saphenous varicose vein surgery without saphenofemoral junction disconnection. Br J Surg. 2010;97(6):820–5.
7. Camilli S, Guarnera G. L' insufficienza venosa primaria e le possibilità della chirurgia ricostruttiva. Padova: Piccin; 1993.
8. Hallberg DA. A method for repairing incompetent valves in deep veins. Acta Chir Scand. 1972;138:143–5.
9. Corcos L, Peruzzi GP, Romeo V, Procacci T, Zamboni P, Dini S. Valvuloplastia de la union safeno-femoral. Video-revista de cirugia. 1992;9:17–30.
10. Corcos L, Zamboni P, Liboni A. External valvuloplasty of the s-f junction in early varicose veins of the lower limbs. In: Davy A, Stemmer R, editors. Phlebologie-Phlebology, vol. 89. Paris: Libbey; 1989. p. 1025–7.
11. Lane RJ, McMahon C, Cuzzilla M. The treatment of varicose veins using the venous valve cuff. Phlebology. 1994;9:136–45.
12. Schanzer H, Skladany M, Peirce ECIII. The role of external valvuloplasty in the surgical management of chronic deep venous disease. Phlebology. 1994;9:8–12.
13. Zamboni P, Marcellino MG, Cappelli M, Feo CV, Bresadola V, Vasquez G, Liboni A. Saphenous vein sparing surgery: principles, techniques and results. J Cardiovasc Surg. 1998;39(2):151–62.
14. Zamboni P, Gasbarro V, Marcellino MG. External valvuloplasty of the sapheno-femoral junction. Vasc Surg. 1994;28:327–36.
15. Zamboni P, Liboni A. External valvuloplasty of the s-f junction using perforated prosthesis. Phlebology. 1991;6:141–7.
16. Zamboni P, Gasbarro V, De Anna D, Liboni A, Donini I. External valvuloplasty of the SFJ with intraoperative angioscopy. J Vasc Surg. 1993;17:438.
17. Belcaro G, Ricci A, Laurora G, Cesarone MR, De Sanctis MT, Incandela L. Superficial femoral vein valve repair and limited anterior plication. Phlebology. 1994;9:146–9.
18. Mendoza E, Blättler W, Amsler F. Great saphenous vein diameter at the saphenofemoral junction and proximal thigh as parameters of venous disease class. Eur J Vasc Endovasc Surg. 2013;45(1):76–83.
19. Rutheford RB, Sawyer JD, Jones DN. The fate of residual saphenous vein after partial removal or ligation. J Vasc Surg. 1990;12:422–6.
20. Fligelstone L, Carolan G, Pugh N, Shandall A, Lane I. An assessment of the long saphenous vein for potential use as a vascular conduit after varicose vein surgery. J Vasc Surg. 1993;18:836–40.

Part IV

How to Treat a Patient in a Modern Phlebologic Setting

14 Treatment Options Depending on the Patient's Presentation

Erika Mendoza

14.1 Introduction

There are very different types of personalities behind varicose veins. Some consult in despair when observing a little spider—which is only found by the doctor after the patient shows it with the fingertip. Others never ever consult, even though the leg turns brown and hard and finally bursts open with an ulceration. The same as with the personalities we can observe with the symptoms. There are typical venous symptoms with swelling and beginning corona at the ankle, and the only duplex finding is a thin refluxive saphenous vein from the groin (mostly with competent terminal valve) to the ankle. And persons with meandering thick tributaries all over the leg and calf live without any symptoms.

And then we have lots of treatment options with little evidence. We never studied if compression is better than surgery in early stages. Nobody investigated how long it will take an asymptomatic vein with no skin changes to develop to a symptomatic vein or to produce complications. All of us know patients since years or even decades that consult with visible veins, no complaints, no skin changes (asymptomatic C2), and we see little or no evolutivity. We recommend just to wear stockings and to come back after some years, because there still is no need to perform any intervention. The only proven so far is that people with symptoms and skin changes have entered the evolutivity phase and will suffer progression if no treatment is performed [1].

This variability in the presentation and evolution of the illness and variety of treatment options makes phlebology that thrilling speciality. There are no real evidence-based protocols to be followed. In this chapter, the author aims to give an orientation to the diagnostic approach and treatment options in a number of typical situations, working out which ones could be the options in each situation in case we decide for a treatment.

Decisions depending on the patient's comorbidities are discussed in Chap. 11.

To be able to apply the topic "choosing wisely" in phlebology, we do need to have a certain minimal setting in our unit concerning diagnostic possibilities and treatment options. We need to know if the venous disease is only cosmetically bothering or it is already provoking clinically visible consequences that might have an evolution to irreversible skin changes.

In theory, we do need to be independent of the reimbursement when recommending options to the patient. As this is not the reality in lots of countries, at least we should always contrast our recommendation to our patients with what we would offer our relatives in the same situation.

E. Mendoza, M.D., Ph.D.
Venenpraxis, Wunstorf, Germany
e-mail: erika.mendoza@t-online.de

P. Zamboni et al. (eds.), *Saphenous Vein-Sparing Strategies in Chronic Venous Disease*,
https://doi.org/10.1007/978-3-319-70638-2_14

14.1.1 Diagnostic Facilities

An appropriate diagnostic result is impossible without asking the patient about the history of his disease and about the concerns he has. Often patients consult, because visible veins are thought to be the reason of spinal nerve-induced pain in the leg. A simple anamnesis will sort this out. Our commitment is not only to find a varicose vein but also to put the vein in the correct context of the patient's concerns. Important examples of questions are as follows:

- Is the pain relieved with compression stockings—probably venous origin?
- Is the pain also present at night—mostly not venous origin?
- Does the pain start at the back and follow neural pathways alongside the inner or lateral part of the leg—mostly not venous origin?
- Do numbness and tingling mostly have neurologic reasons?

We must inform the patient if the problems he suffers will be relieved after a treatment of the varicose veins.

Physical exploration is important to sort out other, like neuromuscular, diseases. Through the exploration, we will detect the degree of skin affection due to venous disease. Even though the clinics in CEAP classification allow large discussions [2–4], it is clear that skin changes classified as C4–6 are obvious alarming signals if combined with visible or detectable varicose veins. Oedema has multiple reasons, and not every oedema is an alarming sign if coexisting with varicose veins. Patients with lipoedema might suffer from varicose veins; the same happens with obesity-induced oedema and lymphoedema. In these cases, it is the personal experience of the treating team together with the patient that must decide which treatment options are possible and do make sense. It is only the physical exploration that gives the hint to the clinical severity of the varicose vein illness.

Duplex ultrasound is available since late 1980s. Today the devices have become as accessible to every phlebologist that it can be asked as mandatory to use a duplex investigation in the diagnostics of a patient affected with varicose veins. When using duplex in experienced hands, no phlebography is necessary—and hand-held Doppler devices are no more appropriate as single diagnostic tool, except for those regions where other technical possibilities are not available. In case of complex varicose veins after deep venous thrombosis, further investigations might be necessary (see Chap. 5).

Basic diagnostic tools to define the presence and extent of venous disease:

- Anamnesis
- Physical exploration
- Duplex ultrasound with colour and PW mode

Supplementary diagnostic tools:

- Plethysmographic methods to quantify deep venous impairment and as a global parameter of venous function
- CW Doppler to exclude arterial disease
- MRI/CT to examine complex post-thrombotic diseases

14.1.2 Therapeutic Options

Fifty years ago, there was only one surgical option in the treatment of truncal varicose veins: high ligation and stripping of the affected vein or wait and see—with or without compression.

Things have changed—and will go on changing in the future. This means that we have developed from one disease, one treatment to a patient-oriented, finding-tailored treatment [5]. But we will only be able to offer this to our patients if we are able to perform all the available techniques and strategies—in our team or in another unit, where we can send our patients in certain cases.

When we inform patients about therapeutic options, we must inform about the consequences as well; that means the side effects of the proposed treatment and the alternative options and the long-term results and recidives. And we should inform the patient about the consequences of doing nothing or at least only compression stockings. And we should confess that there is a huge lack of information concerning lots of long-term results in the new techniques. We have to inform the patient that we do not know about the evolution time of uncomplicated varicose veins—we do only know about the progressivity of complicated varicose veins on treatment waiting lists [1] and about the recidives after applying a treatment [6].

So today we should be able to give our patients different options from wait and see, compression stockings and treatment—which should involve surgery (of saphenous veins, perforators and tributaries), foam sclerotherapy (ultrasound guided for saphenous veins and perforators) and endoluminal devices. The optimum setting is a team with skilled persons in all these options. But often the national health services are built in categories: the basic ones with the diagnostics and the specialised ones with the therapeutic options. A good feedback in the form of discussion of patients allows a better understanding of which strategy and which technique would fit which patient best and help the patients to be sent to the specialist at the perfect moment.

Obligate therapeutic options:

- Surgical options:
  - Possibility to perform surgery of the junctions and perforators with or without stripping of the saphenous veins
  - Tributary phlebectomy
- Ultrasound-guided foam sclerotherapy
- Compression stockings
- Endoluminal treatment options with at least one of the following devices:
  - Laser
  - Radio frequency
  - Glue

14.1.3 Personal Experience

Treatment of varicose veins is suffering quick evolution. Nobody is able to have large personal experience in every treatment option. Therefore, phlebologists need to have good continued formation possibilities and need to be humble enough to tell the patient that they personally do not have experience with some technique or strategy—but are willing to send him to an experienced colleague. The author is aware of the fact that waiting lists and structures in some healthcare systems or extreme poverty in some countries counteract this vision.

14.2 Legs with Varicose Veins and No Truncal Reflux

Some studies suggest that there is an evolution from distal to proximal, from refluxive R3 to refluxive R2 and ascending along the R2 [7–9]. Other theories state that it is the vein wall that has an incorrect function and this fact induces the varicose vein. As long as nobody knows exactly what happens in the evolution of varicose veins, a way to decide in each situation has to be found. Only when the real processes have been analysed, perhaps physicians will have the opportunity to learn how to interact with them to prevent varicose vein formation.

This part of the chapter deals with patients with competent saphenous veins, competent deep veins and visible tributaries. In the vast majority of cases, there are no signs of chronic venous insufficiency; that means no oedema and no skin changes. Symptoms of heavy legs in summer and itching are possible.

14.2.1 Tributaries Not Related to the Saphenous Veins or the Pelvic System

Figure 14.1 shows the haemodynamic situation with competent saphenous veins and no connection between the visible tributaries (or spider veins) and the saphenous vein. No reflux

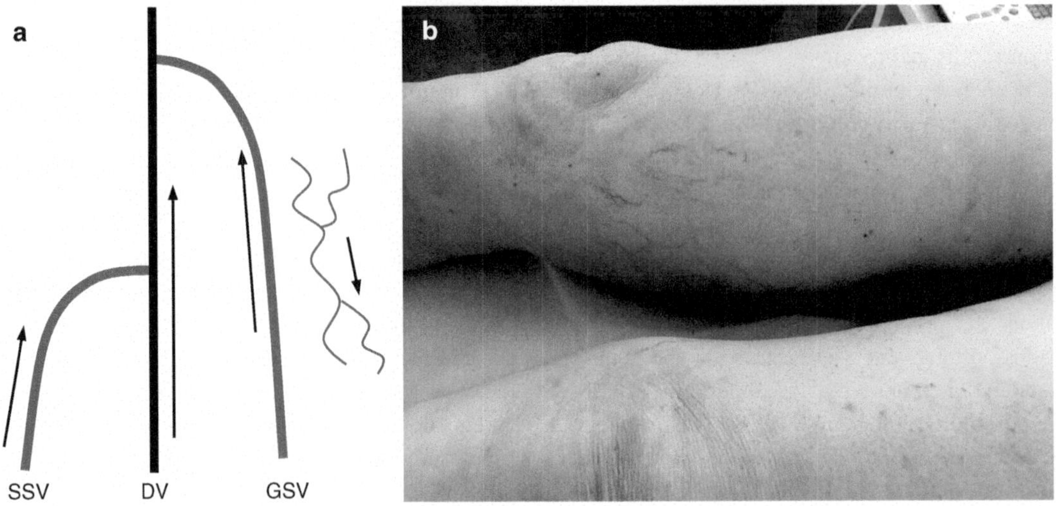

Fig. 14.1 (**a**) Schematic view of the refluxive tributary (N3) without connection to saphenous or deep veins. (**b**) Typical finding with thin veins, most often under 2 mm of diameter and forming profuse networks. *SSV* small saphenous vein, *GSV* great saphenous vein, *DV* deep veins. Deep veins, N1: dark blue. Superficial veins, N2: blue. Refluxive vein: red

source is found like refluxing pelvic vessels (reflux in I-point or P-point; see Chap. 8) or perforators.

The patient usually has no complaints, only seldom itching. The treatment is done under cosmetic considerations. Experience tells us that untreated spider veins or reticular varicosities progress over time and will become more and more visible. So, it might be helpful to treat the visible veins with the least possible invasiveness. We do not know if a treatment in this situation prevents from progression of disease to a higher-level vein (saphenous vein, perforator). After explaining this to the patient, the tributary can be treated either with mini-phlebectomies or sclerotherapy. A treatment of the—competent!—saphenous vein is not indicated.

14.2.2 Tributaries Fed by Reflux Originating in the Pelvic System

In some cases, we find varicose veins emerging from the groin cease or the pudendal region. In ultrasound examination, we discover competent deep leg veins, competent saphenous veins and no reflux at the level of the sapheno-femoral junction. But a refluxing vein emerges from the P-point or the I-point (see Chap. 8) or just from superficial epigastric vessels running from the abdominal wall to the ventral aspect of the thigh. The insufficiency starts mostly in the pelvic network. It looks like better results with surgery are achieved, if the phlebectomy is performed up to the trans-fascial exit point (I- or P-point; see Chap. 8). Another effective possibility is the foam sclerotherapy next to the emerging points of the visible veins and with injection direction to the pelvis. Foam will reach into the trans-fascial veins and could achieve a better occlusion of the connection to the network. Nevertheless, these veins are very prone to recidives after sclerotherapy. Again, any treatment of the—competent!—saphenous vein is not indicated (Fig. 14.2).

14.2.3 Tributaries Fed by Competent Saphenous Veins

Sometimes visible tributaries are fed by a competent saphenous vein. The saphenous vein has only orthograde flow, but feeds the tributary, which is refluxive starting at the point it leaves the saphenous vein. This is the situation we find in shunt type 2 after Franceschi (see Fig. 14.3). The tributary usually is not very dilated, as there is no real recirculation (open shunt when draining through a perforator

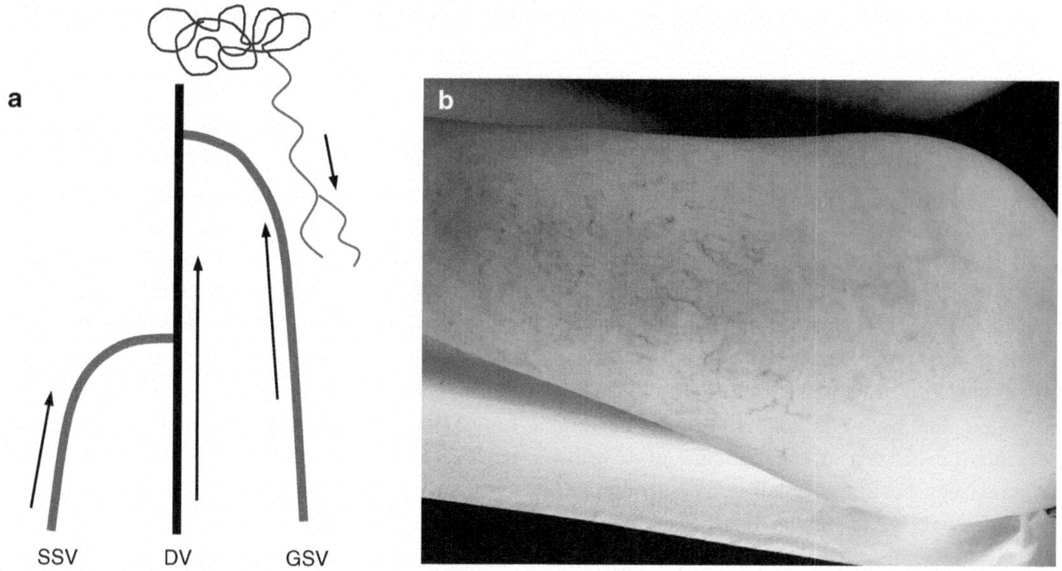

Fig. 14.2 (**a**) Schematic view of the refluxive tributary filled by pelvic network, without connection to saphenous or deep veins. (**b**) Typical finding with thin veins, at the ventral aspect of the thigh, emerging lateral of the sapheno-femoral junction. *SSV* small saphenous vein, *GSV* great saphenous vein, *DV* deep veins. Deep veins, N1: dark blue. Superficial veins, N2: blue. Refluxive vein: red. Pelvic network: dark red

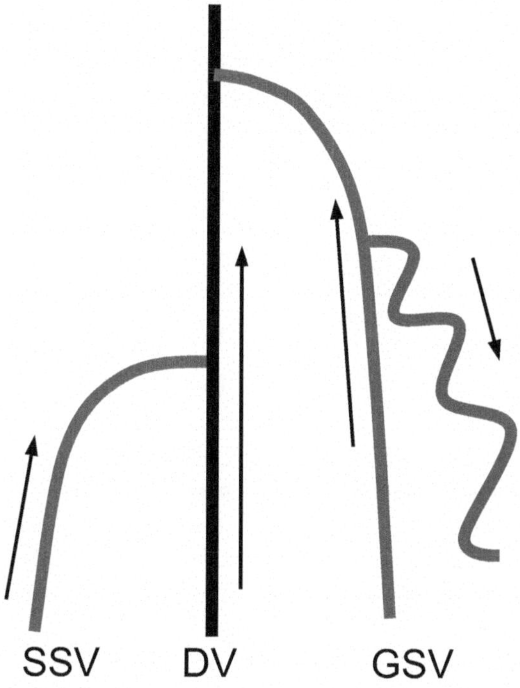

Fig. 14.3 Schematic view of the refluxive tributary fed by a competent saphenous vein. Open shunt, if the drainage is via a perforator; closed shunt, if the drainage is via the same saphenous vein, closing the circle of recirculation [16]. *SSV* small saphenous vein, *GSV* great saphenous vein, *DV* deep veins. Deep veins, N1: dark blue. Superficial veins, N2: blue. Refluxive vein: red

or the other saphenous vein; see Fig. 3.19b). In case of a closed shunt with drainage of the superficial blood (N3) into the same saphenous vein further down (see Fig. 3.19a) this could lead to a more prominent refluxive tributary. Possibly this situation is the first step in the evolution to a retrograde flow in the saphenous vein (ascending theory).

In these cases, a treatment of the tributary might stop a progression of reflux into the saphenous vein. Even if the philosophy fitting to venous-sparing treatments might be to harm as little as possible, we do not know if in these cases the early treatment with little invasiveness could bring a benefit to the patient in the long run. A flush ligation of the tributary at the emerging point of the saphenous vein—with or without phlebectomy of the tributary itself could be the surgical option or a foam sclerotherapy with digital compression of the saphenous vein to avoid passing of foam to the healthy trunk ([10]; see Sect. 7.12). In the experience of the author, these cases have a very good evolution. They must be differentiated from those with little reflux in the saphenous vein fed by proximal, healthy tributaries (shunt "0"), described in Sect. 3.7.4, which might have a poorer evolution in the long term.

14.2.4 Tributaries Fed by Refluxive Perforators

Some varicose veins are fed by perforators without having a saphenous vein involved in the recirculation. It can be the perforator located at the posterior or lateral aspect of the thigh (see Fig. 14.4), an isolated perforator in the knee-fold or a perforator at any place of the leg connecting the deep veins (N1) with a superficial tributary (N3). Another option is a trans-osseal perforator filling varicose veins mostly at the shin [11] (Fig. 3.13). Depending on the diameter of the perforator and the history of the patient, large reflux amounts can be found, leading to skin changes and signs of chronic venous insufficiency. In case of venous symptoms, there is an obvious treatment indication to avoid progression. Other cases might be treated under cosmetic points of view or to meet the patient's wish to avoid progression.

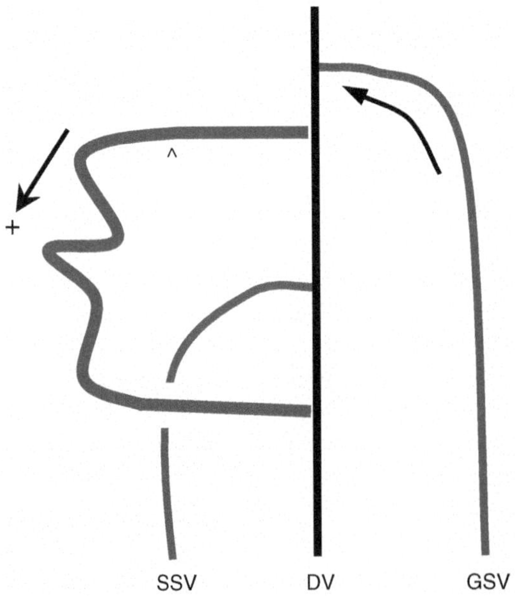

Fig. 14.4 Schematic view of the refluxive tributary (red, +) fed by a refluxive perforator (^) at the dorsal part of the thigh. Drainage into the deep vein of the calf through a terminalising perforating vein, not touching the saphenous vein (Image with kind permission from Schattauer, Phlebologie [10]. *SSV* small saphenous vein, *GSV* great saphenous vein, *DV* deep veins. Deep veins, N1: dark blue. Superficial veins, N2: blue. Refluxive vein: red

One exception should be made in case of trans-osseal perforators (see below).

Depending on the further drainage paths of the reflux, e.g. through saphenous veins, other combinations of treatments will be necessary. In this paragraph, we deal exclusively with those refluxes that are not touching saphenous veins, corresponding with the shunt type 6.

Depending on the flow through the incompetent perforating vein, a foam sclerotherapy might be enough (thinner veins, diameter less than 5 mm in standing position, reflux velocity not too fast) [10]. Alternatively, the interruption of the perforator at subfascial level is necessary, either surgically or if the anatomy does allow it with endoluminal devices.

Again, the treatment of the competent saphenous veins is not indicated in this situation.

In case of bone perforators, most frequently trans-tibial ones (see Fig. 3.13), there is little data about aetiology and evolution. A hole in the bone wall connects with a perforator that feeds the varicose vein. No connection to the deep venous system or saphenous system is observed at this level; the bone marrow is possibly fed by a tributary of the posterior tibial vein [11]. The first observations of evolution after treatment suggest that a surgical interruption is technically difficult, because there is a real hole in the bone wall impeding a classical ligature. So, it looks like foam sclerotherapy is the unique solution and should be applied as soon as possible, because the larger the vein, the more sessions of sclerotherapy seem to be needed.

14.3 Legs with Truncal Reflux and Little Disease (C1–C2n)

Visible varicose tributaries (N3) without other clinical complaints can be fed by an incompetent saphenous vein or other sources (see Sect. 14.2). A saphenous vein treatment is only indicated if there is a reflux in the saphenous vein—thus all the cases described in Sect. 14.2 do not need any saphenous vein treatment.

Some schools defend the theory that by the time a reflux is detected in any saphenous vein, a surgery indication is given. Looking at the statistics, we know that up to 50% of patients suffer a recidive 5–10 years after stripping and still 26% after venous sparing surgery (see literature, Chap. 10). We do not know how many patients with little disease will have an evolution to clinical deterioration in the next 5–10 years. So, we really do not know what to recommend patients with little disease. If the patient has no cosmetic complaints, a wait-and-see strategy (with or without compression stockings) and a new investigation in case of visible progress or new symptoms can be a recommendation. Lots of patients stay in this situation for many years.

If the patient is bothered by the optical impairment, a treatment option with minimal invasiveness and recidives should be chosen, regarding there is little disease. As seen in Sects. 6.4.1 and 6.11.4, the results depend on some factors, worthwhile to be summarised here. The main differentiation at the moment of the decision might be the competence of the terminal valve [12].

14.3.1 Competent Terminal Valve

Little disease and great saphenous vein reflux are often the case, when the terminal valve is competent. Lesser saphenous vein diameters are found [13]. According to Bernardini [7] and Caggiati [8], there is an ascending evolution of varicose disease, meaning that a saphenous reflux with competent terminal valve will evolve to terminal valve incompetence throughout the years.

On the other hand, we know that in case of no draining perforator on the saphenous vein (shunt type 5; see Sect. 6.11.4.4), 97% of patients treated with interruption of the tributary at the level of the saphenous vein achieve a flow correction with orthograde flows in the saphenous vein after 3 years (Fig. 14.5) [12]. If the "untreated" evolution is to develop incompetent terminal valves—and the long-lasting good result for the evolution after treatment of the saphenous trunk depends on the competence of the terminal valve—the treatment in this situation could be performed under a preventive aspect.

Even in case of little reflux amounts, competent terminal valve and draining perforator on the saphenous vein, a disconnection of the tributary (ASVAL or CHIVA; that means tributary disconnection with or without phlebectomies) could induce a situation with a persisting little reflux in the great saphenous vein but without clinics and without visible tributaries (Fig. 14.6).

Foam sclerotherapy of the tributary with digital compression of the saphenous vein is an

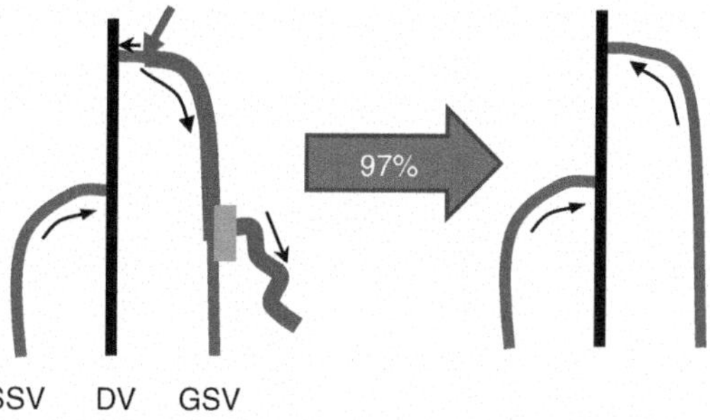

Fig. 14.5 Left: schematic view of a reflux in the GSV with competent terminal valve. Reflux source: groin tributary. Reflux leaves the GSV through a tributary, no draining perforator (reflux elimination test positive; see Sect. 3.8.9), green line: point of surgical interruption. Right: situation after interruption of the distal draining tributary at its origin (GSV), with or without phlebectomy. This situation is stable in 97% after 3 years [12, 16]. *SSV* small saphenous vein, *GSV* great saphenous vein, *DV* deep veins. Deep veins, N1: dark blue. Superficial veins, N2: blue. Refluxive vein: red

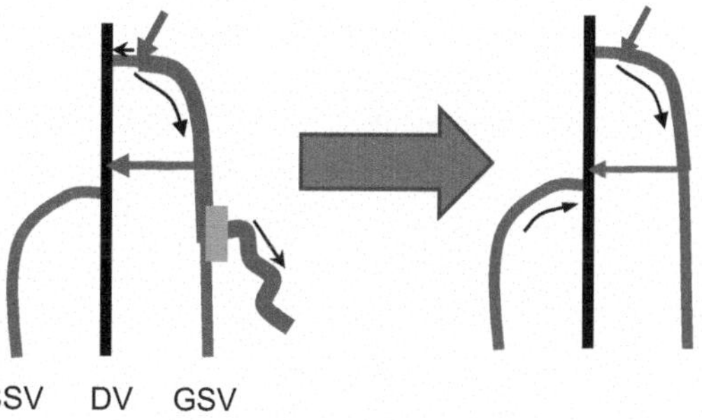

Fig. 14.6 Left: schematic view of a reflux in the GSV with competent terminal valve. Reflux source: groin tributary. Reflux leaves the GSV through a tributary and a draining perforator (reflux elimination test negative), green line: point of surgical interruption. Right: situation after interruption of the distal draining tributary at its origin (GSV), with or without phlebectomy. No data available about how stable the situation might be [16]. *SSV* small saphenous vein, *GSV* great saphenous vein, *DV* deep veins. Deep veins, N1: dark blue. Superficial veins, N2: blue. Refluxive vein: red

alternative option in case of very thin saphenous vein or little reflux and cosmetic complaints; there are no studies of long-term results (see Sect. 7.12).

Of course, the treatment option in case of competent terminal valve and incompetent preterminal valve will be the same, if the clinical presentation is with oedema or skin changes.

14.3.2 Incompetent Terminal Valve

In case of incompetent terminal valve, saphenous reflux and little disease, we have the option to achieve a flow correction in the saphenous vein when performing a distal, draining tributary ligation in about 40% at 1 year and 20% in about 3 years—which is very little [12]. Saphenous vein treatment of any kind can be offered (stripping, endoluminal treatment—thermal, glue or foam—of the saphenous vein, extraluminal valvuloplasty in case of diameter less than 10 mm at the groin or CHIVA with treatment of the SFJ). The question still not resolved is what will be better in the long term—treating or waiting. So, in case the patient has no complaints, a wait-and-see option seems to be a good option in this situation, at least an option to be offered to the patient.

When deciding the treatment strategy, the patient is to be informed about different treatment options and the recidives rate of each.

14.3.3 Reflux Escaping Through Accessory Anterior Saphenous Vein (AASV)

In these cases, the saphenous vein itself is only refluxive between the terminal and the preterminal valve, but the cosmetic situation is usually bothering. In case of thin diameter of the AASV, the refluxive vein might be treated with foam sclerotherapy, starting with ultrasound guidance and perhaps a higher concentration next to the sapheno-femoral junction and applying foam along the visible tributary. It might be good to treat the vein before an evolution to larger diameters.

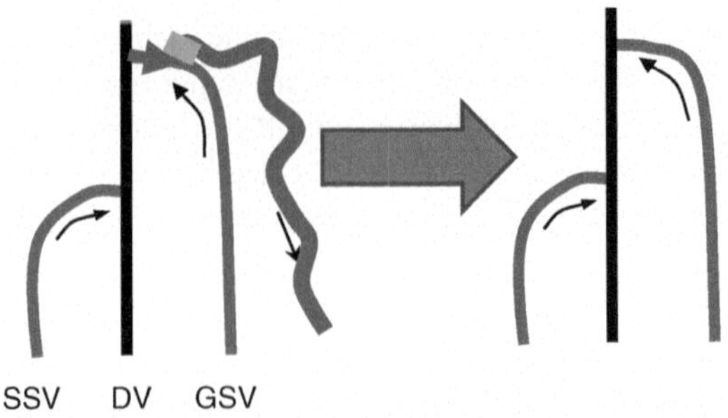

Fig. 14.7 Left: schematic view of a reflux in the GSV with competent terminal valve. Reflux source: groin tributary. Reflux leaves the GSV through a tributary and a draining perforator, green line: point of surgical interruption. Right: situation after interruption of the distal draining tributary at its origin (GSV), with or without phlebectomy. No data available about how stable the situation might be [16]. *SSV* small saphenous vein, *GSV* great saphenous vein, *DV* deep veins. Deep veins, N1: dark blue. Superficial veins, N2: blue. Refluxive vein: red

The "lateral crossectomy" or surgical ligation of the AASV at the level of the GSV is an option in case of larger diameters, as well as endoluminal catheter-assisted techniques in case there is an interfascial rectilinear segment of the AASV. The very short segment of refluxive GSV between the deep vein and the raising of the AASV reverts its flow in the clear majority of cases (Fig. 14.7) in the experience of the authors (data not published).

14.4 Legs with Truncal Reflux and Venous Complaints (C2s, C3–C6)

Usually, in case of venous complaints, the terminal valve is incompetent, or a greater perforator feeds the saphenous vein.

Clinics are also possible, though seldom, in case of terminal valve competence. Treatment options are described in Sect. 14.3.1 and apply also to symptomatic patients.

As described in Sect. 14.3.2, in these cases and depending on the specialisation of the surgeon and the wishes of the patients, sclerotherapy (best in smaller diameters), stripping, endoluminal therapies and CHIVA (possible in all diameters) are possible options. ASVAL is also described for large diameters if the refluxive segment of GSV is not too long. Extraluminal valvuloplasty is only possible, when a certain diameter at the groin is given. If a saphenous ablation option is discussed, the patient must be informed about the possibility of saving the saphenous vein and the lesser amount of complications and recidives when choosing a venous sparing option, as evidenced by the Cochrane review [6].

14.4.1 Treatment Options in Case of Thin Great Saphenous Vein

Seldom we find a long-lasting reflux in thin saphenous veins with oedema, very seldom with skin changes. The first impression of the vein in ultrasound is that its calibre is so thin that a reflux seems unlikely—sometimes the reflux is only visible after a dependency manoeuvre (see Sect. 4.3.3.1). This type of reflux is defined as "non-drained" reflux (see Sect. 3.5.6). Venous diameter is so thin that a reduction of diameter will not improve the valve function. That is why a sclerotherapy of the saphenous vein seems to be the less invasive option with good probabilities of occlusion in one session due to the small diameter. Of course, all the other therapeutic options are possible (crossectomy and stripping, endoluminal heat or glue ablation. CHIVA will not be the optimum choice in this situation, as multiple interruptions of the course of the saphenous trunk are necessary to reach a fractioning of the pressure column). The invasiveness-effectiveness ratio is surely best with sclerotherapy—though no studies were performed in these seldom situation.

14.4.2 Treatment Options in Case of Skin Changes at the Calf or Ulceration

As described above, patients with skin changes usually suffer axial reflux. Depending on the preferences of the surgeon, every treatment option with saphenous vein flow correction could be chosen: CHIVA (interruption of the escape point(s), fractioning of the column), stripping or endoluminal ablation of the saphenous vein. As the incisions in the skin with dermatoliposclerosis (C4–6) is often followed by poor healing, in these cases the venous-sparing options are preferable: only interruption of the most important escape point (mostly the saphenofemoral junction), waiting for a regression of skin changes—which might take months. If there is still a therapy necessity afterwards, further steps like phlebectomies or sclerotherapy or further interruptions could be taken.

These patients are especially prone to minimal invasive interventions, like CHIVA—other than postulated in the past [14]—because CHIVA offers the possibility to treat in different sessions according to the necessities of the patient.

14.5 Superficial Reflux After Superficial Vein Thrombosis

Thrombosis of superficial veins might occur in saphenous veins and/or tributaries; the treatment options depend on the localisation.

14.5.1 Treatment Options in Case of Post-thrombotic Changes in Saphenous Veins

In the acute phase of thrombosis of a superficial vein, the international consensus recommends fondaparinux 2.5 mg a day s.c. for 42 days, in case of thrombi next to the junction anticoagulation for weeks to months. After a good regression of the thrombus, a treatment of the varicose vein should be planned [15].

Large scars after thrombosis of saphenous veins will make it impossible to pass a stripping or endoluminal device through a saphenous vein. Residual thrombi could be displaced and provoke emboli when touched with an endoluminal device. In case of competent terminal valve but post-thrombotic lesions in the proximal saphenous vein, an interruption of the tributary with the goal to achieve a competent saphenous vein (see Sect. 6.4.1) has a theoretic higher risk of recidivant saphenous vein thrombosis and should therefore be avoided, the same as ASVAL or extraluminal valvuloplasty. A new thrombus with progression to the deep vein could end up in a pulmonary embolism, as the sapheno-femoral junction is not closed.

For the reasons explained above, a crossectomy/crossotomy seems to be the most rationale option in these cases, especially to avoid a thrombus dislocation during a manoeuvre. As a vein with scars after superficial vein thrombosis might develop new thrombi after the crossotomy, a longer postioerative anticoagulation should be installed. In addition the vein should be treated with sclerotherapy foam simultaneously to surgery or some days to weeks after the surgery.

14.5.2 Treatment Options After Thrombosis of Tributaries

Thrombi in tributaries usually keep a long time until they are resorbed from the vein by physiologic thrombolysis. After the acute phase treatment depending on the extension and the symptoms of the thrombosis [15], any chosen treatment (stripping, endoluminal or foam ablation, CHIVA or extraluminal valvuloplasty) can be applied to the saphenous veins. After an interruption of the reflux into the tributary, the blood flow in relation to the diameter will be less. As the vein wall is damaged by thrombosis, it will not react in a proper calibre reduction and could reactivate the thrombosis due to the stasis. Thus, the post-thrombotic superficial vein segment should be separated from the saphenous trunk by disconnection, as otherwise a new thrombus could enter the saphenous vein destroying it. Usually sclerotherapy of the post-thrombotic tributary (N3) is the optimum solution, as a phlebectomy can be difficult due to adherences.

Conclusion

In every situation, patient context and venous illness degree offer the possibility to apply saphenous vein-saving surgery. The choice has to be taken after informing the patient about all the options, the advantages and disadvantages and the personal experience of the surgeon.

Literature

1. Sarin S, Shields DA, Farrah J, Scurr JH, Coleridge-Smith PD. Does venous function deteriorate in patients waiting for varicose vein surgery? J R Soc Med. 1993;86(1):21–3.
2. Eklöf B, Rutherford RB, Bergan JJ, Carpentier PH, Gloviczki P, Kistner RL, Meissner MH, Moneta GL, Myers K, Padberg FT, Perrin M, Ruckley CV, Coleridge Smith P, Wakefield TW. Revision of CEAP classification for chronic venous disorders (CVD). J Vasc Surg. 2004;40:1248–52.
3. Lattimer CR, Kalodiki E, Azzam M, Geroulakos G. An international survey on the interpretation of pigmentation using the C class of the Clinical, Etiological, Anatomical, Pathophysiological Classification. Veins Lymphat. 2013;2:e1.
4. Vasquez MA, Rabe E, McLafferty RB, Shortell CK, Marston WA, Gillespie D, et al. Revision of the clinical severity score: venous outcomes consensus statement: special communication of the American Venous Forum Ad Hoc Outcomes Working Group. J Vasc Surg. 2010;52:1387–96.
5. van der Velden SK, Pichot O, van den Bos RR, Nijsten TEC, de Maeseneer MGR. Management strategies for patients with varicose veins (C2-C6): results of a worldwide survey. Eur J Vasc Endovasc Surg. 2015;49:213–20.
6. Bellmunt-Montoya S, Escribano JM, Dilme J, Martinez-Zapata MJ. CHIVA method for the treatment of chronic venous insufficiency. Cochrane Database Syst Rev. 2012;(2):CD009648. https://doi.org/10.1002/14651858.CD009648.
7. Bernardini E, De Rango P, Piccioli R, Bisacri C, Pagliuca V, Genovese G. Development of primary superficial venous insufficiency: the ascending theory. Observational and hemodynamic data from a 9 year experience. Ann Vasc Surg. 2010;24:709–20.
8. Caggiati A, Rosi C, Heyn R, Franceschini M, Acconcia MC. Age-related variations of varicose veins anatomy. J Vasc Surg. 2006;44(6):1291–5.
9. Chastanet S, Pittaluga P. Patterns of reflux in the great saphenous vein system. Phlebology. 2013;28(Suppl 1):39–46. https://doi.org/10.1177/0268355513477021.
10. Mendoza E, Cappelli M. Sclerotherapy technique in CHIVA strategy. Phlebology. 2017;46:5–12.
11. Ramelet AA, Crebassa V, Carlos D, Alotto C, Buero G, Gillet JL, Grenot-Mercier A, Kuepfer S, Mendoza E, Monsallier JM, Obermayer A, Pacheco K, Pros N, Rastel D, Soulie D. Anomalous intraosseous venous drainage: bone perforators? Phlebology. 2017;32(4):241–8.
12. Zamboni P, Gianesini S, Menegatti E, Tacconi G, Palazzo A, Liboni A. Great saphenous varicose vein surgery without saphenofemoral junction disconnection. Br J Surg. 2010;97:820–5.
13. Cappelli M, Molino Lova R, Ermini S, Zamboni P. Hemodynamics of the sapheno-femoral junction. Patterns of reflux und their clinical implications. Int Angiol. 2004;23(1):25–8.

14. Zamboni P, Cisno C, Marchetti F, Mazza P, Fogato L, Carandina S, De Palma M, Liboni A. Minimally invasive surgical management of primary venous ulcers vs. compression treatment: a randomized clinical trial. Eur J Vasc Endovasc Surg. 2003;25(4):313–8. Erratum in: Eur J Vasc Endovasc Surg. 2003;26(3):337–8.
15. Kalodiki E, Strvrtinova V, Allegra C, Andreozzi GM, Antignani PL, Avram R, Brkljacic B, Cadariou F, Dzsinich C, Fareed J, Gaspar L, Geroulakos G, Javien A, Kozak M, Lattimer CR, Minar E, Partsch H, Passariello F, Patel M, Pécsvárady Z, Poredos P, Rotocil K, Scuderi A, Sparovec M, Szostek M, Skorski M. Superficial vein thrombosis: a consensus statement. Int Angiol. 2012;31:203–16.
16. Mendoza E. Handbuch CHIVA. Arrien GmbH; 2002.

The manufacturer's authorised representative in the EU is Springer Nature Customer Service Centre GmbH, Europaplatz 3, 69115 Heidelberg, Germany. If you have any concerns regarding our products, please contact ProductSafety@springernature.com

Printed and bound by CPI Group (UK) Ltd, Croydon, CR0 4YY
05/10/2026
02228142-0001